EDUCATION IN HEART
Volume 1

Series Editor

PETER MILLS
Consultant Cardiologist, London Chest Hospital

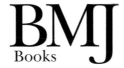

© BMJ Books 2001
BMJ Books is an imprint of the BMJ Publishing Group

First published in 2001
by BMJ Books, BMA House, Tavistock Square,
London WC1H 9JR

www.bmjbooks.com

British Library Cataloguing in Publication Data
A catalogue record for this book is available from the British Library

ISBN 0-7279-1620-3

Cover design by Marritt Associates, Harrow, Middlesex
Typeset by BMJ Electronic Production and Scribe Design, Gillingham, Kent
Printed in Malaysia by Times Offset

Contents

Contents

SECTION VIII: GENERAL CARDIOLOGY

Contributors

Lindsey Allan
Director of the Echocardiography Laboratory, New York Presbyterian Hospital, New York, USA

Robert H Anderson
Cardiac Unit, Institute of Child Health, University College London, UK

Cristina Basso
Department of Pathology, University of Padua Medical School, Padua, Italy

N A Boon
Department of Cardiology, Royal Infirmary of Edinburgh, Edinburgh, UK

Paolo G Camici
MRC Cyclotron Unit, Imperial College School of Medicine, Hammersmith Hospital, London, UK

Domenico Corrado
Department of Cardiology, University of Padua Medical School, Padua, Italy

Michael J Davies
St George's Hospital Medical School, BHF Cardiovascular Pathology, London, UK

P J de Feyter
Department of Cardiology, Erasmus Medical Centre Rotterdam, Rotterdam, The Netherlands

Etienne Delacretaz
University of Lausanne, Division of Cardiology, CHUV, Lausanne, Switzerland

Christina Donnellan
Department of Geriatric Medicine, University of Liverpool, Liverpool, UK

Perry Elliott
Department of Cardiological Sciences, St George's Hospital Medical School, London, UK

Keith A A Fox
Department of Cardiology, The Royal Infirmary, Edinburgh, UK

Enrique Galve
Servicio de Cardiologia, Hospital General Universitari Vall d'Hebron, Barcelona, Spain

Michael D Gammage
Department of Cardiovascular Medicine, Queen Elizabeth Hospital, University Hospital Birmingham NHS Trust, Birmingham, UK

Raymond J Gibbons
Division of Cardiovascular Diseases and Internal Medicine, Mayo Clinic and Mayo Foundation, Rochester, Minnesota, USA

John L Gibbs
Yorkshire Heart Centre at the Leeds General Infirmary, Leeds, UK

Christa Gohlke-Bärwolf
Herz Zentrum, Bad Krozingen, Germany

Bernard Iung
Cardiology Department, Bichat Hospital, Paris, France

Marjo-Riitta Järvelin
Department of Public Health Science and General Practice, University of Oulu, Finland and Department of Epidemiology and Public Health, Imperial College School of Medicine, London, UK

Michael Lye
Department of Geriatric Medicine, University of Liverpool, Liverpool, UK

John J McMurray
Clinical Research Initiative in Heart Failure, Wolfson Building, University of Glasgow, Glasgow, UK

Bernhard Meier
Swiss Cardiovascular Center Bern, University Hospital, Bern, Switzerland

K Nieman
Erasmus Medical Centre Rotterdam, Rotterdam, The Netherlands

Robin M Norris
Royal Sussex County Hospital, Brighton, East Sussex, UK

Celia M Oakley
Imperial College School of Medicine, Hammersmith Hospital, London, UK

Catherine M Otto
Division of Cardiology, University of Washington, Seattle, USA

M Oudkerk
Erasmus Medical Centre Rotterdam, Rotterdam, The Netherlands

René Prêtre
Cardiovascular Surgery, University Hospital, Zürich, Switzerland

Dan M Roden
Vanderbilt University School of Medicine, Nashville, Tennessee, USA

Contributors

Jordi Soler-Soler
Servicio de Cardiologia, Hospital General Universitari Vall d'Hebron, Barcelona, Spain

William G Stevenson
Harvard Medical School, Brigham and Women's Hospital, Boston, Massachusetts, USA

Simon Stewart
Clinical Research Initiative in Heart Failure, Wolfson Building, University of Glasgow, Glasgow, UK

Allan D Struthers
Department of Clinical Pharmacology & Therapeutics, Ninewells Hospital, Dundee, UK

Gaetano Thiene
Department of Pathology, University of Padua Medical School, Padua, Italy

David R Thompson
British Heart Foundation Rehabilitation Research Unit, Department of Health Studies, University of York, UK

Adam Timmis
Department of Cardiology, Royal Hospitals NHS Trust, London, UK

Andrew M Tonkin
National Heart Foundation of Australia, Austin and Repatriation Medical Centre, Melbourne, Australia

Eric J Topol
Department of Cardiology, The Cleveland Clinic Foundation, Cleveland, Ohio, USA

A D Toft
Endocrine Clinic, Royal Infirmary of Edinburgh, Edinburgh, UK

Tom Treasure
St George's Hospital, London, UK

Marko I Turina
Cardiovascular Surgery, University Hospital, Zürich, Switzerland

P van Ooijen
Erasmus Medical Centre Rotterdam, Rotterdam, The Netherlands

Albert L Waldo
Department of Medicine, Division of Cardiology, Case Western Reserve University/University Hospitals of Cleveland, Cleveland, Ohio, USA

Peter L Weissberg
School of Clinical Medicine, University of Cambridge, Cambridge, UK

Stephen Westaby
Oxford Heart Centre, John Radcliffe Hospital, Headington, Oxford, UK

Stephen Windecker
Swiss Cardiovascular Center Bern, University Hospital, Bern, Switzerland

Introduction

During 1999, the *Heart* journal recognised we had a role to play in the important arena of continuing postgraduate education. In response, we commissioned a series of articles that would collectively cover the field of knowledge that usefully informs practising cardiologists. This includes coronary disease, heart failure, cardiomyopathy, valve disease, electrophysiology, congenital heart disease, imaging techniques, and general cardiology.

Our aim was to help meet the worldwide need for educational material for established consultants in cardiology, so they can remain up to date with clinical and scientific aspects of the specialty. We were more concerned with providing timely summaries of the latest thinking than elaborate discussions of published original research. We stipulated that each article was to have no more than 20 annotated references. As an additional benefit, we hoped the articles would prove useful to trainee cardiologists, by providing an authoritative exposition on subjects that are also relevant to them.

After the encouraging feedback we received on their initial publication, we have decided to re-issue the articles in book form. We hope that gathering all the articles into one volume will make it even easier for cardiologists to use them. Nothing beats a book for communicating and absorbing large amounts of information.

We purposely selected authors from a broad geographical base to reflect the best thinking from around the world and to appeal to the journal's UK and worldwide readership. Each author is a respected international authority on their subject, so the relevance and pertinence of his or her views is guaranteed.

The complete series of articles will be published over three years. This volume contains the first year's worth; the articles will continue to appear each month in *Heart* throughout 2001 and 2002 with collected volumes published at the end of each of these years. As when the articles were initially published, all feedback is welcome – please email heartjournal@bmjgroup.com.

The commitment and inspiration of the section editors is obvious and I would like to express my sincere gratitude to them. I would also like to thank the project manager, Mr John Weller, for all his hard work and excellent advice in developing this series.

In short, this volume of collected articles represents the best way of staying up to date in all areas of cardiology. We hope you will find it invaluable.

PETER MILLS
SERIES EDITOR

Section editors:
Michael J Davies (cardiomyopathy), Christopher Davidson (general cardiology) , John L Gibbs (congenital heart disease), Roger Hall (valve disease), David Lefroy (heart failure, imaging techniques, electrophysiology), Janet M McComb (electrophysiology), R Gordon Murray (coronary disease)

SECTION I: CORONARY DISEASE

1 The pathophysiology of acute coronary syndromes

Michael J Davies

Virtually all regional acute myocardial infarcts are caused by thrombosis developing on a culprit coronary atherosclerotic plaque. The very rare exceptions to this are spontaneous coronary artery dissection, coronary arteritis, coronary emboli, coronary spasm, and compression by myocardial bridges. Thrombosis is also the major initiating factor in unstable angina, particularly when rest pain is recent and increasing in severity. Necropsy studies suggest that a new thrombotic coronary event underlies 50–70% of sudden deaths caused by ischaemic heart disease.

The culprit plaque

Given the importance of thrombosis as the trigger for acute myocardial ischaemia, it is necessary to know something about the structure of plaques before thrombotic events occur and why there should be a sudden change from a stable state (no thrombus) to an unstable state (thrombus).

The fully developed human fibrolipid plaque, designated by the American Heart Association (AHA) as type IV or type Va,[1] has a core of lipid surrounded by a capsule of connective tissue (fig 1.1). The core is an extracellular mass of lipid containing cholesterol and its esters, some of which is in a crystalline form. The core is surrounded by numerous macrophages, many of which contain abundant intracytoplasmic droplets of cholesterol (foam cells). These macrophages are derived from monocytes which crossed the endothelium from the arterial lumen. They are not inert or end stage cells, but are highly activated, producing procoagulant tissue factor and a host of inflammatory cell mediators such as tumour necrosis factor α (TNF α), interleukins, and metalloproteinases. The connective tissue capsule which surrounds this inflammatory mass is predominantly collagen synthesised by smooth muscle cells. The portion of the capsule separating the core from the arterial lumen itself is the plaque cap.

The early stages of plaque development (AHA types I–III) are not associated with evidence of structural damage to the endothelium. Once plaque formation has progressed to stage IV, however, structural changes in the endothelium become almost universal.[2] The endothelium over and between plaques shows enhanced replication compared to normal arteries, implying a degree of endothelial cell immaturity and abnormal physiological function. Focal areas of endothelial denudation occur over the plaque, exposing the underlying connective tissue matrix and allowing a monolayer of platelets to adhere at the site. Such ultramicroscopic thrombi are far too small to be visible on angiography or to impede flow, but may contribute to plaque smooth muscle cell growth by release of platelet derived growth factor.

Mechanisms of thrombosis

Thrombosis over plaques occurs because of two somewhat different processes. One is caused by an extension of the process of endothelial denudation so that large areas of the surface of the subendothelial connective tissue of the plaque are exposed. Thrombus forms which is adherent to the plaque surface (fig 1.2). This process has become known as endothelial erosion. Observational studies have linked endothelial cell loss to the proximity of macrophages. These macrophages are highly activated and cause endothelial cell death by apoptosis, and also by the production of proteases which cut loose the endothelial cells from their adhesion to the vessel wall.

The second mechanism for thrombus formation is plaque disruption (synonyms rupture, fissuring) (fig 1.3). Here the plaque cap tears to expose the lipid core to blood in the arterial lumen. The core area is highly thrombogenic, containing tissue factor, fragments of collagen, and crystalline surfaces to accelerate coagulation. Thrombus forms initially in the plaque itself which is expanded and distorted from within; thrombus may then extend into the arterial lumen (fig 1.4).

Plaque disruption, like endothelial erosion, is a reflection of enhanced inflammatory activity within the plaque.[3] The cap is a dynamic structure within which the connective tissue matrix, upon which its tensile strength depends, is constantly being replaced and maintained by

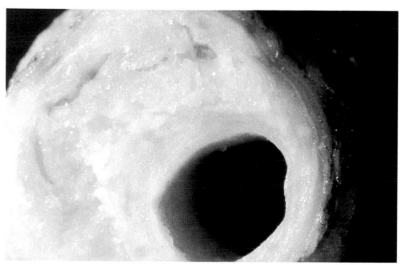

Figure 1.1. The established stable plaque. In this cross section of a human coronary artery there is an established fibrolipid plaque with a core of lipid. The lipid core is separated from the lumen by the plaque cap. The plaque only occupies part of the circumference of the artery, leaving a segment of normal arterial wall.

the smooth muscle cell. The inflammatory process both reduces collagen synthesis by inhibiting the smooth muscle cell and causes its death by apoptosis. Macrophages also produce a wide range of metalloproteinases capable of degrading all the components of the connective tissue matrix, including collagen. These metalloproteinases are secreted into the tissues in an inactive form and then activated by plasmin. Metalloproteinase production by macrophages is upregulated by inflammatory cytokines such as TNFα. Plaque disruption is therefore now seen as an auto-destruct phenomenon associated with an enhanced inflammatory activation.

The relative importance of disruption and erosion as triggers of thrombosis may vary between different patient groups. Disruption is the predominant cause (> 85%) of major coronary thrombi in white males with high plasma concentrations of low density lipoprotein (LDL), and low concentrations of high density lipoprotein (HDL). In contrast, in women endothelial erosion is responsible for around 50% of major thrombi.[4-6] The distinction between erosion and disruption is not necessarily of major clinical importance. Both processes depend on enhanced inflammatory activity within the plaque and appear equally responsive to lipid lowering. Disruption has an intraplaque component more resistant to fibrinolytic treatment, while in erosion the thrombus is more accessible. This potential advantage is, however, offset by erosion related thrombi tending to occur at sites where the pre-existing stenosis was more severe. In women there is also a form of thrombosis caused by endothelial erosion over plaques which do not contain lipid or have a major inflammatory component.[6] This type of disease is rare and arguably distinct from conventional atherosclerosis, and may be smoking related.

The vulnerable plaque concept

Analysis of plaques which have undergone disruption has been used to determine characteristics which may indicate currently stable plaques whose structure and cell content makes them likely to undergo an episode of thrombosis in the future (vulnerable plaques).

There is widespread unanimity[7] in the belief that these features are:
- a large lipid core occupying at least 50% of the overall plaque volume
- a high density of macrophages
- a low density of smooth muscle cells in the cap
- a high tissue factor content
- a thin plaque cap in which the collagen structure is disorganised.

All of these markers of plaques at future risk are likely to be the direct result of macrophage activity, which enlarges the core and thins the cap.

The risk of any subject with coronary artery disease having a future acute event will depend on the number of these vulnerable plaques which are present rather than on the total number of plaques. Patients, however, vary in the number of vulnerable plaques which are present in the coronary arteries—this variation explains why one individual has a series of infarcts at regular intervals while another individual has an infarct without further events for 10 or even 20 years.

The sequence of thrombotic events

The thrombi which occur either in disruption or erosion circumstances are dynamic and evolve in stages. In disruption the initial stage occurs within the lipid core itself and is predominantly formed of platelets. As thrombus begins to protrude into the lumen the fibrin component increases, but any surface exposed to the blood in the lumen will be covered by activated platelets. While antegrade flow continues over this exposed thrombus, clumps of activated platelets are swept down into the distal intramyocardial arteries as microemboli (fig 1.5). Thrombus may grow to

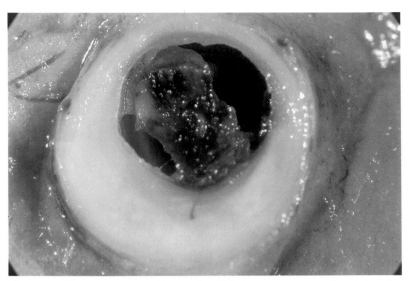

Figure 1.2. Thrombosis caused by erosion. This human coronary artery is largely occluded by a mass of thrombus which is adherent to the surface of a plaque. The plaque itself is intact.

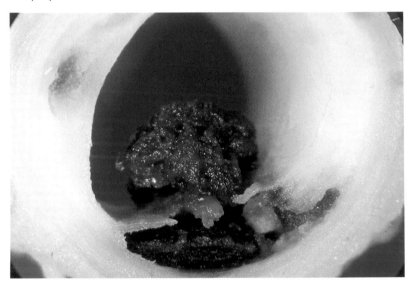

Figure 1.3. Thrombosis caused by disruption. The cap of a plaque has torn and projects up into the lumen. Thrombus has formed within the original lipid core from where it projects into, but does not totally occlude, the lumen. This is the typical lesion of unstable angina.

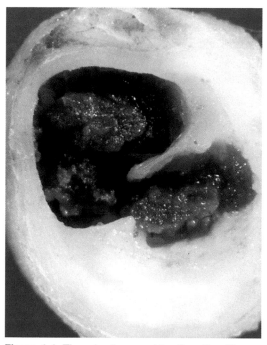

Figure 1.4. Thrombosis caused by disruption. The cap of the plaque has torn and thrombus within the lipid core extends into and occludes the lumen. This is the typical lesion of acute myocardial infarction.

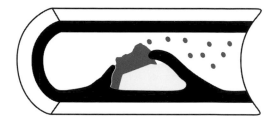

Figure 1.5. Platelet embolisation. Any thrombus (red) which protrudes into the arterial lumen but does not occlude has the surface covered by a layer of activated platelets strongly expressing the IIb/IIIa receptor. Clumps of these platelets are swept down into the myocardium vascular bed.

occlude the artery, leading to a final stage in which there is a loose network of fibrin containing large numbers of entrapped red cells. This third and final stage thrombus may propagate distally after the onset of myocardial infarction. The final stage of occlusive thrombus has a structure making it very susceptible to either natural or therapeutic lysis, but this will expose the deeper and earlier thrombus which is more resistant to lysis.

Symptomology in relation to coronary thrombi

Episodes of plaque disruption which are almost entirely associated with intraplaque thrombus are associated with the onset or exacerbation of stable angina caused by a sudden increase in plaque volume.

Thrombi which project into but do not occlude the lumen (mural thrombi) are the basis of unstable angina. The intermittent attacks of myocardial ischaemia at rest are caused by several potential mechanisms.

- The thrombus may intermittently wax and wane in size and become occlusive for relatively short periods of time.
- There may be intense local vasoconstriction. Many disrupted plaques are eccentric, with the retention of an arc of normal vessel wall in which constriction can reduce blood flow.
- Platelet deposition is a known potent stimulus for local smooth muscle constriction.
- Embolisation of platelet aggregates into the intramyocardial vascular bed both block smaller arteries in the size range of 50–100 μm external diameter and cause vasoconstriction within the myocardium. Necropsy studies show a strong correlation between such platelet thrombi and microscopic foci of myocyte necrosis.[8][9]

Clinical correlations

Much of the work described so far is based on necropsy observations but these have been extended and amplified by observations made in life to give the dynamic dimension.

Acute myocardial infarction

It is difficult now to perceive why coronary thrombosis was regarded 25 years ago as an inconstant and irrelevant consequence of acute infarction rather than its prime cause. Once angiography was carried out soon after the onset of infarction, and it was realised that the subtending artery was totally blocked but spontaneously reopened with time in many cases (and that this reopening was accelerated by fibrinolytic treatment), thrombosis was seen as a major causal factor in occlusion. Suddenly the clinical world found thrombi to be both dynamic and important. Pathologists had thought thrombi were important but did not realise how dynamic they could be. Sequential angiograms taken over some years in patients with chronic ischaemic heart disease also changed perceptions. It was realised that a significant proportion of the thrombotic occlusions causing infarction did not develop at sites where there was pre-existing high grade stenosis, or even a plaque identified at all. Sixty eight per cent of the occlusions leading to acute infarction were judged to have caused less than 50% diameter stenosis previously, while only 14% developed on high grade stenoses of more than 70% diameter in a recent review of the literature.[10]

The advent of intravascular ultrasound has confirmed that many stable coronary plaques are angiographically invisible because of arterial remodelling. In this process, described so well by Glagov,[11] the artery is seen to respond to plaque growth by increasing its cross sectional area while retaining normal lumen dimensions. Angiography cannot and does not predict the sites and risk of future infarction. It is true that chronic high grade stenoses do progress to occlude, but this is a slow process and is often caused by erosion type thrombosis, and is not associated with acute infarction due to collateral flow. For example, 24% of lesions occluding more than 80% by diameter will progress to chronic total occlusion by five years.

6

The magnitude of episodes of disruption varies widely. At one extreme the plaque has a crack or fissure only, and the large thrombotic response appears out of proportion to the stimulus. Such events are easily treated by lysis to give a lumen size which is little different from the previous state or event taken to be a normal artery. At the other extreme a plaque undergoes complete disintegration, occluding the lumen with a mixture of plaque content and thrombus. Another form is where the artery is occluded by the thrombus expanding the plaque from within. These more complex types of disruption occlusion will be more likely to respond to primary angioplasty. The exact morphology of disrupted plaques causing occlusion cannot, however, be determined in vivo by any current methodology.

Transmural regional acute myocardial infarction is caused by a coronary artery occlusion which develops over a relatively short time frame of a few hours and persists for at least 6–8 hours. The infarcted tissue is structurally suggestive of a homogenous entity—that is, all the myocardium involved died at around the same time. Non-transmural regional infarcts (non-Q wave) have a different structure which is built up by the coalescence of many small areas of necrosis of very different ages. This pattern of necrosis characteristically follows crescendo unstable angina and appears to be caused by repetitive episodes of short lived occlusion or platelet embolisation, or both. A further factor in limiting the spread of necrosis and preserving the subpericardial zone is the existence of prior collateral flow in the affected artery.

Unstable angina

The challenge of understanding the pathophysiology of unstable angina is the wide spectrum of clinical severity.[12] Necropsy studies are inevitably biased toward the worst outcome, but within this limitation show unstable angina to be caused by disrupted plaques with exposed mural thrombus and retention of antegrade flow in the artery. This feature of some persistent antegrade flow is all that separates the vascular lesion of unstable angina from that of acute infarction. The persistence of the thrombotic process so that it neither progresses to occlude nor resolves to heal represents a balance between prothrombotic and antithrombotic factors. Confirmation of plaque disruption and thrombosis as the basis for severe unstable angina has come from angiography in vivo where type II lesions with irregular overhanging edges and intraluminal filling defects (fig 1.6) representing thrombus are found.[13] These angiographic appearances are rare in stable angina. Type II lesions have been shown to be disrupted plaques by pathology studies. Angioscopy has directly observed torn plaque caps in vivo and intravascular ultrasound has also identified disrupted plaques in vivo. Atherectomy studies comparing tissue from plaques thought to be responsible for stable and unstable angina have shown very consistent results. A significant proportion, but not all, of samples from unstable

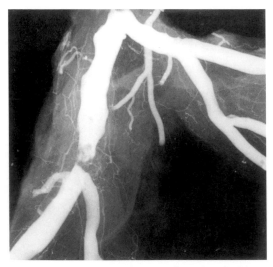

Figure 1.6. Angiogram of plaque disruption. In this postmortem angiogram there is a typical type II eccentric ragged stenosis with an overlying intraluminal filling defect indicating thrombus over the plaque.

angina contain thrombus, while most samples from stable angina, but not all, do not contain thrombus. The absence of thrombus in unstable angina is in part related to the time delay between acute symptoms and atherectomy.[14]

Samples taken some weeks after the last episode of rest pain often show accelerated smooth muscle proliferation—that is, the healing process rather than the acute thrombotic process. The presence of thrombus in plaque causing stable angina highlights the role of subclinical disruption or erosion in plaque growth. The pathological changes in plaques causing unstable angina expose thrombus in an artery in which antegrade flow continues. Platelet emboli into the myocardium cause microscopic foci of necrosis which are the basis of the increased concentrations of troponin T found in the blood in a proportion of cases of unstable angina.

The problem of the pathophysiology of unstable angina lies in patients who have milder and persistent rest pain over months or even years. The perception is that these cases are related to vasomotor tonal abnormalities often occurring at specific sites in the coronary artery tree. Why one such plaque should lead to local spasm is unclear—one suggestion is that there is local endothelial damage and repetitive ultramicroscopic thrombosis. The preponderance of literature reports of such vasospastic angina from Japan suggests there may be racial or geographic differences in the pathogenesis of this form of unstable angina.

Plaque disruption: the healing process

The great majority of episodes of plaque disruption do not cause a major event such as infarction or death. Minor episodes of erosion or disruption are often clinically silent but do contribute to the episodic progression of coronary artery disease seen on sequential angiography.

Thrombus will be removed by natural lysis to some extent and is also associated with "passi-

Plaques at risk of future thrombotic events are characterised by:

- Large lipid cores (> 50% overall plaque volume)

- Thin caps

- High densities of macrophages and high levels of expression of tissue factor and metalloproteinases

- Low densities of smooth muscle cells

fication", a term implying that the exposed collagen becomes less active in causing platelet adhesion probably due to being coated by natural heparinoids. Any residual thrombus which is still present after 36 hours will provoke smooth muscle cell migration into the area, with the production of new connective tissue which smooths out the surface and restores plaque integrity. The final result will be a stable lesion which may cause anything from chronic total occlusion to only a minor increase from the pre-existing degree of stenosis. The process, however, takes weeks and residual thrombi in the base of the exposed lipid core act as a nidus for a further thrombotic event at the same site for up to six months.

The risk of progressing to complete occlusion on angiography within a year of an episode of unstable angina, or after lysis for acute myocardial infarction, is far higher if the culprit lesion has an irregular outline on the initial angiogram taken immediatcly after the acute event.[15]

Inflammation and coronary atherosclerosis

Atherosclerotic plaques are the site of an inflammatory reaction which is of equal intensity to that found in the synovium in acute rheumatoid arthritis. The volume of any individual plaque in the coronary arteries is small, but most individuals have many plaques in the carotid artery and aorta which can be up to 2 cm in length. It is therefore not surprising that there may be elevation in systemic markers of inflammation such as fibrinogen and C reactive protein in subjects with chronic coronary atherosclerosis. The physicians health study shows that the difference between the lowest and highest quartiles of C reactive protein concentration is a threefold increase in the risk of a future acute event.[16] The actual concentrations of C reactive protein are not, however, high and such estimates give assessment of group rather

Mechanisms of myocardial ischaemia in non-occluding coronary thrombosis

- Distal embolisation of aggregates of platelets

- Intermittent total occlusion

- Spasm at thrombus site

than individual risk. One explanation is that the subjects with the highest concentrations of C reactive protein have the largest plaque mass. The link between systemic markers of chronic inflammation and acute coronary events may, however, be more complex. There is experimental evidence that upregulation of systemic inflammation will have a secondary affect of enhancing inflammatory activity in the plaque.[17 18] On this basis any factor which increases systemic inflammation would potentially trigger plaque instability and increase the risk of unstable angina. Causes of such systemic low grade inflammation include infection by chlamydia or helicobacter, diseases such as rheumatoid arthritis, and chronic dental sepsis.

Lipid lowering, infection, and acute coronary events

The current view of atherosclerosis is that the prime stimulus for plaque inflammation is the reaction between oxidised LDL and the macrophage. Significant reduction of plasma lipids in animal models of atherosclerosis has a profound effect on the plaque morphology, with a reduction in both macrophage numbers and activation products including metalloproteinases. The resultant plaque will be less inflammatory, and smooth muscle cell numbers and the collagen content rise. Although not reduced greatly in size, the plaque would be at far less risk of thrombosis. Similar changes in human plaques would explain the consistent benefit observed in a reduction of acute events in all the statin based trials.

Even allowing for poor patient compliance, the need for at least 18 months for the benefit to appear, and inadequate lipid lowering, acute ischaemic events still occur in treated patients. This suggests there may be non-lipid dependent factors enhancing plaque inflammation. One such factor is direct invasion of the plaque by chlamydia. These organisms exist within macrophages and potentially could upregulate the production of inflammatory mediators within the plaque.[18] Therapeutic trials of antichlamydial drugs to reduce acute coronary event rates are currently underway but results so far are contradictory. It seems likely that there are many other factors which enhance the inflammatory activity of the plaque, but the primary stimulus remains the conversion of plasma LDL in the intima to a proinflammatory product.[19] In keeping with this view is the consistent message from animal models of atherosclerosis that reducing plasma lipid concentrations strikingly reduces all the inflammatory processes in the plaque.[20]

1. **Stary H, Chandler A, Dinsmore R,** *et al.* A definition of advanced types of atherosclerotic lesions and a histological classification of atherosclerosis. A report from the committee on vascular lesions of the council on atherosclerosis, American Heart Association. *Circulation* 1995;**92**:1355–74.
- *Atherosclerotic plaques are morphologically diverse. This AHA committee report is the best nomenclature so far produced to describe the different forms and highlights the importance of a lipid core and fibrous cap in plaques at risk of thrombotic compliations.*

2. **Davies M, Woolf N, Rowles P,** *et al.* Morphology of the endothelium over atherosclerotic plaques in human coronary arteries. *Br Heart J* 1988;**60**:459–64.

3. **Ross R.** Atherosclerosis—an inflammatory disease. *N Engl J Med* 1999;**340**:115–26.

4. **Burke A, Farb A, Malcom G,** *et al.* Coronary risk factors and plaque morphology in men with coronary disease who died suddenly. *N Engl J Med* 1997;**336**:1276–82.

5. **Davies M.** The composition of coronary artery plaques. *N Engl J Med* 1997;**336**:1312–13.

6. **Arbustini E, Dal Bello P, Morbini P,** *et al.* Plaque erosion is a major substrate for coronary thrombosis in acute myocardial infarction. *Heart* 1999;**82**:269–72.
• *Thrombosis over a plaque is either caused by erosion or disruption. This paper illustrates endothelial erosion and highlights its contribution to acute myocardial infarction.*

7. **Davies M.** Stability and instability: two faces of coronary atherosclerosis. The Paul Dudley White Lecture 1995. *Circulation* 1996;**94**:2013–20.
• *A review of the concept of plaque thrombosis being caused by erosion or disruption and highlighting the role that plaque inflammation plays. The concept that collagen production and smooth muscle proliferation are essential in maintaining plaque stability (resistance to thrombosis) is described.*

8. **Davies M, Thomas A, Knapman P,** *et al.* Intramyocardial platelet aggregation in patients with unstable angina suffering sudden ischaemic cardiac death. *Circulation* 1986;**73**:418–27.

9. **Falk E.** Unstable angina with fatal outcome: dynamic coronary thrombosis leading to infarction and/or sudden death. *Circulation* 1985;**71**:699–708.
• *This paper describes the characteristic non-occluding thrombi that cause unstable angina and explains that distal embolisation of platelets is an important mechanism for intermittent myocardial ischaemia.*

10. **Falk E, Shah P, Fuster V.** Coronary plaque disruption. *Circulation* 1995;**92**:656–71.

11. **Glagov S, Weisenberd E, Zarins C,** *et al.* Compensatory enlargement of human atherosclerotic coronary arteries. *N Engl J Med* 1987;**316**:1371–5.
• *This article should be compulsory reading for everyone who carries out coronary angiography. It explains that the usual response of a coronary artery to the formation of a plque is to increase its cross sectional area to preserve lumen size. Most plaques therefore remain angiographically occult. Stenosis occurs when this compensatory mechanism fails.*

12. **Braunwald E.** Unstable angina. An etiologic approach to management. *Circulation* 1998;**98**:2219–22.

13. **Ambrose J, Winters S, Stern A,** *et al.* Angiographic morphology and the pathogenesis of unstable angina. *J Am Coll Cardiol* 1985;**5**:609–16.

14. **Mann J, Kaski J, Pereira W,** *et al.* Histological patterns of atherosclerotic plaques in unstable angina patients vary according to clinical presentation. *Heart* 1998;**80**:19–22.

15. **Chen L, Chester M, Redwood S,** *et al.* Angiographic stenosis progression and coronary events in patients with "stabilised" unstable angina. *Circulation* 1995;**91**:2319–24.

16. **Ridker P, Cushman M, Stampfer M.** Inflammation aspirin and the risk of cardiovascular disease in apparently healthy men. *N Engl J Med* 1997;**336**:973–9.

17. **Libby P, Egan D, Skarlatos S.** Roles of infectious agents in atherosclerosis and restenosis: an assessment of the evidence and need for future research. *Circulation* 1997;**96**:4095–103.

18. **Libby P, Ridker PM.** Novel inflammatory markers of coronary risk, theory and practice. *Circulation* 1999;**100**:1148–50.

19. **Witztum J.** The oxidation hypothesis of atherosclerosis. *Lancet* 1994;**344**:793–5.

20. **Aikawa M, Voglic SJ, Sugiyama S,** *et al.* Dietary lipid lowering tissue factor expression in rabbit atheroma. *Circulation* 1999;**100**:1215–22.

2 Atherogenesis: current understanding of the causes of atheroma

Peter L Weissberg

Until recently, atherosclerosis was thought of as a degenerative, slowly progressive disease, predominantly affecting the elderly, and causing symptoms through its mechanical effects on blood flow, particularly in the small calibre arteries supplying the myocardium and brain. Thus the approach to treatment has traditionally been surgical and focused on the largest and most visible or symptomatic lesions, coupled with a somewhat nihilistic belief that there was little likelihood of medical management affecting such a longstanding "end stage" process. However, recent research into the cellular and molecular events underlying the development and progression of atherosclerosis, prompted by careful descriptive studies of the underlying pathology, has shown that atherosclerosis is a dynamic, inflammatory process that is eminently modifiable. Support for this view comes from clinical trials of lipid lowering agents, particularly the "statins", which have shown only minor effects on the size of existing lesions, but major reductions in clinical events caused by plaque rupture, implying a beneficial stabilising effect on plaque composition. This calls for a change from a quantitative (how many and how tight are the stenoses?) to a more qualitative (how active are the plaques we cannot see?) approach to atherosclerosis. Also, a better understanding of the molecular and cellular basis of atherosclerosis will inevitably lead to the design of better diagnostic and therapeutic approaches. The purpose of this review is to summarise current understanding of the pathogenesis and progression of atherosclerosis with particular reference to potential new diagnostic or therapeutic approaches.

The atherosclerotic plaque

Atherosclerosis begins as a subendothelial accumulation of lipid laden, monocyte derived foam cells and associated T cells which form a non-stenotic fatty streak. With progression, the lesions take the form of an acellular core of cholesterol esters bounded by an endothelialised fibrous cap containing vascular smooth muscle cells (VSMC) and inflammatory cells, predominantly macrophages with some T cells and mast cells, which tend to accumulate at the shoulder regions of the plaque. Also present in advanced lesions are new blood vessels and deposits of calcium hydroxyapatite. Thus atherosclerotic lesions are complex and it is the dynamic interaction between the different components of the plaque that dictates outcome of the disease.

The endothelium

Since the discovery of endothelium dependent relaxation, and its biochemical entity, nitric oxide (NO), it has been recognised that the endothelium plays an important role in vascular biology. Several roles have been ascribed to vascular NO including modulation of tone, inhibition of platelet aggregation, inhibition of VSMC proliferation, and production of potentially destructive free radicals, in particular peroxynitrite. The earliest detectable physiological manifestation of atherosclerosis is reduced production of NO in response to pharmacological or haemodynamic stimuli. This phenomenon is present even in children with hypercholesterolaemia,[1] and is consistent with the hypothesis that high circulating concentrations of atherogenic lipoproteins lead to endothelial dysfunction and (by unknown mechanisms) subendothelial lipid accumulation. Importantly, however, it remains unclear whether this manifestation of endothelial dysfunction is a cause or a consequence of lipid accumulation, since fatty streaks are also present from a young age. Interestingly, a number of drugs that are known to influence beneficially the outcome of vascular disease, including statins and angiotensin converting enzyme (ACE) inhibitors, have been shown to improve endothelial function in studies of brachial artery dilatation in response to increased forearm blood flow.

In addition to reduced NO bioavailability, and possibly partly because of it, endothelial cells in atherosclerosis express surface bound molecules (selectins and adhesion molecules) that attract and capture circulating inflammatory cells and facilitate their migration into the subendothelial space. The importance of these molecules in the development of atherosclerosis is demonstrated in mice deficient in molecules such as intercellular adhesion molecule 1 (ICAM 1) and P selectin, which develop smaller lesions with less lipid and fewer inflammatory cells than control mice when fed a high lipid diet. Thus recruitment of inflammatory cells is important for plaque development, but since inflammatory cells do not accumulate in the intima in the absence of lipid, these data suggest that lipid accumulation is the initiating event and that inflammatory cells play a permissive role in lesion progression. The predisposition for atherosclerosis at particular sites in the vascular tree may be influenced by subtle, local effects on endothelial function, particularly shear stress which is known to regulate expression of a number of endothelial cell genes including ICAM 1 and eNOS. It remains to be seen whether new treatments being designed, for example, to enhance deficient NO bioavailability or to reduce adhesion molecule expression will have any impact on atherosclerosis or its consequences in man.

10

Inflammatory cells

Accumulated subendothelial lipid, particularly if oxidised, exacerbates the local inflammatory reaction and maintains activation of the overlying endothelium. This results in continued expression of selectins and adhesion molecules and also expression of chemokines, in particular monocyte chemoattractant proteins-1 (MCP-1). Chemokines are proinflammatory cytokines that function in leucocyte chemoattraction and activation. Atheroma prone mice lacking MCP-1 develop smaller atherosclerotic lesions than mice expressing MCP-1, providing further evidence that inflammatory cells play an important part in lesion development. Once captured, the inflammatory cells migrate into the subendothelial space where, under the influence of local chemokines, they become activated. The monocytes mature into macrophages and express the necessary scavenger receptor to ingest modified lipids and become macrophage foam cells. The predominant role of the macrophage in atherosclerosis is to ingest and dispose of atherogenic lipids. However, activated macrophages and T cells also express a variety of proinflammatory cytokines and growth factors that contribute to the evolution of the plaque. The progression of an atherosclerotic plaque is best understood in terms of the dynamic interaction between a subendothelial inflammatory stimulus and the local reactive "wound healing" response of surrounding VSMCs.

Vascular smooth muscle cells

Medial VSMCs contain large amounts of contractile proteins since their predominant role is to maintain vascular tone. This "contractile" VSMC phenotype is maintained particularly by the influence of extracellular proteins in the media on VSMC surface integrins. However, if medial VSMCs are taken out of this environment, for example into cell culture, they undergo a change in phenotype characterised by a reduction in content of contractile proteins and an increase in synthetic organelles. VSMCs undergo a similar change when they move from the media to the intima in vivo. This change in phenotype from "contractile" to "synthetic" was once thought of as being a key initiating event in the pathogenesis of an atherosclerotic lesion.[2] However, recent studies have shown a remarkable similarity in gene expression between intimal VSMCs in atherosclerosis and VSMCs in the early developing blood vessel,[3] consistent with the view that intimal VSMCs are more likely to be performing a reparative than a permissive role in atherosclerosis. In adopting a "repair" phenotype VSMCs express the proteinases that are required to break down the surrounding basement membrane to facilitate their migration to the site of injury; they produce growth factors that facilitate their proliferation at the site of injury, and they produce

the necessary matrix proteins, in particular collagens and elastin, to repair the vessel. Indeed, expression of this repertoire of genes is essential for the formation of a fibrous cap over the lipid core of an atherosclerotic plaque. Since the fibrous cap separates the highly thrombogenic lipid rich core from circulating platelets and proteins of the coagulation cascade and confers structural stability to an atherosclerotic lesion, and since the VSMC is the only cell capable of synthesising the cap, it follows that VSMCs play a pivotal role in maintaining plaque stability and protecting against plaque rupture and consequent thrombosis.[4]

Cellular interactions and plaque stability

Atherosclerotic lesions are ubiquitous in most adults in the developed world, but they are largely asymptomatic. There are two mechanisms by which atherosclerosis leads to symptoms. If the lesion becomes sufficiently large to restrict blood flow, such that nutrient supply cannot meet demand, then tissue ischaemia will occur, as in chronic stable angina pectoris. However, plaque growth does not always lead to lumen stenosis, since atherosclerotic arteries can remodel to accommodate the expanding atherosclerotic lesion while still maintaining a normal or near normal lumen diameter.[5] Thus large atherosclerotic lesions may be, and often are, clinically silent.

If the lesion ruptures or erodes platelets rapidly accumulate and intravascular thrombosis can occur, leading to the acute coronary syndromes of unstable angina and myocardial infarction. Plaques with a large lipid pool and a thin fibrous cap are much more prone to rupture than those with a thick cap, partly because a thick fibrous cap is more able to resist local mechanical stresses. However, the most important determinant of plaque stability is the composition of the fibrous cap, in that a preponderance of inflammatory cells and a relative paucity of VSMCs leads to plaque rupture.[6]

There are several mechanisms by which inflammatory cells can weaken the fibrous cap. Firstly, they affect matrix protein turnover by producing specific metalloproteinases that degrade matrix proteins in the cap[4] and proinflammatory cytokines, in particular interferon γ (INF γ), that inhibit VSMC proliferation and collagen synthesis. Secondly, they secrete inflammatory cytokines, in particular interleukin 1β, tumour necrosis factor α (TNF α) and INF γ, that are synergistically cytotoxic for VSMCs. Thirdly, it has recently been shown that activated macrophages can induce VSMC apoptosis (programmed cell death) by direct cell-cell contact. All this is further compounded by the phenotype of the VSMCs within the fibrous cap of a mature plaque which have a reduced ability to proliferate and an enhanced susceptibility to apoptosis.[7] [8] Thus inflammatory cells can destroy the fabric of the fibrous cap and resident VSMCs are poorly equipped to compensate. Importantly, these features can be and often are present in small, haemodynamically insignificant atherosclerotic plaques that are clinically silent and angiographically invisible. Thus plaque composition is far more important than plaque size in determining outcome.

Consequences of plaque rupture

Rupture or erosion of the fibrous cap exposes the highly thrombogenic collagenous matrix and lipid core to the circulation and leads inevitably to platelet accumulation and activation. This, in turn, leads to fibrin deposition, thrombus formation and, at its most extreme, vessel occlusion. However, vessel occlusion is not inevitable, and it is now clear that episodes of silent, subclinical plaque rupture occur frequently in patients with atherosclerosis. In one study up to 70% of plaques causing high grade stenosis had evidence of previous plaque rupture and repair in the absence of vessel occlusion or a corresponding clinical event.[9] These episodes of non-occlusive plaque rupture induce recruitment of new VSMCs under the influence of mitogens, in particular platelet derived growth factor and thrombin[10] in the thrombus. Thrombus also contains large quantities of transforming growth factor β which is a potent stimulator of VSMC matrix synthesis. These factors therefore drive formation of a new fibrous cap over the thrombus, thereby increasing the size of the lesion (fig 2.1). Thus the size of atherosclerotic lesions increases as a consequence of repeated episodes of rupture and repair. The chief implication of this is that pharmacological inhibition of silent plaque rupture would be expected to reduce progression of atherosclerotic lesions. It also serves to explain and emphasise the value of antiplatelet drugs in atherosclerosis.

Diagnostic implications of plaque biology

Imaging
The mainstay of clinical diagnosis of coronary disease is the coronary angiogram. Angiography can only detect lesions that impinge significantly on the lumen, however, and provide little or no information on the composition of a stenotic lesion. Since it is composition rather than size that determines the likelihood of plaque rupture, it follows that angiography is likely to be a poor predictor of clinical events. Thus, Falk and colleagues[11] showed that most of the lesions that cause myocardial infarction produce less than a 50% stenosis. This important observation explains why myocardial infarction occurs so commonly in patients who have experienced no previous symptoms and emphasises why better diagnostic tools are required. Thus, despite its continuing pivotal role in evaluation and management of symptomatic coronary disease, angiography has little to offer in risk prediction or therapeutic monitoring in the asymptomatic population. The same is true for intravascular ultrasound, even though it provides much more information than angiography on the extent and composition of targeted plaques. Ideally, what is required is an imaging technique that can be used repeatedly to identify and monitor asymptomatic atherosclerosis.

The extent of coronary calcification, as quantified by electron beam computed tomography, has been shown to predict clinical events, and an absence of calcification can be taken to indicate an absence of significant coronary disease. The precise relation between calcification and plaque progression remains to be determined, however, and monitoring calcification will only be of value if it proves to be reversible as indicated by recent studies.[12]

The most promising emerging imaging techniques are magnetic resonance imaging (MRI) and radionucleide based techniques, in particular positron emission tomography (PET). MRI can differentiate some plaque components in animal models and human vessels.[13] However, image resolution and movement artefact remain substantial obstacles to the use of MRI to monitor coronary disease and while MRI may provide fine anatomical detail, it is unlikely to provide information on inflammatory activity within plaques. In contrast, PET provides little anatomical information but offers the potential to measure and monitor plaque inflammatory cell content and activity. Early animal studies using [^{18}F]FDG-PET to measure plaque metabolic activity have been encouraging, but as with MRI, resolution is a major obstacle to imaging coronary atheroma in man. Despite these obstacles, it seems inevitable that non-angiographic imaging of atherosclerosis will be developed in the foreseeable future.

Risk factor evaluation
The realisation that atherosclerosis is essentially an inflammatory process has prompted the search for measurable biochemical markers of plaque inflammation, some of which are non-specific, such as serum amyloid A (SAA), C reactive protein (CRP) and TNF α, while others, such as ICAM 1 and VCAM 1, are thought to be more specific for vascular inflammation. Most prominent of these is the use of highly sensitive assays to measure low concentrations of CRP—that is, below the limit of detection of assays used in routine clinical practice—which have shown a strong correlation between CRP and risk of myocardial infarction and stroke.[14] Furthermore, those patients with highest CRP concentrations (albeit within the conventional normal range) derived most benefit from prophylactic aspirin treatment. Also, benefit derived from pravastatin treatment in the CARE study was associated with a reduction in CRP and SAA concentrations. It is likely that in the near future biochemical measures of inflammation, in combination with measurement of conventional risk factors, will be used to guide selection of patients at highest risk for primary

12

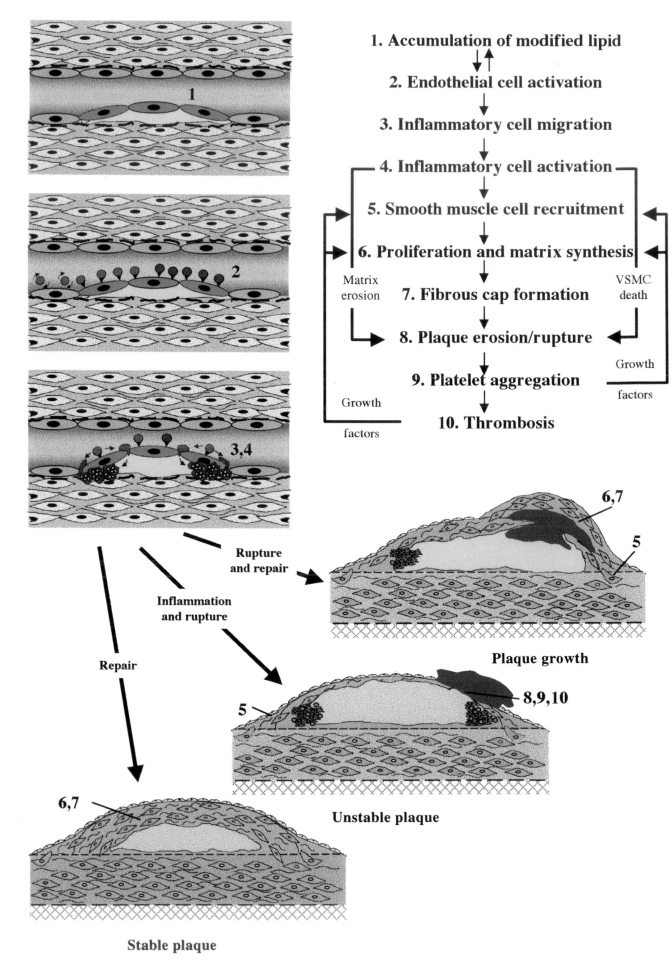

Figure 2.1. Cellular interactions in the development and progression of atherosclerosis. VSMC, vascular smooth muscle cells.

prevention treatment and to monitor their progress. Also, it is likely that a better understanding of the molecular interactions that dictate plaque instability will lead to the discovery of more specific circulating markers of disease activity.

Therapeutic implications of plaque biology

Angiographic studies have shown that effective lipid lowering with statins reduces the incidence of new lesion formation and produces a significant, but haemodynamically unimportant (0.04–0.07 mm), improvement in established stenoses.[15] Importantly, however, they also reduce the rate of progression of preexisting lesions and the number of new vessel occlusions. Both of these beneficial effects are likely to be due to prevention of plaque rupture since, as discussed above, lesions grow by repeated episodes of subclinical rupture and repair, and silent occlusion arises when plaque rupture and thrombosis occur in the context of a well collateralised myocardial circulation such that no significant ischaemia results from the occlusion. Despite the modest effects of statins on size of pre-existing lesions, several outcome studies, both in primary and secondary prevention settings, have shown a substantial (30–40%) reduction in cardiovascular events in the statin treated groups.[16–18] Taking the angiographic and outcome data together, these results argue strongly that statins stabilise plaques.

The balance of atherosclerosis

Atherosclerosis is a dynamic balance between the destructive influence of inflammatory cells and the reactive, stabilising effects of VSMCs. The balance is biased in favour of plaque rupture by factors such as high low density lipoprotein (LDL) cholesterol, lipid peroxidation and, probably, genetic variability in the inflammatory molecules involved. For example, there is a correlation between plaque progression and a polymorphism in the stromelysin-1 gene promoter. Also, it is entirely plausible that infective agents, in particular *Chlamydia pneumoniae*, which can be found in plaque macrophages, may exacerbate the inflammatory process and tip the balance in favour of plaque rupture; this hypothesis is currently being tested in clinical trials.

In contrast, the balance will be biased towards repair and stability by a reduction in plaque inflammation. Lipid lowering, by whatever means, is associated with a reduction in clinical events and animal studies have shown dramatic reductions in plaque inflammatory cell content during statin treatment, even in the absence of lipid lowering.[19] These observations, coupled with a greater benefit from pravastatin treatment than was predicted by the achieved reduction in LDL cholesterol in the West of Scotland coronary prevention study,[16]

- Atherosclerosis is not thought to represent an inflammatory reaction to the subendothelial accumulation of modified lipid

- Atherosclerosis is invariably associated with abnormal endothelial cell function. Vascular smooth muscle cells are the only cells capable of protecting against plaque rupture and its consequences

- The outcome of atherosclerosis is determined much more by plaque composition than plaque size

- Atherosclerotic lesions frequently enlarge as a consequence of repeated subclinical episodes of rupture and repair. The only logical conclusion to be drawn from the angiographic and outcome studies of statin treatment is that statin treatment stabilises atherosclerotic lesions

- Atherosclerosis is a dynamic process capable of being modified

have led to the suggestion that some statins may exert effects on plaque stability which are additional to and independent of lipid lowering. Laboratory studies have shown that statins can exert direct effects on endothelial cell function, inflammatory cell activity, VSMC proliferation, platelet aggregation, and thrombus formation.[20 21] Since the effects of different stains are not equivalent, it has been suggested that some may afford more or less protection than others for an equivalent lipid lowering effect. Such observations argue strongly for robust outcome studies to prove overall efficacy and safety.

Understanding of the non-lipid associated events in atherogenesis raises the prospect of developing drugs targeted at specific events in its pathogenesis which might act synergistically with lipid lowering drugs to enhance plaque stability. Possible targets include endothelial NO and adhesion molecule production, the matrix metalloproteinases, inflammatory cytokines and their receptors, and angiogenesis, since mice lacking specific angiogenic factors develop smaller atherosclerotic lesions than controls. If oxidised lipids are the major stimulus for atherogenesis, then antioxidants, such as vitamin E, might be expected to reduce the inflammatory drive in atherosclerosis and thereby promote plaque stability. However, despite early promise, recent large scale studies have cast doubt on the integrity of this hypothesis.

In addition to reducing inflammation, stimulation of the VSMC repair process should result in increased stability. For example, balloon angioplasty stimulates a vigorous VSMC repair response. This may contribute to restenosis and the re-emergence of angina, but the resulting lesion is always fibrotic and stable and rarely if ever precipitates an acute coronary event, even when the original target lesion was unstable. It is feasible therefore that better understanding of the molecular regulators of

VSMC behaviour may lead to drug treatments aimed at enhancing fibrous cap formation. Modulators of TGF β activity may have a particularly important role to play in this context.

Summary

Atherosclerosis is a dynamic balance between lipid driven inflammatory cells and their cytokines within the substance of the plaque, and the natural stabilising properties of the surrounding VSMCs. That plaque composition is much more important than size is illustrated by clinical and laboratory studies with statins which have little effect on plaque size yet have a major influence on plaque composition and clinical outcome. In future, cardiologists will need to re-focus their attention away from angiographic appearances in symptomatic patients towards potential measures of inflammatory atherosclerotic activity in asymptomatic patients with subclinical disease. Our evolving knowledge of the cellular and molecular interactions that lead to plaque development and progression is likely to lead to novel imaging strategies and novel biochemical measures of disease progression, and potentially also to the development of drugs aimed specifically at stabilising atherosclerotic lesions. That this is achievable has already been demonstrated.

PLW is the British Heart Foundation Professor of Cardiovascular Medicine.

1. **Sorensen KE, Celermajer DS, Georgakopoulos D,** *et al.* Impairment of endothelium-dependent dilation is an early event in children with familial hypercholesterolemia and is related to the lipoprotein(a) level. *J Clin Invest* 1994;**93**:50–5.

2. **Ross R, Glomset J.** The pathogenesis of atherosclerosis. Part 1. *N Engl J Med* 1976;**295**:369–77.
• *This was the first of a number of very influential reviews published by Ross on the pathogenesis of atherosclerosis. Although this review focuses very much on the role of platelets and smooth muscle cells in the development of an atherosclerotic lesion, subsequent reviews published in the same journal in 1986 and 1999 demonstrate the evolution of the field towards the recognition that atherosclerosis is fundamentally an inflammatory condition.*

3. **Shanahan C, Weissberg P.** Smooth muscle cell heterogeneity—patterns of gene expression in vascular smooth muscle cells in vitro and in vivo. *Arterioscler Thromb Vasc Biol* 1998;**18**:333–8.

4. **Libby P.** Molecular bases of the acute coronary syndromes. *Circulation* 1995;**91**:2844–50.
• *This article encapsulates the link between the cellular and molecular interactions thought to be taking place within atherosclerotic lesions and the clinical syndromes that result. In particular it emphasises the fundamental role of smooth muscle cells in protecting against plaque rupture.*

5. **Glagov S, Weisenberg E, Zarius C,** *et al.* Compensatory enlargement of human atherosclerotic coronary arteries. *N Engl J Med* 1987;**316**:371–5.

6. **Davies MJ.** Stability and instability—2 faces of coronary atherosclerosis. The Paul-Dudley-White lecture 1995. *Circulation* 1996;**94**:2013–20.
• *In this paper Davies elegantly sets out the fundamental pathological observations on which our current understanding of the pathogenesis and progression of atherosclerosis is founded. By quantifying the contribution of inflammatory cells to plaque rupture, Davies changed the whole approach to atherosclerosis research and treatment.*

7. **Ross R, Wight TN, Strandness E,** *et al.* Human atherosclerosis. I. Cell constitution and characteristics of advanced lesions of the superficial femoral artery. *Am J Pathol* 1984;**114**:79–93.

8. **Bennett MR, Macdonald K, Chan SW,** *et al.* Cooperative interactions between RB and p53 regulate cell proliferation, cell senescence, and apoptosis in human vascular smooth muscle cells from atherosclerotic plaques. *Circ Res* 1998;**82**:704–12.

9. **Davies MJ.** Acute coronary thrombosis—the role of plaque disruption and its initiation and prevention. *Eur Heart J* 1995;**16**(suppl L):3–7.

10. **McNamara CA, Sarembock IJ, Bachhuber BG,** *et al.* Thrombin and vascular smooth muscle cell proliferation: implications for atherosclerosis and restenosis. *Semin Thromb Hemost* 1996;**22**:139–44.

11. **Falk E, Shah P, Fuster V.** Coronary plaque disruption. *Circulation* 1995;**92**:657–71.
• *This important publication demonstrates quite clearly that plaques that rupture and cause an acute myocardial infarction are most commonly those which do not cause the most significant stenoses when viewed angiographically. These observations confirm that the size of atherosclerotic lesions is less important than their content in determining outcome.*

12. **Callister TQ, Raggi P, Cooil B,** *et al.* Effect of HMG-CoA reductase inhibitors on coronary artery disease as assessed by electron-beam computed tomography [see comments]. *N Engl J Med* 1998;**339**:1972–8.

13. **Toussaint JF, LaMuraglia GM, Southern JF,** *et al.* Magnetic resonance images lipid, fibrous, calcified, hemorrhagic, and thrombotic components of human atherosclerosis in vivo. *Circulation* 1996;**94**:932–8.

14. **Ridker P, Cushman M, Stampfer M,** *et al.* Inflammation, aspirin, and the risk of cardiovascular disease in apparently healthy men. *N Engl J Med* 1997;**336**:973–9.
• *This paper firmly establishes the link between measurements of a circulating inflammatory marker, in this case a C reactive protein, and risk of a clinical event caused by atherosclerosis. Importantly, it shows that patients with the highest levels of CRP gain most benefit from aspirin treatment.*

15. **MAAS Investigators.** Effect of simvastatin on coronary atheroma: the multicentre anti-atheroma study (MAAS). *Lancet* 1994;**334**:633–8.

16. **Shepherd J, Cobbe S, Ford I,** *et al.* Prevention of coronary heart disease with pravastatin in men with hypercholesterolemia. *N Engl J Med* 1995;**333**:1301–7.

17. **LIPID Study Group.** Prevention of cardiovascular events and death with pravastatin in patients with coronary heart disease and a broad range of initial cholesterol levels. The long-term intervention with pravastatin in ischaemic disease (LIPID) study. *N Engl J Med* 1998;**339**:1349–57.
• *This is the largest and most recent of the secondary prevention studies with a statin, in this case pravastatin. The results prove beyond any reasonable doubt that statins prevent heart attacks and strokes in patients with established coronary artery disease, but effectively "normal" cholesterol concentrations.*

18. **Scandinavian Simvastatin Survival Study Group.** Randomised trial of cholesterol lowering in 4444 patients with coronary heart disease: the Scandinavian simvastatin survival study (4S). *Lancet* 1994;**344**:1383–9.

19. **Williams JK, Sukhova GK, Herrington DM,** *et al.* Pravastatin has cholesterol-lowering independent effects on the artery wall of atherosclerotic monkeys. *J Am Coll Cardiol* 1998;**31**:684–91.

20. **Treasure CB, Klein JL, Weintraub WS,** *et al.* Beneficial effects of cholesterol-lowering therapy on the coronary endothelium in patients with coronary artery disease [see comments]. *N Engl J Med* 1995;**332**:481–7.

21. **Rosenson RS, Tangney CC.** Antiatherothrombotic properties of statins: implications for cardiovascular event reduction [see comments]. *JAMA* 1998;**279**:1643–50.

website
extra

Additional references appear on the Heart website

www.heartjnl.com

3 Acute coronary syndromes: presentation—clinical spectrum and management

Keith A A Fox

Acute coronary syndromes define a spectrum of clinical manifestations of acute coronary artery disease. These extend from *acute myocardial infarction* through *minimal myocardial injury* to *unstable angina*. This spectrum shares common underlying pathophysiological mechanisms. The central features consist of fissuring or erosion of atheromatous plaque with superimposed platelet aggregation and thrombosis. This is complicated by microfragmentation and distal embolisation with alterations in vascular tone in affected myocardium. As a consequence, clinical manifestations are dependent upon the severity of obstruction in the affected coronary artery (fig 3.1), the presence or absence of collateral perfusion, and the volume and myocardial oxygen demand within the affected territory. Thus, the spectrum extends from abrupt occlusion with acute ischaemia leading to infarction, through partial coronary obstruction and distal ischaemia with minor enzyme release (minimal myocardial injury), to non-occlusive thrombosis with normal cardiac enzymes (unstable angina) (table 3.1).

The distinction between acute myocardial infarction and minimal myocardial injury is of immediate practical importance as emergency reperfusion treatment is indicated for acute infarction but not for the remainder of the acute coronary syndromes.[1] Acute infarction patients are identified by the combination of a typical clinical syndrome and electrocardiographic changes of ST elevation, new bundle branch block or posterior infarction. Such patients usually evolve Q waves and the release of cardiac enzymes with elevations to more than twice the upper limit of normal. In contrast, those with minimal myocardial injury do not have sustained ST segment elevation or the evolution of Q waves, and cardiac enzyme release is no more than twice the upper limit of normal. The terms "non-Q wave myocardial infarction" and "subendocardial myocardial infarction" refer to retrospective or pathological features and they are of little value as a guide to management in the acute clinical setting. It is impossible to characterise infarctions accurately into Q wave and non-Q wave at the time of presentation. In contrast, those with minimal myocardial injury/unstable angina can be defined at presentation and include individuals with a spectrum of electrocardiographic changes (table 3.1), but no features to indicate the need for immediate reperfusion. The management of such patients consists of anti-ischaemic treatment (β blockers, nitrates, calcium antagonists) in combination with antiplatelet treatment (aspirin, adenosine diphosphate antagonists, glycoprotein IIb/IIIa inhibitors) and antithrombin treatment (heparin and low molecular weight heparin) (fig 3.2).

The most frequently cited classification of patients with unstable angina is that proposed by Braunwald (table 3.2) and it describes the time course and mode of presentation. Relations have been demonstrated between classification categories and outcome, but this system excludes ECG information and it pre-dates modern enzymatic measures including troponins and the important prognostic information that both measures convey. Furthermore, the classification pre-dates current treatment strategies and hence we lack an evidence base upon which to differentiate management according to the Braunwald classification.

An alternative is to separate patients into high, intermediate, and low risk categories. These categories are important for the choice of pharmacological and interventional treatment as the relations between risks and outcome have been defined in trials. Risk status requires regular review, and documentation, as patients may change risk status as ECG, haemodynamic, and enzyme findings evolve. Specific prediction of cumulative risk can be derived from registry and trial data (that is, the six month risk of death/myocardial infarction or death/myocardial infarction/refractory an-

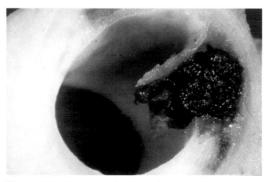

Figure 3.1. Macroscopic view of ruptured coronary plaque with intraplaque thrombosis and intraluminal extension. Superficial platelet rich thrombus (pale colour). This lesion would not produce flow limitation, at rest, and may not be detectable on coronary angiography.(High resolution colour slide; reproduced with permission from Professor Michael Davies).

Table 3.1   Acute coronary syndromes

Clinical syndrome	ECG features	Enzyme features
● Acute myocardial infarction (MI)	ST elevation New bundle branch block ECG changes of posterior MI Evolution of Q waves	> 2 × upper limit of CK-MB, CK Troponins T > 0.2 ng/dl Troponin I* > 1.0–1.5 ng/dl
● Minimal myocardial injury	Aborted ST elevation MI Transient ST elevation ST depression T inversion Minor non-specific ECG changes	< 2 × elevation CK-MB, CK Troponins T 0.01–0.2 ng/dl Troponin I* 0.1 or 0.4 ng/dl to 1.0–1.5 ng/dl
● Unstable angina	Transient ST elevation ST depression T inversion Minor non-specific ECG changes Normal ECG	CK-MB, CK below upper limit of normal Troponins T < 0.01 ng/dl Troponin I* < 0.1 or 0.4 ng/dl

*Troponin I cut off values depend upon assay system

16

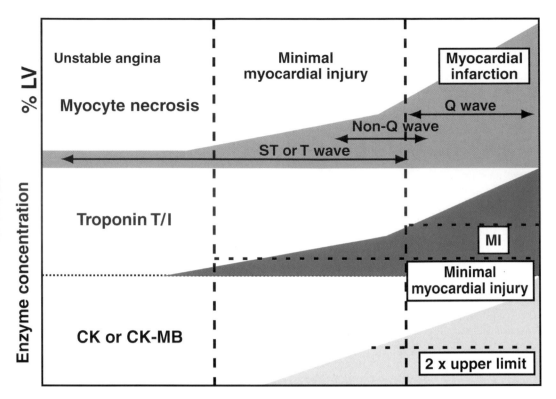

Figure 3.2. Spectrum of acute coronary syndromes. Schematic of the relation between the extent of myocardial necrosis, electrocardiographic markers, and cardiac enzymes (CK-MB and troponins). Troponins provide a more sensitive indicator of myocardial injury with a lower threshold indicating adverse prognostic outcome (troponin T 0.01 ng/dl, troponin I 0.1–0.4 ng/dl depending on assay system), than for myocardial infarction (table 3.1).

gina), but for clinical purposes tertiles of risk are more straightforward (see below) as they do not require complex algorithms for their derivation.

Outcome: unstable angina and minimal myocardial injury

Previously, the hazards associated with unstable angina and minimal myocardial injury have been underestimated. Imprecise definitions of the syndrome and inconsistency in the need for corroborative evidence of acute coronary disease (enzyme markers and ECG change) have led to the inclusion of patients with chest pain and low prospective risk. For example, applying the Braunwald criteria, various forms of subacute rest pain, including that more than 48 hours previously, could classify the patient as class 2 unstable angina. This could include patients with entirely normal ECGs, normal cardiac enzymes, and low risk subsequent stress tests. Not surprisingly the outcome of such a heterogeneous population is more benign than for those with diagnostic features of the syndrome.

Definition of the syndrome
Based upon trial data and prospective registries the following features define patients with an acute coronary syndrome:
- Ischaemic chest pain (discomfort) at rest or on minimal exertion or emotion (2×5 minute episodes or 1 episode > 10 minutes).
and

- Evidence of underlying coronary artery disease (at least one of the following):
  - ECG: ST segment depression, T wave inversion or transient ST elevation
  - Enzyme elevation: troponin I or T, creatine kinase (CK) or CK-MB
  - Evidence of coronary artery disease on angiography or perfusion scanning.

Patients with typical clinical features of unstable angina but a normal ECG and no prior documented coronary disease have a suspected acute coronary syndrome until enzymes and further ECGs confirm or refute the diagnosis.

Those with persistent ST elevation have suspected acute myocardial infarction and their management is considered elsewhere.

Overall outcome in unstable angina/non-ST elevation myocardial infarction
Based upon prospective international registry data among 8000 patients in six countries, the risk of death or myocardial infarction is approximately 10% at six months and almost a quarter of patients sustain these events or acute refractory angina within six months of initial presentation (OASIS registry).[2] Overall, half of these events occur within the first seven days of presentation. Based on those included

Table 3.2   Braunwald classification of unstable angina

Classification		A. Secondary unstable angina	B. Primary unstable angina	C. Postinfarction (< 2 weeks) unstable angina
I	New onset, severe or accelerated angina	IA	IB	IC
II	Subacute rest angina (> 48 hours ago)	IIA	IIB	IIC
III	Acute rest angina (within 48 hours)	IIIA	IIIB	IIIC

in clinical trials, and excluding those with normal ECGs, about 10% suffer death or myocardial infarction at 30 days (GUSTO II data).[3] These events occur despite aspirin treatment and antianginal medications. Recent data from the PRAISE UK registry indicate rates of death/myocardial infarction of 12.2% at six months.[4]

Identification of high risk and low risk patients

There are two main components to the risk carried by an individual patient: *prior risk* and *acute ischaemic risk*.

Prior risk is determined by systemic risk factors such as age, diabetes, hypertension, smoking, heart failure, and previous infarction. Such factors influence the extent of underlying coronary artery disease and left ventricular dysfunction, and their impact may be revealed by echocardiography, stress testing, perfusion scanning or coronary angiography.

Acute ischaemic risk is determined by the severity of impaired perfusion, the volume of myocardium affected, and the consequent changes in mechanical and electrical function. The distinction is important because a patient with a minor ischaemic event may nevertheless have extensive underlying coronary artery disease, and management strategies need to address both aspects of care. The converse may also occur.

The most powerful discriminators of acute ischaemic risk are:

- refractory angina with electrocardiographic evidence of ischaemia;
- ischaemia associated with haemodynamic instability or arrhythmia;
- recurrent ST segment change with positive troponin release;
- either positive troponin release or recurrent ST segment change.

A detailed discussion of risk prediction in acute coronary syndromes has been covered elsewhere.[5] The key factors predicting adverse risk are summarised in the adjacent box. Readily available clinical characteristics can be used to separate patients into high, medium, and low risk based upon independent predictors of adverse outcome (prior risk characteristics and ECG changes). In consequence, the rates of death/myocardial infarction/stroke at six months are 7.4%, 10.1%, and 17.9%, respectively.[2] Risk prediction is further improved by inducing troponin/CK-MB data and ST analysis.

Management of unstable angina and minimal myocardial injury

Presentation and general measures

Patients with an acute coronary syndrome may present de novo with new onset angina CCS (Canadian Cardiovascular Society) class III or IV, or following abrupt deterioration of previously stable angina with more severe and prolonged symptoms and diminished responsiveness to glyceryl trinitrate. The

---

Predicting adverse risk in unstable angina and minimal myocardial injury (summary)

- Prior risk
  - older age (> 65 years)
  - prior myocardial infarction or heart failure
  - comorbidity: diabetes, hypertension
  - impaired renal function

- Acute ischaemic risk
  - refractory or recurrent ischaemic pain
  - ECG: ST segment depression or transient ST elevation during pain
  - ECG: T wave inversion (lower risk than ST segment depression or transient ST elevation)
  - impaired left ventricular function with ischaemia
  - release of cardiac enzymes: CK, CK-MB, troponin T or troponin I
  - raised C reactive protein (high sensitivity assay)

---

symptoms may be present at rest or may be precipitated by minor exertion or emotion. Where such symptoms develop within the first two weeks following acute myocardial infarction, there is an increased risk of acute occlusion.

Patients with acute coronary syndromes may present directly to emergency departments (especially with acute infarction or severe ischaemia) but they may also present to chest pain clinics, care of the elderly units or to primary care physicians. On presentation a 12 lead ECG should be performed whenever possible during an episode of pain. This provides valuable diagnostic information.

Patients with diagnostic features of acute infarction or those of acute ischaemia with characteristic pain require emergency hospitalisation and management in a cardiac care unit or high dependency unit with continuous ECG monitoring. Repeat ECGs are required in those with suspected evolving infarction but in whom the initial features are non-diagnostic. Those with a suspected acute coronary syndrome should also be admitted directly to hospital (emergency admissions unit or chest pain assessment unit) to differentiate low risk patients for early discharge and intermediate/high risk patients for appropriate treatment. In current practice recent registry studies in the UK (PRAIS)[4] and elsewhere (ENACT)[6] suggest that low and high risk patients have similar lengths of stay; across Europe these averaged eight days of hospitalisation with approximately three days of care in a high dependency area.[6] Patients in whom cardiac enzymes remain non-elevated at baseline and eight hours after presentation are at very low risk of subsequent cardiac events (99% remain free of cardiac events, 95% confidence interval 96% to 100%). Additional tests did not improve predictive accuracy.[7]

Presentation and diagnosis of acute coronary syndromes: summary

Ischaemic chest pain $> 2 \times 5$ minutes or > 10 minutes at rest or minimal exertion or persistent symptoms of myocardial infarction ($\pm$ autonomic features).

- Evolving acute myocardial infarction
    - ECG: ST$\uparrow$, bundle branch block, posterior myocardial infarction
    Manage for acute myocardial infarction

- Abnormal ECG
    - transient ST$\uparrow$, ST$\downarrow$, T$\downarrow$
    Diagnosis: *unstable angina/minimal myocardial injury*
    - elevated troponin T/I or CK, CK-MB
    Diagnosis: *minimal myocardial injury*
    - enzymes not elevated
    Troponin T < 0.2, troponin I < upper limit for laboratory
    CK, CK-MB < 2 × upper limit for lab
    Diagnosis: *unstable angina*

    ECG: persistence of previously abnormal ECG (conduction defect, Q waves, T$\downarrow$)
    Diagnosis: *suspected acute coronary syndrome*
    a) Repeat ECG, especially during pain
    b) Troponin T/I, or CK, CK-MB
    If (a) or (b) diagnostic: acute coronary syndrome confirmed.
    If neither (a) nor (b) diagnostic: *unstable angina or non-acute coronary syndrome diagnosis*. Requires stress test $\pm$ angiography to confirm or refute diagnosis.

- Normal ECG
    ECG normal at baseline and 8–12 hours after pain. Troponins normal at 8–12 hours after pain.
    Diagnosis: *low risk patient or non-cardiac diagnosis*

Antiplatelet treatment

Aspirin

The critical role of platelets and of thrombus formation in the pathophysiology of this condition is discussed elsewhere.[8] Although aspirin is an irreversible inhibitor of platelet cyclo-oxygenase, and can inhibit the formation of thromboxane A_2 and inhibit platelet aggregation, its effects can be overcome in the presence of potent thrombogenic stimuli. Nevertheless, the benefits of aspirin are substantial and clearly defined; the antiplatelet trialist collaboration demonstrated a 36% reduction in death or myocardial infarction with antiplatelet treatment (predominantly aspirin) versus placebo in unstable angina trials.[9] Four key studies have demonstrated that aspirin almost halves the risk of cardiac death or non-fatal MI in patients with unstable angina. Thus, aspirin treatment is indicated in all patients with acute coronary syndromes unless there is good evidence of aspirin allergy. A starting dose of 300 mg (chewed) and a maintenance dose of 75 mg daily is recommended.

Adenosine diphosphate antagonists

The platelet adenosine diphosphate inhibitor clopidogrel has been employed as an adjunctive antiplatelet agent during coronary stenting. It appears to offer similar benefits to those of ticlopidine but with a more favourable safety profile (severe neutropenia as infrequent as that of aspirin: 0.04% clopidogrel v 0.02% aspirin). Chronic treatment with clopidogrel offers approximately a 9% risk reduction compared with aspirin treatment and it is specifically indicated in those with aspirin intolerance. The use of combination aspirin and clopidogrel in acute coronary syndromes is currently under evaluation.

Glycoprotein IIb/IIIa inhibitors

Despite the undoubted benefits of aspirin, patients with acute coronary syndromes nevertheless suffer important risks of subsequent cardiac events. In the presence of a potent thrombogenic stimulus, like that which follows rupture of an atheromatous plaque, the effects of aspirin may be overcome and platelet aggregation ensues. Cross linking of platelets occurs via the glycoprotein IIb/IIIa receptor, with fibrinogen acting as the bridge.[10]

Large scale clinical trials have been conducted with three glycoprotein IIb/IIIa inhibitors: abciximab, tirofiban, and eptifibatide. More than 32 000 patients have been randomised in clinical trials of glycoprotein IIb/IIIa inhibitors (16 trials) and a highly significant benefit is observed for the combined end point of death or myocardial infarction at 48 hours, 30 days, and six months. Overall, there are approximately 20 fewer events per thousand patients treated.[11] A highly significant benefit is also observed on the combined end point of death/myocardial infarction or revascularisation. The net impact on mortality is modest and not observed at 30 days and beyond, except in a pooled analysis of abciximab trials. It is convenient to group glycoprotein IIb/IIIa inhibitors together, and undoubtedly there is a class effect, but there are biological and pharmacological differences between the agents and important differences in trial design when comparing studies. No direct head to head trials have been conducted.

Studies have been performed on the use of glycoprotein IIb/IIIa inhibitors in high risk groups, including those undergoing percutaneous intervention; these studies reveal more pronounced treatment effects than seen for the unstable angina population as a whole (27 fewer events per 1000 patients treated compared with 13 fewer events per 1000 treated for those studied where percutaneous intervention was not mandatory). In addition, post-hoc analyses have been conducted on the CAPTURE, PRISM PLUS, and PRISM studies and these indicate that almost all of the benefit is seen among patients with troponin release.

Thus, glycoprotein IIb/IIIa inhibitors are indicated in patients with elevated troponins and in whom percutaneous intervention is scheduled. Irrespective of revascularisation strategy, evidence supports the use of glycoprotein IIb/IIIa inhibitors in those with recurrent or refractory ischaemia (despite heparin and aspirin treatment) and in whom intervention is delayed or contraindicated.

Antithrombin treatment

Unfractionated heparin is widely used in the management of patients with unstable angina or minimal myocardial injury, although the evidence supporting its use in the absence of aspirin treatment is less robust than in the presence of aspirin. Maintaining accurate antithrombin control with unfractionated heparin is unpredictable because of plasma proteins binding, including that induced by acute phase proteins. There is reduced effectiveness in the presence of platelet rich and clot bound thrombin. Nevertheless, unfractionated heparin has formed the reference standard against which other antithrombins have been compared.

Low molecular weight heparins
The FRISC trial demonstrated that low molecular weight heparin is superior to placebo in aspirin treated patients.

Trials have also been conducted of low molecular weight heparin versus unfractionated heparin and two of these trials (ESSENCE and TIMI 11b, both using enoxaparin) have indicated superiority, with an absolute reduction of 30 events per 1000 patients treated (death/myocardial infarction/refractory angina). These benefits are seen without excess major bleeding but with some increase in minor bleeding including bruising at puncture sites. Other trials of low molecular weight heparins have not shown benefit over unfractionated heparin, but the overall conclusions are as follows:
- low molecular weight heparin is superior to placebo in aspirin treated patients;
- low molecular weight heparin is at least as effective as unfractionated heparin;
- low molecular weight heparin can be used in place of unfractionated heparin and with practical advantages.
- The use of low molecular weight heparin with intervention and/or glycoprotein IIb/IIIa inhibitors is still being defined.

Anti-ischaemic treatment

The aim of anti-ischaemic treatment is to reduce myocardial oxygen demand and to induce vasodilatation and hence reduce ischaemia. Both antithrombotic treatment and mechanical revascularisation may also reduce ischaemia, and these treatments are considered separately.

Nitrates
Nitrates act predominantly by venodilatation and in higher doses by arteriolar dilatation;

Anti-ischaemic treatment: summary

The following conclusions are based upon pharmacologic and clinical trial evidence of anti-ischaemic treatment:

- Patients with suspected acute coronary syndromes (without persistent ST elevation) should be initiated on a β blocker (unless contraindicated) and a nitrate

- In those with contraindications to β blockers, a heart rate slowing calcium antagonist should be employed

- The combination of calcium antagonist and β blocker is superior to either agent alone

- In patients with recurrent ischaemia (with ECG abnormalities) despite anti-ischaemic treatment, urgent revascularisation should be considered rather than the addition of a third or fourth anti-ischaemic agent

---

hence they reduce preload and afterload, thereby decreasing oxygen demand. Large outcome trials have been conducted using nitrates in acute myocardial infarction but not in the remainder of acute coronary syndromes. Their major limitation is the induction of tolerance, and increased doses of nitrates may be required with dose titration on the basis of the heart rate and blood pressure response, and relief of symptoms. Following the acute phase, patients may be switched to oral nitrates, but if tolerance has been induced such treatment may have reduced effectiveness.

Calcium entry blockers
Calcium antagonists act by inhibiting the slow inward current induced by the entry of extracellular calcium through the cell membrane. They lower myocardial oxygen demand and reduce arterial pressure and contractility. Some agents induce a reflex tachycardia and these are best administered in combination with a β adrenoceptor antagonist. In contrast, diltiazem and verapamil are suitable for patients who cannot tolerate a β blocker because they slow conduction through the atrioventricular node and tend to cause bradycardia. Calcium entry blockers have been shown to reduce the frequency of angina. A meta-analysis of calcium entry blockers in acute coronary syndromes indicates a nonsignificant trend towards higher mortality versus control patients (5.9% v 5.2% in 7551 patients). In individual trials, diltiazem has been compared with propranolol and both agents produced a similar reduction in anginal episodes. In summary, patients unable to tolerate β blockers should have a heart rate slowing calcium antagonist. Short acting dihydropyridines should not be used in isolation in acute coronary syndromes.

19

β Blockers

β Adrenoceptor antagonists reduce heart rate, blood pressure, and myocardial contractility. They are mainly used to reduce ischaemia, and large scale outcome trials have not been conducted in unstable angina. A meta-analysis of five trials involving 4700 patients with threatened myocardial infarction (treated with intravenous β blockers followed by oral therapy) resulted in approximately 13% reduction in the risk of myocardial infarction. In summary, β blockers are the antianginal agents of choice in those without contraindications.

Potassium channel activators

Potassium channel activators (for example, nicorandil) have both arterial and venous dilating properties and do not exhibit the same tolerance as seen with nitrates. They have been shown to be better than placebo in relieving symptoms of angina, but little evidence exists in comparison with other antianginal agents. Nicorandil possesses both potassium channel and nitrate like properties and may be considered as an alternative to nitrate administration.

Revascularisation

Revascularisation may be required in the acute phase on account of refractory or recurrent symptoms; it may also be required following stabilisation in high risk patients (those with troponin release and/or ST segment depression). In addition, non-high risk patients should undergo stress testing during the recovery phase in order to detect those with severe underlying coronary artery disease. Such patients may also require revascularisation for prognostic indications (those with left main or three vessel disease, or severe two vessel disease and impaired left ventricular function). In addition, revascularisation may be required for the relief of symptoms in those in whom medical treatment proves inadequate.

Registry studies have demonstrated that although consistency exists for some aspects of management of patients with acute coronary symptoms, wide discrepancies occur from hospital to hospital and regionally with respect to revascularisation.[2 6] Prospective registry studies have demonstrated that countries or regions with high revascularisation rates do not necessarily have improved outcomes compared with countries with lower revascularisation rates.[2] Higher rates are associated with more periprocedural complications including stroke and bleeding. Counter-intuitively, most procedures are performed in lower risk rather than higher risk patients.

Limited randomised trial data exist. Trials in the 1970s and 1980s of coronary artery bypass surgery, in patients admitted with unstable angina, produced inconclusive results, and one of the two trials was non-randomised by design. The TIMI IIIb trial conducted in the early 1990s randomised 1473 patients to an early invasive or an early conservative strategy. However, it was rather underpowered and suf-fered from high crossover rates from the conservative to the invasive strategy (61% revascularisation in the invasive arm versus 49% in the conservative arm). Death or myocardial infarction occurred in 7.2% of patients in the invasive arm versus 7.8% in the conservative arm (six weeks) and the corresponding rates at one year were 10.8% versus 12.2%, with both comparisons being non-significant. The invasive strategy was associated with a lower rate of rehospitalisation.

In the VANQWISH trial there were 916 patients with evolving non-ST segment elevation myocardial infarction randomised to an aggressive or a more conservative strategy. These patients had a high prevalence of comorbidity and the death/reinfarction rate was 24% in the revascularisation group at one year versus 19% in the medical group. The excess mortality was primarily seen in those randomised to surgical revascularisation, but a substantial number of the deaths occurred in patients in whom the procedure was not performed. Nevertheless, the conclusions of the study suggested a net hazard with more aggressive surgical revascularisation.

In the FRISC II trial an effective separation of treatment strategies was achieved. Patients were stabilised on low molecular weight heparin for six days, and revascularisation performed in 71% of those in the invasive arm and only 9% in the non-invasive arm, within 10 days. At six months, death or myocardial infarction occurred in 9.4% of the invasive group compared to 12.1% of the non-invasive group (a risk ratio of 0.78, p = 0.031), and the results remained significant at one year. Greatest benefits were demonstrated in those with the most pronounced ST segment change. However, the risk ratios were no greater for those with troponin release than those without.

In conclusion, taking all the trial data, the findings are not consistent. However, caution must be exercised in comparing older trials with more modern treatment strategies. FRISC II does provide evidence of benefit with revascularisation following an early period of stabilisation, but the findings need confirmation in other large trials (TACTICS and RITA-3). FRISC II has not tested aggressive *early* revascularisation (that is, within 72 hours) and the results should not be interpreted as such. Furthermore, the use of glycoprotein IIb/IIIa inhibitors was low and adjunctive treatment may further reduce complications.

Integrated approach to the management of unstable angina, minimal myocardial injury

There are three components:
- Identification of patients with suspected acute coronary syndromes.
- Establishing the diagnosis and risk category.
- Management.

Patients with a suspected acute coronary syndrome may present to their primary care physician, a hospital based emergency receiv-

Management of unstable angina/minimal myocardial injury

All patients: aspirin, antianginal treatment, heparin/low molecular weight heparin, oxygen if required, manage arrhythmic and mechanical complications.

Highest risk

- Refractory angina with ischaemic ECG changes

- Ischaemia with haemodynamic instability or arrhythmia

- Recurrent ECG change and troponin elevation

Management: Optimise anti-ischaemic treatment. Heparin/IV glycoprotein IIb/IIIa inhibitor. Heparin. Emergency angiography/revascularisation unless contraindicated or patient unfit to transfer

High risk

- Troponin elevation (or CK, CK-MB) but no ST elevation nor new Q waves. ± ECG change (ST↓ or T↓)

Management: Optimise anti-ischaemic treatment. Heparin/low molecular weight heparin. Consider glycoprotein IIb/IIIa inhibitor
Clinically stable: pre-discharge angiography if candidate for revascularisation
If recurrent symptoms or haemodynamically unstable, see *highest risk* above

Intermediate or indeterminate risk

- Recurrent symptoms without ECG change
  Consider alternative diagnoses
  Stress testing or angiography

- Persistence of previously abnormal ECG

Management: stress test—perfusion/echo/exercise tolerance test
- reversible perfusion defect/ischaemia: consider revascularisation
- no defect: alternative diagnosis
- fixed defect: prior myocardial infarction

Low risk

- Clinically stable, normal ECG, normal troponins (> 12 hours after pain)

Management: Discharge plus elective stress test (pre- or postdischarge)

Trial acronyms

CAPTURE: Chimeric 7e3 AntiPlatelet Therapy in Unstable angina Refractory to standard treatment
ENACT: European Network for Acute Coronary Treatment
ESSENCE: Efficacy and Safety of Subcutaneous Enoxaparin in unstable angina and Non-Q wave myocardial infarction
FRISC: FRagmin during InStability in Coronary artery disease
GUSTO: Global Use of Strategies To open Occluded coronary arteries
OASIS: Organisation to Assess Strategies for Ischaemia Syndromes
PRAIS: Prospective Registry of Acute Ischaemic Syndromes
PRISM: Platelet Receptor Inhibition for Ischaemic Syndrome Management
RITA: Randomised Intervention Treatment of Angina Trial
TACTICS: Treat Angina with Aggrastat (tirofiban) and determine Cost of Therapy with Invasive or Conservative Strategy
TIMI: Thrombolysis In Myocardial Infarction
VANQWISH: Veterans Affairs Non-Q Wave Infarction Strategies in Hospital

Following identification of those with suspected acute coronary syndrome, such patients are further categorised on the basis of their clinical syndrome plus the ECG changes, cardiac enzyme markers, and stress testing. This allows the identification of those with evidence of evolving acute infarction, those with suspected or confirmed unstable angina/minimal myocardial injury, and low risk patients, and those with non-cardiac or non-acute coronary syndrome diagnoses.

Conclusions

Previously, the hazards of acute coronary syndromes (especially unstable angina or minimal myocardial injury) have been underestimated. This is mainly because of inconsistencies in diagnosis and the inclusion of patients with chest pain but without confirmatory evidence of an acute coronary syndrome.

Recent data from large scale clinical trials, and from registry studies, demonstrate that patients can be identified on the basis of the clinical syndrome plus electrocardiographic and enzyme criteria. These tools should be available in all hospitals.

Characterisation of patients with acute coronary syndromes firstly identifies those with suspected evolving acute infarction, for reperfusion treatment. Among the remainder, those with unstable angina or minimal myocardial injury are identified on the basis of ECG

ing unit (including care of the elderly) or an acute cardiology unit. A clinical history of ischaemic chest pain is central to establishing the diagnosis. As a minimum, chest pain is present for at least two, five minute episodes or one, 10 minute episode at rest or on minimal exertion or emotion. In those with evolving infarction the pain may be persistent and accompanied by autonomic features.

abnormalities or cardiac enzyme elevation, or both. This strategy allows the separation of high, intermediate, and low risk patients. Such stratification permits the targeting of more potent pharmacological treatment at those at highest risk, and the identification of patients with the most to gain from revascularisation strategies. Registry studies across Europe currently show that such stratification is not systematically performed, and that it does not currently guide management strategies. The above strategy has the further advantage that it allows the separation of low risk patients for early discharge. Thus diagnostic and risk stratification is based upon the underlying pathophysiology of the syndrome, it is validated in prospective clinical trials and registry studies, and it provides a rational basis for pharmacological and interventional treatment.

1. **White HD.** Unstable angina. In: Topol EJ, ed. *Comprehensive cardiovascular medicine.* Philadelphia: Lippincott-Raven, 1998.
• *Comprehensive review of acute coronary syndromes.*

2. **Yusuf S, Flather M, Pogue,** *et al* **for the OASIS Registry Investigators.** Variations between countries in invasive cardiac procedures and outcomes in patients with suspected unstable angina or myocardial infarction without initial ST elevation. *Lancet* 1998;**352**:507–14.
• *OASIS registry study demonstrating risks of death, myocardial infarction, and recurrent angina among patients admitted with stable angina or non-ST elevation myocardial infarction.*

3. **The Global Use of Strategies to Open Occluded Coronary Arteries (GUSTO IIb) Investigators.** A comparison of recombinant hirudin with heparin for the treatment of acute coronary syndromes. *N Engl J Med* 1996;**335**:775–82.
• *Large scale trial comparing hirudin and heparin in acute coronary syndromes and providing outcome data for this population.*

4. **Collinson J, Flather MD, Fox KAA,** *et al* **for the PRAIS-UK Investigators.** Clinical outcomes, risk stratification and practice patterns of unstable angina and myocardial infarction without ST elevation: prospective registry of acute ischaemic syndromes in the UK (PRAIS-UK). *Eur Heart J* In press.
• *Prospective UK registry of unstable angina and non-ST elevation myocardial infarction. 12.2% rate of death/myocardial infarction at six months and 30% rate of death/myocardial infarction, refractory angina or readmission for unstable angina.*

5. **Timmis A.** Acute coronary syndromes: risk stratification. *Heart* 2000;**83**:241–6.
• *Education in Heart series article on risk stratification in acute coronary syndromes.*

6. **Fox KAA, Cokkinos DV, Deckers JW,** *et al.* The ENACT study: a pan-European survey of acute coronary syndromes. *Eur Heart J* In press.
• *The first pan-European data on the management and in-hospital events for patients admitted with the full spectrum of acute coronary syndromes.*

7. **Hillis GS, Zhao N, Taggart P,** *et al.* Utility of cardiac troponin I, creatine kinase-MB$_{mass}$, myosin light chain 1, and myoglobin in the early in-hospital triage of "high risk" patients with chest pain. *Heart* 1999;**82**:614–20.
• *The role of specific cardiac enzymes in the triage of high risk patients with chest pain.*

8. **Davies MJ.** The pathophysiology of acute coronary syndromes. *Heart* 2000;**83**:361–6.
• *Education in Heart series on the pathophysiology of acute coronary syndromes.*

9. **Anti-platelet Trialists Collaboration.** Collaborative overview of randomised trials of antiplatelet therapy - I: prevention of death, myocardial infarction, and stroke by prolonged antiplatelet therapy in various categories of patients. *BMJ* 1994;**308**:81–106.
• *Key combined analysis of all of the trials of antiplatelet therapy up to 1994. Major impact of aspirin demonstrated.*

10. **Fox KAA.** Comparing trials of glycoprotein IIb/IIIa receptor antagonists. *Eur Heart J* 1999;**1**(suppl R):R10–17.
• *Review of the trials of glycoprotein IIb/IIIa antagonists for acute coronary syndromes.*

11. **Kong DF, Califf RM, Miller DP,** *et al.* Clinical outcomes of therapeutic agents that block the platelet glycoprotein IIb/IIIa integrin in ischemic heart disease. *Circulation* 1998;**98**:2829–35.
• *Pooled analysis of the trials of glycoprotein IIb/IIIa inhibitors for acute coronary syndromes with or without mandated intervention. Sustained impact on myocardial infarctions, especially in those undergoing percutaneous intervention.*

4 Acute coronary syndromes: risk stratification

Adam Timmis

Risk stratification in acute coronary syndromes aims to identify those patients at greatest risk of recurrent ischaemic events who might benefit prognostically from further investigation and treatment. Unfortunately, however, none of the clinical or investigative markers currently available has sufficient diagnostic power to identify all high risk patients while excluding those at negligible risk. Moreover, for patients judged to be at high risk, the value of specific treatment may be poorly defined. Nevertheless, high event rates and finite facilities for invasive management emphasise the clinical and logistical importance of risk stratification which should play a central role in the management of acute coronary syndromes.

What is the risk and when is it greatest?

Our own database in east London shows that about 30% of patients with acute myocardial infarction and 20% with unstable angina experience a major event (death or non-fatal coronary syndrome) during the first year after hospital admission. Risk, however, is not a linear function of time, and as fig 4.1 shows, 66% of all major events during the first six months after myocardial infarction occur in the first 30 days. Moreover, the determinants of risk may change with time, acute phase arrhythmias and myocardial rupture in the first 48 hours giving way to reinfarction, heart failure, and secondary arrhythmias later after presentation. Thus assessment of risk, using strategies tailored to address its changing determinants, is an essential part of the management of acute coronary syndromes and must be applied at an early stage to identify successfully patients with most to benefit. Recognition of this fact has rendered obsolete old arguments about the appropriate timing of stress testing and other non-invasive tests which must be performed as early as possible (certainly before discharge) to be of significant value for risk stratification.

Determinants of risk

The major determinant of risk in the acute phase of ischaemic syndromes is ventricular fibrillation, which probably accounts for > 80% of out of hospital deaths. For hospital populations, risk is determined by the cumulative impact of a variety of clinical, pathophysiological, and coronary anatomical factors.

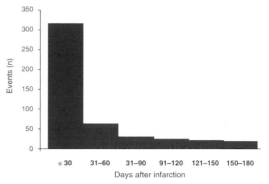

Figure 4.1. Recurrent ischaemic events in the first six months after acute myocardial infarction (unpublished data of 1829 patients on Newham General Hospital database). Among 1829 patients with acute myocardial infarction, recurrent ischaemic events (death, non-fatal acute coronary syndromes) occurred in 481 patients during the first six months. Of these recurrent events, 66% occurred in the first 30 days.

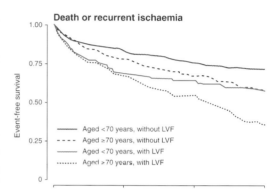

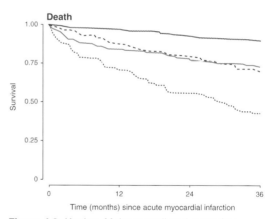

Figure 4.2. Kaplan–Meier overall and event free survival by age for 1225 patients with acute myocardial infarction surviving to hospital discharge. LVF, left ventricular failure. Reproduced from Barakat et al[2] with permission of The Lancet.

Most important are advanced age and ventricular dysfunction (fig 4.2), with residual myocardial ischaemia and cardiac arrhythmias also contributing significantly.[1] Thus, the mortality risk within one year of acute myocardial infarction is 14.8 times greater in men aged ≥ 70 years with heart failure than in men aged < 60 years without heart failure.[2] Clinical factors variably related to advanced ventricular dysfunction include diabetes, heart failure, Q wave development, and bundle branch block, while ongoing chest pain and fluctuating ST segment change usually reflect important residual ischaemia.

> **Major determinants of risk in acute coronary syndrome**
>
> - Electrical instability
> - Advanced age
> - Left ventricular dysfunction
> - Residual ischaemia

Making risk assessments

Faced with these multiple determinants of risk, the clinician must decide which to measure and which to apply in the stratification process. Clinical determinants are, of course, readily available and are often sufficient to define risk and management options without the need for additional tests. Cardiac chest pain that fails to settle, for example, indicates that the risk of further ventricular injury is high and provides clear indication for angiography with a view to revascularisation. Similarly, intractable heart failure confirms a high level of risk, and additional tests aimed merely at refining risk status will not always provide significant incremental information. In many patients, however, particularly those who make an uncomplicated initial recovery, risk status is difficult to define based solely on clinical criteria and in this group further tests are necessary. These will usually include an evaluation of left ventricular function, or residual myocardial ischaemia, or both. Interpretation of these tests should take account of clinical, electrocardiographic, and biochemical data already available, recognising that risk stratification is an incremental process and the predictive value of non-invasive investigation is influenced importantly by the pretest assessment of risk.

Risk stratification in the acute phase of coronary syndromes

Ventricular fibrillation, the major determinant of risk in the acute phase, requires immediate electrical cardioversion to avoid death. Because it is largely unpredictable, electrocardiographic monitoring and ready access to a defibrillator are the most important management strategies for saving lives in acute coronary syndromes. Also important is antithrombotic treatment which should be given to all patients acutely, with daily aspirin continuing thereafter. In other respects, management in the acute phase of coronary syndromes is largely determined by the perceived risk as judged by clinical, electrocardiographic, metabolic, and biochemical factors.

Clinical factors
Severe hypertension in the acute phase that does not respond promptly to opiate analgesia, heightens risk by intensifying ischaemia and predisposing to myocardial rupture. Intravenous β blockade may protect against rupture and should be used in acute infarction if systolic blood pressure is > 160 mm Hg. Heart failure also heightens risk and identifies a group that may benefit prognostically from angiotensin converting enzyme inhibition and β blockade. The risk is particularly high in cardiogenic shock which remains the leading cause of hospital death despite reperfusion treatment; primary angioplasty does not appear to offer any short term benefit but may improve survival in the longer term. For most patients, emergency cardiac catheterisation is reserved for patients with ongoing or recurrent chest pain, although this policy is largely pragmatic and may be overly conservative, particularly for patients with unstable angina.[3]

Electrocardiographic factors
When regional ischaemia is sufficiently severe to produce ST segment depression or elevation, risk increases significantly.[4] Thus, in unstable angina ST depression, particularly when recurrent, identifies a group at risk of infarction and provides indication for urgent cardiac catheterisation.[5] In myocardial infarction, ST elevation increases risk substantially but its prompt resolution, either spontaneously or in response to thrombolytic treatment and aspirin (fig 4.3), may reflect successful reperfusion and is a good prognostic sign, particularly if Q waves do not develop.[6] Failure of ST resolution, on the other hand, or recurrent episodes of ST elevation indicate failed reperfusion or coronary reocclusion, which increase risk and may provide indication for urgent angiography with a view to rescue angioplasty. Risk also increases progressively with increasing degrees of atrioventricular block, and is particularly high when advanced bundle branch block complicates anterior infarction, probably reflecting the adverse consequences of extensive myocardial injury. Primary ventricular arrhythmias in the first 48 hours of acute coronary syndromes do increase the risk of hospital death although there is no evidence that prophylactic antiarrhythmic treatment is helpful. Secondary arrhythmias later after admission are commonly associated with advanced left ventricular dysfunction and identify a group at high risk of death in the first year. If secondary arrhythmias fail to respond to treatment cardiac catheterisation is recommended to define revascularisation options, with electrophysiological investigation in reserve for tailored antiarrhythmic treatment or deployment of an implantable defibrillator.

Metabolic factors
The heightened risk associated with diabetes requires measurement of blood glucose concentration. Patients known to be diabetic or with a blood glucose concentration > 11 mmol/l should receive insulin and glucose infusion during the acute phase which improves prognosis in acute myocardial infarction, although whether similar benefit occurs in unstable angina is not known. Hypercholesterolaemia also increases long term risk and lipid profiles should be measured at the time of admission, patients with a total cholesterol

Electrocardiographic determinants of risk in acute coronary syndromes

- ST elevation or depression
- Failure of prompt ST resolution in response to treatment
- Q wave development
- Intraventricular conduction defects
- Secondary arrhythmias

≥ 5.0 mmol/l benefiting from treatment with statins.

Biochemical factors

Enzymes released from cardiac myocytes have long been used as markers of injury to confirm myocardial infarction in patients presenting with acute coronary syndromes (fig 4.3). Creatine kinase and its more specific MB fraction remain widely used, but in recent years a number of novel biochemical markers (myoglobin, troponin I and T) have been developed that are more sensitive and appear in the blood earlier after the onset of symptoms. Almost regardless of which biochemical marker is used, increased concentrations are associated with an increased risk of recurrent ischaemic events. Myoglobin peaks particularly early and is reliably detected within four hours of injury, making it potentially useful for very early diagnosis. However, myoglobin is relatively non-specific and it is troponin I and T (regulatory proteins with isoforms found only in cardiac myocytes) that have emerged as the most useful biochemical markers for diagnostic and prognostic purposes. Raised concentrations of troponins are reliably detected within 12 hours of injury, and are highly specific for myocardial infarction and for the "minimal myocardial damage" that may occur following transient or subocclusive thrombus formation in unstable angina.

Minimal damage of this type is now recognised as a powerful predictor of subsequent ischaemic events. Troponins are there-fore finding special application for risk stratification in unstable angina.[7] A recent study found that troponin T ≥ 0.10 µg/l in patients with acute coronary syndromes was associated with a 30 day mortality rate of 10.4% compared with only 3.2% in troponin negative patients.[8] Similarly, troponin positivity in acute myocardial infarction is associated with a substantially higher risk of future events. These findings are consistent with those of other investigators and have led to recommendations for troponin based risk management in acute coronary syndromes, with troponin positive patients a target for more aggressive strategies.

Predischarge risk stratification

Many high risk patients with coronary syndromes can be clearly identified in the acute phase, but there remains a group that makes a largely uncomplicated early recovery, some of whom remain at high risk. This group, therefore, should be a target for predischarge risk stratification, although identification of high risk individuals may not be easy. Strategies for predischarge risk stratification include non-invasive evaluation of left ventricular function, tests for ongoing myocardial ischaemia (silent or stress induced), and tests for electrical instability.

Left ventricular function

Left ventricular function is one of the major determinants of long term risk. There is now clear evidence that specific treatment with angiotensin converting enzyme (ACE) inhibitors (probably also β blockers) can reduce that risk, and coronary bypass surgery may be particularly beneficial when left ventricular dysfunction is associated with multivessel coronary artery disease. For many patients clinical criteria are sufficient to exclude significant left ventricular dysfunction, and an analysis of data from the GUSTO 1 trial confirmed that in patients presenting with a first infarct, absence of anterior infarction, left bundle branch block, or acute phase pulmonary oedema accurately

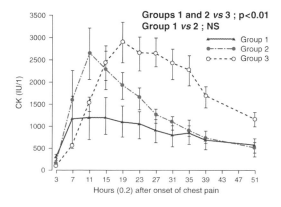
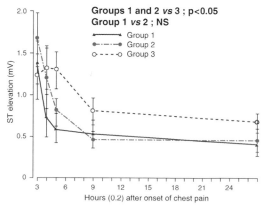

Figure 4.3. Kinetics of creatine kinase (CK) release (left) and ST resolution (right) in response to coronary reperfusion. Sequential coronary arteriograms 90 minutes apart in 41 patients presenting with acute coronary syndromes and ST elevation permitted identification of three groups: group 1—patency of infarct related artery at first arteriogram before thrombolytic treatment (n = 12); group 2—early recanalisation of the infarct related artery within 90 minutes of thrombolytic treatment (n = 10); group 3—persistent occlusion of infarct related artery (n = 19). Serial CK analysis showed early peaking in groups with coronary recanalisation (groups 1 and 2). Cumulative CK release was considerably greater in patients with failed recanalisation (group 3). Serial ECGs showed rapid resolution of ST segment elevation in patients in groups 1 and 2, while in those patients with persistent coronary occlusion (group 3), ST elevation persisted considerably longer. Reproduced from Timmis et al[6] with permission of BMJ Publishing Group.

Clinical criteria associated with an ejection fraction ≥ 40% in acute myocardial infarction

- First myocardial infarction in the absence of:
    - –anterior infarction
    - –left bundle branch block
    - –acute phase pulmonary oedema

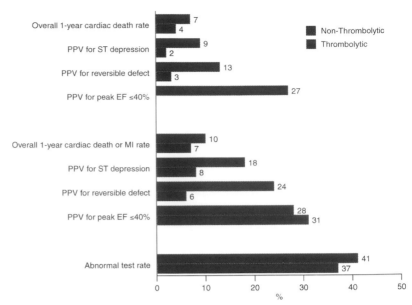

Figure 4.4. Positive predictive value (PPV) of non-invasive tests in non-thrombolytic and thrombolytic treated patients for cardiac death or reinfarction rates, and rates of abnormal tests. EF, ejection fraction. Reproduced from Shaw *et al*[10] with permission.

identified 94% of all patients with an ejection fraction ≥ 40%.[9] For the remainder, non-invasive evaluation of left ventricular function by echocardiography or radionuclide angiography is recommended in order to determine appropriate risk management.

Myocardial ischaemia

Stress testing

Patients with ongoing symptomatic ischaemia early after acute coronary syndromes are usually regarded as a high risk group requiring urgent angiographic investigation. However, many patients who make an uncomplicated early recovery have inducible ischaemia (with or without symptoms) that is variably predictive of recurrent ischaemic events. Thus stress testing has a time honoured role for predischarge risk stratification, particularly in uncomplicated myocardial infarction. A symptom limited test using the Bruce protocol is recommended for most patients although for some, particularly the elderly, modified protocols may be more suitable. An abnormal stress test with ST depression may be predictive of recurrent ischaemic events and provides grounds for coronary arteriography with a view to revascularisation. Other markers of risk include low exercise tolerance (< 7 mets), failure of the blood pressure to rise normally during exercise, and exertional arrhythmias. Unfortunately, recent meta-analysis has shown that inducible ischaemia during treadmill testing has a low positive predictive value for death and myocardial infarction in the first year (fig 4.4), falling below 10% in patients who have received thrombolytic treatment.[10] Nevertheless, when "non-ischaemic" risk criteria are considered, the treadmill may provide added clinical value, inability to perform a stress test and low exercise tolerance both being independently predictive of recurrent events.[11] Moreover, the negative predictive accuracy of predischarge stress testing is high, those with a normal test usually having a good prognosis without the need for additional investigation. Finally, it should be noted that the diagnostic value of exertional ST depression and reversible thallium perfusion defects is equivalent, making the treadmill a more cost effective strategy for risk stratification after myocardial infarction than the gamma camera.[10] Predischarge stress testing has also been recommended in unstable angina, but although an ischaemic response at low work load has been associated with an increased risk, the positive predictive value of an abnormal test is low.

Holter ST monitoring

Ambulatory ischaemia during predischarge Holter monitoring also identifies patients at

---

Treadmill stress testing for predischarge risk stratification

- Positive predictive accuracy of ST depression < 10% after thrombolytic treatment
- Inability to perform a stress test and low exercise tolerance are most useful predictors of recurrent events
- Negative predictive accuracy is high
- Diagnostic value of exertional ST depression and thallium perfusion defects are equivalent, making the treadmill more cost effective than the gamma camera

---

risk of recurrent ischaemic events. In unstable angina its use is well documented; although it provides prognostic information additional to that available from the admission ECG, its incremental value relative to stress testing is not clear. In myocardial infarction ischaemic ST shift during predischarge Holter monitoring has a positive predictive value for recurrent infarction and death of 20%, and provides prognostic information that is additional to and independent of that obtained from stress testing and clinical assessment.[12] Preliminary evidence suggests therefore that ambulatory ischaemia during Holter monitoring may be more useful than stress testing for risk stratification in acute coronary syndromes. It can certainly be applied earlier after admission when risk is greatest, but it is unlikely to become more widely used until further studies are available defining its role.

Electrical instability

Patients at greatest risk of arrhythmic death in the first year are those with extensive myocardial injury evidenced by Q waves, anterior infarction, left bundle branch block, or heart failure. Risk is further increased if late ventricular arrhythmias (frequent ectopy, ventricular tachyarrhythmia, ventricular fibrillation) occur before discharge.[13] Because there are no well defined strategies for reducing the risk of arrhythmic death, routine electrocardiographic monitoring (Holter, telemetry) before discharge is not recommended although patients who declare themselves clinically with sustained ventricular arrhythmias require investigation to identify provocative factors (ischaemia, hypoxaemia, metabolic derangement). Where possible β blockers should be prescribed, based on evidence of efficacy in protecting against sudden death, but resistant life threatening arrhythmias require cardiac catheterisation to examine the potential for revascularisation. Electrophysiological investigation using programmed stimulation, though recommended by certain investigators, has proved unreliable for guiding treatment and predicting mortality.

Heart rate variability analysis
Holter monitoring after myocardial infarction permits analysis of autonomic function by

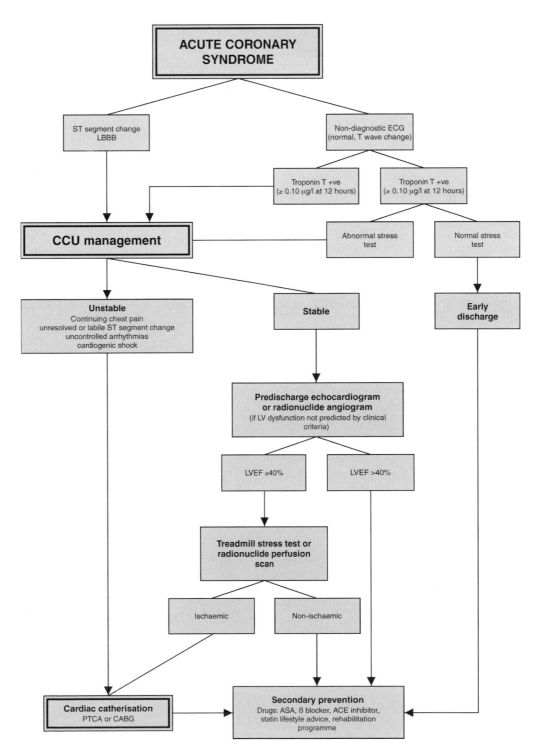

Figure 4.5. Algorithm for risk management in acute coronary syndromes. CCU, coronary care unit; LBBB, left bundle branch block; LVEF, left ventricular ejection fraction; PTCA, percutaneous transluminal coronary angioplasty; CABG, coronary artery bypass grafting; ASA, acetylsalicylic acid (aspirin); ACE, angiotensin converting enzyme.

measurement of heart rate variability. Sympathovagal balance is usually reduced in the postinfarction period, and the severity of the derangement is predictive of outcome, particularly arrhythmic and sudden death, but also all cause mortality.[14] At present, however, it is not clear if heart rate variability analysis provides incremental data for risk stratification, or what the therapeutic implications of reduced heart rate variability should be. Similar considerations apply to unstable angina.

Signal averaged ECG
Ventricular late potentials detected by signal averaging are predictive of arrhythmic events late after myocardial infarction. Again, however, the therapeutic implications of ventricular late potentials are not well defined and the role, if any, in unstable angina is unknown.

Practical recommendations

In patients with acute coronary syndromes, management should be risk based from the time of arrival in the emergency room (fig 4.5). An ECG and troponin assay should be obtained immediately with repeat troponin assay at 12 hours.[15] Patients with regional ST change (elevation or depression) or left bundle branch block are a high risk group requiring admission to the coronary care unit and appropriate antithrombotic treatment. Patients with an ECG that is normal, or shows nondiagnostic T wave changes, should be treated similarly if troponin assay is positive, but if troponins are negative at 12 hours further management should be guided by the results of a stress test. An abnormal stress test requires further cardiac investigation and treatment, but if the stress test is normal then risk is very low, permitting early discharge pending review of the diagnosis.

If ST elevation or depression fails to respond promptly to treatment or recurs after early resolution, the risk of ongoing myocardial injury is considerable and urgent cardiac catheterisation is recommended with a view to revascularisation. Similar considerations apply to patients with unrelieved or recurrent cardiac chest pain. Invasive management may also be required for heart failure and late ventricular arrhythmias, particularly if responses to initial treatment are unsatisfactory or there is evidence of residual ischaemia or stunning.

For patients in whom the hospital course is uncomplicated, discharge at five days is usually possible. If clinical criteria are insufficient to exclude significant left ventricular dysfunction, a predischarge echocardiogram should be obtained, those with an ejection fraction ≤ 40% representing a high risk group requiring ACE inhibition and also cardiac catheterisation if there is residual ischaemia on stress testing. Those with well preserved left ventricular function are a low risk group in whom stress testing is not usually helpful for risk assess-

ment. Nevertheless, for troponin positive patients with unstable angina or non-Q wave infarction, risk is high and a predischarge stress test is recommended.

Regardless of the hospital course, all patients should receive secondary prevention with aspirin and, when possible, β blockers. Aggressive management of diabetes and dyslipidaemia is essential and ACE inhibitors should be given to patients who have had clinical evidence of heart failure. A cardiac rehabilitation course should be available for all patients recovering from acute coronary syndromes.

1. **Deedwania PC, Amsterdam EA, Vagelos RH.** Evidence-based, cost effective risk stratification and management after myocardial infarction. *Arch Intern Med* 1997;**157**:273–80.
   • *A short but useful review that is unusual in considering the cost effectiveness of different strategies for risk stratification in acute myocardial infarction.*

2. **Barakat K, Wilkinson P, Deaner A,** *et al.* How should age affect management of acute myocardial infarction? A prospective cohort study. *Lancet* 1999;**353**:955–9.

3. **Fragmin and Fast Revascularisation During Instability in Coronary Artery Disease (FRISCáll) Investigators.** Invasive compared with non-invasive treatment in unstable coronary artery disease: áFRISC II prospective randomised multicentre study. *Lancet* 1999;**354**:708–15.

4. **Patel DJ, Holdright DR, Knight CJ,** *et al.* Early continuous ST segment monitoring in unstable angina: prognostic value additional to the clinical characteristics and the admission electrocardiogram. *Heart* 1996;**75**:222–8.

5. **Lange RA, Hillis LD.** Use and overuse of angiography and revascularization for acute coronary syndromes. *N Engl J Med* 1998;**338**:1838–9.

6. **Timmis AD, Griffin B, Nelson DJ,** *et al.* The effects of early coronary patency on the evolution of myocardial infarction: a prospective arteriographic study. *Br Heart J* 1987;**58**:345–51.

7. **Luscher MS, Thygesen K, Ravkilde J,** *et al* **for the TRIM Study Group.** Applicability of cardiac troponin T and I for early risk stratification in unstable coronary artery disease. *Circulation* 1997;**96**:2578–85.

8. **Newby LK, Christenson RH, Ohman EM,** *et al.* Value of serial troponin T measures for early and late risk stratification in patients with acute coronary syndromes. The GUSTO-IIa investigators. *Circulation* 1998;**98**:1853–9.

9. **Peterson ED, Shaw LJ, Califf RM.** Clinical guideline: part II. Risk stratification after myocardial infarction. *Ann Intern Med* 1997;**126**:561–82.
   • *An excellent review, emphasising that risk stratification after myocardial infarction is an ongoing process that starts at the time of hospital admission and continues until discharge.*

10. **Shaw LJ, Peterson ED, Kesler K,** *et al.* A meta-analysis of predischarge risk stratification after acute myocardial infarction with stress electrocardiographic, myocardial perfusion, and ventricular function imaging. *Am J Cardiol* 1996;**78**:1327–37.
    • *State of the art meta-analysis of non-invasive testing for predischarge risk stratification.*

11. **Stevenson R, Wilkinson P, Marchant B,** *et al.* Relative value of clinical variables, treadmill stress testing and Holter ST monitoring for post-infarction risk stratification. *Am J Cardiol* 1994;**74**:221–5.
    • *One of few attempts in the literature to quantify the incremental value of non-invasive tests in postinfarction risk stratification.*

12. **Stevenson R, Ranjadayalan K, Wilkinson P,** *et al.* Assessment of Holter ST monitoring for risk stratification in patients with acute myocardial infarction treated by thrombolysis. *Br Heart J* 1993;**70**:233–40.

13. **Maggioni AP, Zuanetti G, Franzosi MG,** *et al.* Prevalence and prognostic significance of ventricular arrhythmias after acute myocardial infarction in the fibrinolytic era. GISSI-2 results. *Circulation* 1993;**87**:312–22.

14. **Farrell TG, Bashir Y, Cripps T,** *et al.* Risk stratification for arrhythmic events in postinfarction patients based on heart rate variability, ambulatory electrocardiographic variables and the signal-averaged electrocardiogram. *J Am Coll Cardiol* 1991;**18**:687–97.

15. **de Winter RJ, Koster RW, Sturk A,** *et al.* Value of myoglobin, troponin T, and CK-MB mass in ruling out an acute myocardial infarction in the emergency room. *Circulation* 1995;**92**:3401–7.

website
extra

Additional references appear on the Heart website

www.heartjnl.com

5 Acute myocardial infarction: thrombolysis

Eric J Topol

Infarction is the most intensively studied medical intervention in the history of clinical investigation, with more than 200 000 patients enrolled in large scale, worldwide trials. The results of these trials have led to an irrevocably altered approach, with routine use of reperfusion treatment. Streptokinase, tissue plasminogen activator (t-PA), and new plasminogen activators have been shown to reduce mortality significantly, and the reduction is inversely proportional to the time that treatment is initiated from symptom onset. For patients treated in the first 60 minutes of symptom onset, the so called "golden hour", mortality is reduced by more than 50%. Even frank prevention of the event can be assured in many patients treated in this very early time frame. Nevertheless, there are some major obstacles to optimal reperfusion treatment that have been increasingly recognised in recent years, which new directions in this field will hopefully circumvent. This paper will review the substantive progress in the field, including recognition of major pitfalls, and lay the groundwork for future improvements in pharmacologic myocardial reperfusion treatment.

"Patency centric" approaches

With the validation of intravenous thrombolytic treatment versus placebo in the classic GISSI 1 and ISIS 2 trials,[1 2] the next step was to determine whether a higher level of early infarct vessel patency would result in improved survival. This was the focus of the GUSTO 1 trial which showed that a significant increase in patency at 90 minutes after treatment was initiated, from 30% with streptokinase to 54% with accelerated t-PA, was associated with a 15% reduction in mortality (fig 5.1).[3] The term "patency" refers to brisk flow and clearance of angiographic contrast dye through the affected epicardial artery.

More recently, trials of new plasminogen activators have gone forward using accelerated t-PA as the "gold" standard for comparison. The new plasminogen activators are bioengineered mutants of wild type t-PA. All have longer half lives and are administered as a single or double bolus. Three new agents, reteplase (r-PA), tenecteplase (TNK), and lanetoplase (n-PA) have each been studied in trials of 15 000 to 17 000 patients. None of these trials have shown superior mortality outcomes with the new plasminogen activators compared with t-PA. For TNK, "equivalence" was demonstrated with virtually the same mortality for TNK as with t-PA,[2] but for r-PA and n-PA there were very small gaps in mortality compared with t-PA (approximately 0.20 absolute per cent) that pre-empt an unequivocal declaration of "equivalency". Nevertheless, the field of thrombolytics has widened greatly from 1987 when the initial commercialisation for acute myocardial infarction was granted with the original choice of either streptokinase or t-PA. r-PA is now registered for use in most countries throughout the world and the approval for TNK is imminent.

Although new plasminogen activators have been shown to achieve more rapid or complete infarct vessel patency than t-PA, this has not resulted in an improvement in survival. Figure 5.2 shows data from the angiographic study known as RAPID 2, which compared r-PA and t-PA, juxtaposed with data from the GUSTO 3 mortality trial which also compared these two agents.[4 5]. Even though RAPID 2 showed better early patency for r-PA, there was not even a trend for less mortality. This strongly suggests that the relation of patency to survival is not as direct and straightforward as had been anticipated.

Unrecognised importance of the microcirculation

A likely explanation for the discrepancy between infarct vessel patency and survival lies in microvascular obstruction. A large number

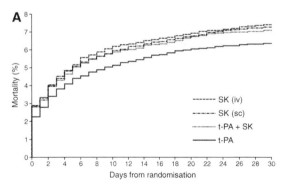

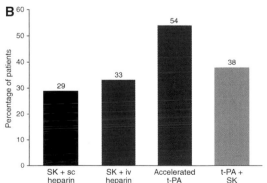

Figure 5.1. (A) Mortality curves in GUSTO 1 by thrombolytic strategy assignment. For streptokinase (SK) the parentheses indicate the heparin strategy, intravenous (iv) or subcutaneous (sc). (B) Patency of the infarct vessel at 90 minutes of treatment in the GUSTO 1 angiographic trial evaluating the four thrombolytic strategies.

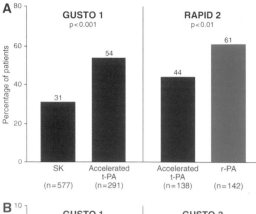

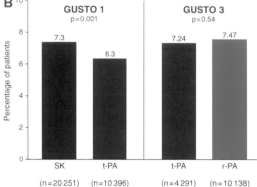

Figure 5.2. (A) Patency of the infarct vessel in two angiographic comparative trials. (B) Mortality at 30 days for each thrombolytic strategy.

of studies have shown that epicardial artery patency does not assure microvascular flow. Indeed, the classic study by Ito and colleagues using contrast echocardiographic tissue imaging showed that at least one in four patients with TIMI 3 flow (brisk epicardial arterial flow) do not have tissue level perfusion.[6] Many groups have independently confirmed these findings and extended the significance of lack of reflow at the tissue level. For example, Porter and colleagues have shown that end systolic cavity size and ejection fraction are impaired in patients with TIMI 3 flow but without tissue level perfusion.[7]

Beyond contrast echocardiography, other investigators have used imaging modalities such as magnetic resonance or intracoronary Doppler flow velocity to assess microvascular obstruction. During extended follow up of a cohort of patients after myocardial reperfusion treatment,[8] the finding of microvascular obstruction carried a fourfold increase in adverse events including death, reinfarction, or the development of congestive heart failure. In a randomised trial of 200 patients undergoing primary stenting for acute myocardial infarction, Doppler assessment of the infarct vessel showed a notable increase in peak velocity with the use of abciximab, a potent platelet glycoprotein IIb/IIIa inhibitor.[9]

These pivotal findings have revamped our understanding of the reperfusion process. Indeed, rather than achieve complete dissolution of the thrombus, our treatments are likely achieving only partial clot dissolution and potentiating embolisation of part of the thrombus into the microcirculation. This sets up the backdrop for the "illusion" or false sense of

achieving reperfusion by improperly focusing on the epicardial artery, when the critical supplier of perfusion to the infarct territory may be obstructed.

Beyond the partial clot dissolution, the constituency of the thrombus is particularly important. Underlying the coronary thrombotic event is a fissured, eroded, or frank atherosclerotic plaque rupture. This breach of the vessel wall first sets up platelet thrombus that is seen angioscopically as "white" thrombus. Quickly surrounding this nidus of platelet aggregation is the "red" thrombus that is fibrin rich. Accordingly, the approach of dissolving the culprit coronary artery thrombus is presently focused on the "red" clot component.

Unfortunately, "thrombolytics" are not really thrombolytics because plasminogen activators are "fibrinolytics"—that is, rather than lysing a coronary thrombus, fibrinolytics can only achieve dissolution of the fibrin strands making up the "red" thrombus (fig 5.3). This leaves thrombin, previously enmeshed in the "red" clot, exposed and leads to a prothrombotic state. Not only can exposed, activated thrombin beget its own formation via an autocatalytic loop in the extrinsic coagulation pathway, but thrombin is the most potent platelet proaggregatory biologic molecule. Thus, the mainstay of our current approach to myocardial reperfusion is narrowly directed to the fibrin–thrombus component and, unfortunately, induces a prothrombotic state.

Evidence for the untoward effect of fibrinolytics may also explain part of the discrepancy seen in the large scale mortality reduction trials. In GUSTO 3, where r-PA failed to provide survival benefit compared with t-PA, r-PA was shown to activate platelets more than t-PA.[10] This would counter the facilitation of

- ADMIRAL: Abciximab associateD with priMary angIoplasty and stenting in acute myocaRdiAL infarction
- CCF: Cleveland Clinic Foundation
- GISSI 1: Gruppo Italiano per lo Studio della Streptochinasi nell'Infarto Miocardico
- GUSTO 1: Global Utilization of Streptokinase and t-PA for Occluded coronary arteries
- INTRO: INTegrilin and Reduced dOse of thrombolysis
- ISIS 2: Second International Study of Infarct Survival
- Munich: See reference 9
- RAPID 2: Reteplase (r-PA) versus Alteplase Patency Investigation During myocardial infarction
- RAPPORT: ReoPro in Acute myocardial infarction and Primary PTCA Organization and Randomized Trial
- SPEED: Strategies for Patency Enhancement in the Emergency Department
- TIMI 14: Thrombolysis in Myocardial Infarction (with abciximab)

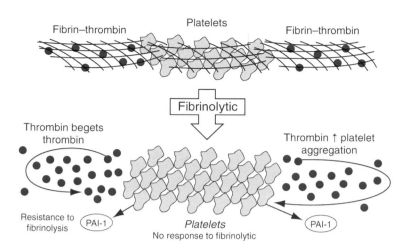

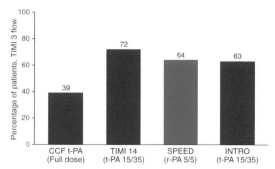

Figure 5.4. Angiographic patency (TIMI 3) of the infarct vessel in four sets of patients using the same core angiographic laboratory t-PA is compared with three trials of combined half dose fibrinolysis and full dose glycoprotein IIb/IIIa inhibition.

Figure 5.3. Prothrombotic effects of fibrinolytic treatment. Coronary thrombus is composed of a platelet core with fibrin–thrombin admixture ("white" and "red" clot). After fibrinolytic treatment, there is exposure of free thrombin, which autocatalytically begets more thrombin and strongly promotes platelet aggregation (note more platelet mass). Platelets themselves are resistant to fibrinolytic treatment and furthermore secrete large amounts of plasminogen activator inhibitor (PAI-1), which is a potent antagonist to fibrinolysis. Reproduced from Topol EJ. *Circulation* 1998;**97**:211–18, with permission.

infarct vessel patency of r-PA, and likely would result in some higher proportion of microvascular obstruction.

More comprehensive thrombolysis

A combined strategy of low dose fibrinolytic and full dose platelet-lytic has been proposed.[10] The advantages of this "fibrinoplatelet" lysis approach would include the ability to reduce the fibrinolytic dose, thereby potentially avoiding the prothrombotic state and the risk of intracerebral haemorrhage. Second, such a strategy is more comprehensive in addressing both the "red" and "white" components of the coronary artery thrombus. Intravenous platelet glycoprotein IIb/IIIa inhibitors are fully capable of rapid dissolution of platelet "white" thrombus. Even though platelet activation is inevitable with the use of a plasminogen activator, this effect would potentially be overridden by concomitant administration of a potent antiplatelet inhibitor. Of course, a theoretical limitation of the combination strategy is serious bleeding complications, as these patients also receive concurrent anticoagulation and are thus "bombarded" with three different classes of agents simultaneously. Nevertheless, since the early use of pharmacologic reperfusion treatment patients have received combined plasminogen activators, heparin, and aspirin. So the proposed approach can be viewed as refinement of each of the limbs of the fundamental strategy.

Pilot studies have been especially encouraging. Combined t-PA or r-PA with abciximab, or eptifibatide, have yielded very high frequencies of early infarct vessel patency. In fig 5.4, data at 60 minutes for three different trials are summarised and compared with full dose t-PA, which is still considered to be the "gold" standard. These findings support a near 50% improvement of epicardial infarct vessel patency for combined half dose fibrinolytic and full dose of glycoprotein IIb/IIIa inhibitors.

Perhaps more important than patency of the infarct vessel is the improvement of microvascular perfusion. Although many new imaging modalities may assess this in an elegant fashion, the easiest and most accessible method is to use a 12 lead ECG. A finding of > 70% resolution of ST segment elevation from baseline is highly indicative of restoration of perfusion at the tissue level. Indeed, in the TIMI 14 trial of t-PA and abciximab, there was a more than 50% increase in resolution of ECG ST segment elevation, reflecting relief of microvascular obstruction. Even so, 90 minutes after treatment was initiated 30% of patients with the combined strategy of low dose t-PA and abciximab did not have > 70% ST segment elevation resolution. These findings have been replicated in other phase II studies of combined lytic strategies, and suggest that the combination should be considered a significant step forward for relief of microvascular obstruction but certainly not viewed as a "be all and end all" treatment. The fact that nearly a third of patients are not having tissue level perfusion from a "comprehensive" lytic strategy suggests the need for additional components of an ideal, futuristic reperfusion approach.

Indeed, one of the most important and fundamental obstacles is time. The excessive time that it typically takes for patients to present to an emergency room, or for the healthcare team to deliver rapid treatment, frequently is relatively late for making a difference in salvaging myocardial tissue. When there is extensive damage, the myocardial oedema, leucostasis, and inflammatory reaction in the subtended myocardium may make tissue level perfusion impossible or futile. No matter what strategy is ultimately developed for improved myocardial reperfusion, the issue of timeliness will certainly remain centre stage.

The longstanding feud with catheter based reperfusion

The early trials of immediate coronary angioplasty following t-PA showed higher mortality

32

and reinfarction rates, and the need for emergency bypass surgery. This was not expected at the time (late 1980s). It was known that most patients have a significant underlying atherosclerotic lesion after fibrinolytic treatment. Furthermore, alleviation of the stenosis early on in the course of treatment was expected to be a more definitive strategy. On the other hand, when primary balloon angioplasty was performed as sole treatment (no antecedent lysis), the adverse events appeared to be considerably less than when this procedure followed intravenous t-PA. What was not understood at the time was the pro-thrombotic "dark" side of fibrinolytic treatment. A literal "feud" was engendered between the "balloonatics" and the "thrombolunatics" that has persisted for more than a decade.

There is no reason for partitioning of the two forms of reperfusion treatment now that we have enhanced understanding of the biological process. Intravenous platelet glycoprotein IIb/IIIa treatment or placebo has been administered on a double blind basis in three catheter based reperfusion trials as summarised in fig 5.5.[9 11 12] In all three trials there was a pronounced reduction of the composite end point of death, reinfarction, or urgent revascularisation. Furthermore, we now know that transcoronary intervention is almost always accompanied by embolisation of atherosclerotic debris, in addition to the dislodgement of thrombotic material. Microvascular obstruction can result as a response to embolisation, and potent platelet glycoprotein IIb/IIIa inhibitor treatment would be expected to relieve or pre-empt the process. The direct Doppler demonstrations of improved microvascular perfusion by Neumann and colleagues strongly support this tenet.[9]

Yet the simple adjunctive use of a glycoprotein IIb/IIIa inhibitor is not taking advantage of a pharmacologic strategy designed to achieve early reperfusion and foster a successful

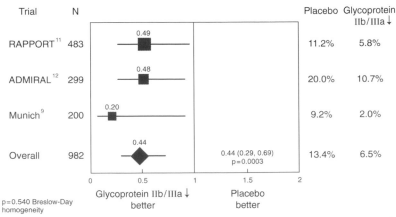

Figure 5.5. Odds ratio and 95% confidence intervals (CI) for 30 day composite of death, myocardial infarction, and urgent revascularisation in three trials of catheter based reperfusion with abciximab or placebo.

catheter based intervention. While intravenous glycoprotein IIb/IIIa inhibition by itself can achieve streptokinase like patency results, the ideal situation would be to achieve "macro" and "micro" vessel patency as quickly as possible. The average time from "door to balloon" is nearly 120 minutes, such that a drug treatment that restores patency long before entering the cardiac catheterisation laboratory, in the highest proportion of patients, would be expected to be of considerable value. In fact, fewer patients have even required catheter intervention in our early experience because of the lack of a significant residual stenosis.

"Connecting the dots"

Many of the concepts described in this review are theoretical, based on experimental models, observational studies, or extrapolation. In order to validate the use of a combined lytic approach, and the implications of microvascular perfusion, data from large scale trials will be necessary. One such trial that is currently ongoing is GUSTO, a 17 000 patient trial comparing r-PA (full dose) as a standard fibrinolytic approach with low dose r-PA (half the usual dose) combined with abciximab. This trial should be completed by the end of 2000 with the primary end point of 30 day mortality. As the event rate for intracerebral haemorrhage is very low (< 1%), only in controlled trials of thousands of patients can the safety of the experimental combined strategy be assured. Substudies, such as the use of continuous 12 lead ECG and conventional ECG assessment for resolution of ST segment elevation, will be helpful to show the link between mortality reduction and microvascular perfusion. Other combination approaches of TNK or t-PA with eptifibatide and TNK with tirofiban will incorporate mechanistic studies using contrast echocardiography and magnetic resonance imaging. Ultimately, in the next couple of years we should have ample evidence that a new standard of myocardial reperfusion has been validated, and that a significant mechanism for improving survival relates to better flow at the tissue level. With acute myocardial infarction as the number 1 killer, and awareness of the

Summary

- The relation of patency to survival is not as direct and straightforward as had been anticipated

- The finding of microvascular obstruction carries a fourfold increase in adverse events including death, reinfection, or the development of congestive heart failure

- Considerable data are emerging to show the ability of low dose fibrinolytics and glycoprotein IIb/IIIa inhibition to relieve or prevent microvascular obstruction

- No matter what strategy is ultimately developed for improved reperfusion, the issue of timeliness will certainly remain centre stage

- In order to validate the use of a combined lytic approach and the implications of microvascular perfusion, data for large scale trials will be necessary

inadequacies of our current treatment, it is vital to continue to refine our approach to the desired goal—that no one with evolving myocardial infarction actually suffers infarction. To that end, we have quite a long way to go.

1. Gruppo Italiano per lo Studio della Streptochinasi nell'Infarto Miocardico (GISSI). Effectiveness of intravenous thrombolytic treatment in acute myocardial infarction. *Lancet* 1986;i:397–401.
• *Classic first large scale trial to show mortality reduction with thrombolysis.*

2. ISIS-2 (Second International Study of Infarct Survival Collaboration Group). Randomized trial of intravenous streptokinase, oral aspirin, both, or neither among 17,187 cases of acute myocardial infarction. *Lancet* 1988;ii:349–60.
• *Confirms the GISSI 1 trial and extends findings by showing importance of aspirin.*

3. GUSTO Investigators. An international randomized trial comparing four thrombolytic strategies for acute myocardial infarction. *N Engl J Med* 1993;**329**:673–82.
• *The largest, confirmed myocardial infarction reperfusion trial that showed a 15% mortality reduction for accelerated t-PA compared with streptokinase and established the mechanism of early patency of the infarct vessel.*

4. Smalling RW, Bode C, Kalbfleisch J, *et al* **for the RAPID Investigators.** More rapid, complete, and stable coronary thrombolysis with bolus administration of reteplase compared with alteplase infusion in acute myocardial infarction. *Circulation* 1995;**91**:2725–32.
• *An angiographic trial showing superiority of reteplase over t-PA for early infarct vessel patency.*

5. GUSTO-III Investigators. An international, multicenter, randomized comparison of reteplase with alteplase for acute myocardial infarction. *N Engl J Med* 1997;**337**:1118–23.
• *The first large scale trial to compare a new bioengineered plasminogen activator r-PA versus t-PA, showing lack of superiority for the new agent.*

6. Ito H, Okamura A, Iwakura K, *et al.* Myocardial perfusion patterns related to thrombolysis in myocardial infarction perfusion grades after coronary angioplasty in patients with acute anterior wall myocardial infarction. *Circulation* 1996;**93**:1993–9.

• *A classic demonstration of no reflow at the tissue level, and its sequelae using myocardial contrast echocardiography.*

7. Porter TR, Li S, Oster R, *et al.* The clinical implications of no reflow demonstrated with intravenous perfluorocarbon containing microbubbles following restoration of thrombolysis in myocardial infarction (TIMI) 3 flow in patients with acute myocardial infarction. *Am J Cardiol* 1998;**82**:1173–7.
• *Impressive evidence for cavity size dilatation and lessened ejection fraction in patients with myocardial contrast echo defect despite TIMI 3 flow.*

8. Wu KC, Zerhouni EA, Judd RM, *et al.* Prognostic significance of microvascular obstruction by magnetic resonance imaging in patients with acute myocardial infarction. *Circulation* 1998;**97**:765–72.
• *Demonstration via magnetic resonance imaging of microvascular obstruction and its impact on prognosis.*

9. Neumann F-J, Blasini R, Schmitt C, *et al.* Effect of glycoprotein IIb/IIIa blockade on recovery of coronary flow and left ventricular function after the placement of coronary-artery stents in acute myocardial infarction. *Circulation* 1998;**98**:2695–701.
• *A landmark myocardial infarction study that showed glyoprotein IIb/IIIa inhibition improved microvascular perfusion of the infarct territory, and that this correlated with improved cardiac function.*

10. Gurbel PA, Serebruany VL, Shustov AR, *et al* **for the GUSTO III Investigators.** Effects of reteplase and alteplase on platelet aggregation and major receptor expression during the first 24 hours of acute myocardial infarction treatment. The GUSTO III platelet study. *J Am Coll Cardiol* 1998;**31**:1466–73.
• *Mechanistic platelet study showing heightened activation after reteplase compared with alteplase.*

11. Brener SJ, Barr LA, Burchenal JEB, *et al* **for the RAPPORT Investigators.** Effect of abciximab on the pattern of reperfusion in patients with acute myocardial infarction treated with primary angioplasty. *Am J Cardiol* 1999;**84**:728–30.
• *The first randomised trial of glycoprotein IIb/IIIa inhibition for acute myocardial infarction, performed in the setting of catheter based reperfusion.*

12 Montalescot G, Barragan P, Wittenberg O, *et al.* Abciximab associated with primary angioplasty and stenting in acute myocardial infarction: the ADMIRAL study, 30-day results [abstract]. *Eur Heart J* 1999;**20**(suppl):170.

33

6 The natural history of acute myocardial infarction

Robin M Norris

The majority of readers of this article are likely to be hospital based clinicians whose experience of acute myocardial infarction is necessarily limited to examination of the survivors of a storm which has already taken its major toll. As has always been the case, most deaths from heart attack occur outside hospital and are medically unattended, as are about one quarter of non-fatal infarctions which are "silent" with no or atypical symptoms. For out-of-hospital deaths, even if a necropsy is carried out, it is in the majority of cases impossible to determine whether death had been caused by a developing infarction or by re-entrant ventricular fibrillation starting at the borders of a myocardial scar. Finally, it is impossible strictly speaking nowadays to speak about "natural" history. The history is inevitably "unnatural" in that it has in many cases been modified by treatment.

Myocardial infarction outside hospital

In the most recent study performed in the UK,[1] 74% of 1589 deaths from acute coronary heart attacks in people under 75 years of age occurred outside hospital; the proportion of out-of-hospital to total deaths varied inversely with age from 91% at age < 55 years to 67% at age 70–74 years (fig 6.1). Had the lives of 5% of potential victims of out-of-hospital sudden death not been saved by advanced life support given by ambulance staff, the proportion of out-of-hospital deaths to total deaths would have been even higher. The finding of three quarters rather than the previously quoted two

thirds of deaths outside hospital may reflect a declining hospital fatality rate owing to better treatment, with no or a lesser reduction in the numbers of early sudden deaths.

Seventy five per cent of out-of-hospital deaths in our study occurred in the home and about 60% were witnessed. Advanced life support given by ambulance personnel was attempted in a little over half the cases. Of the 25% of deaths which occurred away from home, 16% happened in a public place, usually the street, 3% in an ambulance, 3% in nursing homes, 1% in doctors' surgeries, and only 2% at the place of work. Sudden death at mass gatherings such as football stadia or railway stations was unusual.

Pathology of out-of-hospital death

What proportion of out-of-hospital deaths are caused by developing infarction, and what proportion are caused by a re-entrant arrhythmia? Sudden unexpected death in England must be reported to a coroner unless the victim was known to have coronary disease and had been seen by a doctor within the last two weeks. Depending on the practice of individual coroners, the proportion of unexpected deaths coming to necropsy is high. However, developing infarction cannot be recognised in most cases of sudden death because the earliest histological change (invasion by leucocytes) does not develop until 12–24 hours after the onset. Evidence must be sought by examination of the coronary arteries.

Occlusion of the infarct related coronary artery by thrombus is nearly always present in patients with ST elevation myocardial infarction admitted early to hospital[2]; this is almost certainly the event which causes the infarct, so that the presence of occlusive thrombus at necropsy is almost pathognomonic of developing infarction. In a consecutive series of 168 sudden coronary deaths (within six hours of onset of symptoms)[3] in which the coronary arteries were examined by postmortem arteriography and histology of sections made at 3 mm intervals, occlusive thrombus was present in 30% of cases, and mural thrombus in 43%. In 8% of cases plaque fissuring only was present, and there was no acute lesion in

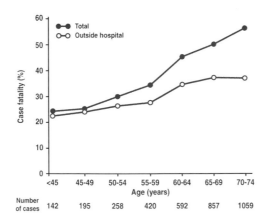

Figure 6.1. Total case fatality in the UK heart attack study and case fatality outside hospital by age group. Reproduced from Norris[1] with permission of BMJ Publishing Group.

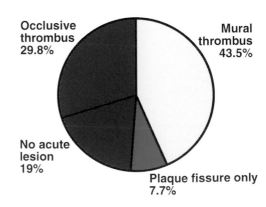

Figure 6.2. Necropsy findings in 168 cases of sudden coronary death in which the coronary arteries were examined by post mortem arteriography and histology of sections made at 3 mm intervals. Reproduced from Davies[3] with permission of the American Heart Association.

19% (fig 6.2). Thus from this series it appeared that perhaps 30% of sudden cardiac deaths were definitely caused by developing infarction, and in an additional 45% infarction was highly likely (because the finding of intraluminal thrombus is unusual in definite non-coronary death). In the remaining 25% infarction was unlikely because plaque fissuring is quite common in people who die from an unrelated cause.[3]

Postmortem arteriography and serial sectioning of the coronary arteries is not carried out routinely by hospital pathologists who frequently limit the procedure, as far as the heart is concerned, to cursory section of the coronary arteries. Histological examination is not routine, and in these circumstances neither non-occlusive thrombus nor plaque fissuring are often commented upon. In the UK heart attack study (UKHAS)[4] 1037 (83%) of the 1247 out-of-hospital coronary deaths which we recognised in people up to 75 years of age came to necropsy. Occlusive thrombus was recognised by hospital pathologists in 23% of cases, recent myocardial infarction in 20%, and an old myocardial scar in 56%. Stenoses of one or more coronary arteries were present in all cases.

CLINICOPATHOLOGICAL CORRELATIONS
In about half of the victims of out-of-hospital coronary death in the UKHAS study we were able to discover whether death had been truly sudden or if there had been prodromal symptoms (usually chest pain) before death. Of particular interest was that necropsy evidence of old infarction was more common and recent infarction less common in 124 victims who apparently had had no prodromal symptoms before death (70% and 11%) than in the 386 who had had prodromal chest pain (45% and 29%) (p < 0.001). However, occlusive thrombus was no more common in people with symptoms (26%) than in those without symptoms (29%). This latter finding is at variance with that of Davies[3] who was able to show a much higher number of thrombi with serial sectioning of the arteries. Of the 168 cases of sudden cardiac death mentioned earlier, occlusive thrombus was more common when prodromal pain had been present than when it had been absent. To summarise the evidence from necropsies, it is impossible to give any reliable estimate of the proportion of sudden coronary deaths which were caused by developing infarction and what proportion were caused by "electrical" death. However, both the detailed anatomical studies of Davies[3] and our own larger series of routine necropsies do support the existence of at least two separate mechanisms for out-of-hospital coronary death.

RESUSCITATION FROM OUT-OF-HOSPITAL ARREST
Further evidence does, however, come from one of the earliest studies of patients resuscitated from out-of-hospital cardiac arrest.[5] In Seattle, Washington, between 1970 and 1973, 146 patients were resuscitated from out-of-hospital ventricular fibrillation and were fol-

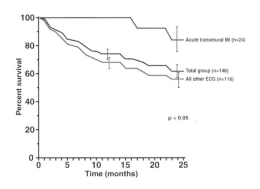

Figure 6.3. Two year survival after resuscitation from out-of-hospital arrest according to whether or not new pathological Q waves developed. Reproduced from Baum and colleagues[5] with permission of the American Heart Association.

lowed for two years. The subsequent survival of the 17% of patients whose arrest was caused by Q wave infarction was significantly better (p < 0.005) than the survival of the 83% who did not develop new pathological Q waves (fig 6.3).[5] It was this seminal observation that led to the recognition of "electrical" coronary death as a distinct pathological entity and its consequent electrophysiological investigation and treatment with implantable defibrillators. The Seattle findings also suggested that the majority of sudden deaths were "electrical". However, this conclusion, based on findings in a subset of survivors, may be incorrect in view of those from the detailed pathological examinations described above.[3]

EPIDEMIOLOGICAL STUDIES
The final arbiter of the classification of acute coronary events, both fatal and non-fatal, is the epidemiologist. Discussion of global differences in incidence of new coronary events and prevalence of the disease is not the purpose of this article. However, methods used by the World Health Organisation MONICA (monitoring trends and determinants in cardiovascular disease) investigators[6] highlight the difficulties in exact definition. MONICA recognised both fatal and non-fatal events in the two categories of "definite" and "probable", and constructed their main analyses of incidence, mortality, and case fatality on "definite" only non-fatal events and "definite" plus "probable" fatal events. A third category of "unclassifiable" fatal events was also encountered; these were unexpected deaths in which no necropsy had been carried out and cause of death had been certified as coronary disease in the absence of definite evidence for or against the diagnosis. These deaths too were included in the analyses. MONICA definitions are not in dispute, but the problems in applying them to differing cultures with differing legal requirements for death certification are immense. From the epidemiologists' perspective the problem of "unclassifiable" deaths and the frequent unreliability of death certificates, particularly in the elderly, is very real. Different counting methods used by clinicians and epidemiologists yield differing results; this problem is discussed in a recent editorial.[7] Of

**Problems in defining the true natural
history of myocardial infarction**

- Two thirds to three quarters of fatal events
occur outside hospital. Such deaths may be
caused by infarction or may be electrical.
Although it may be possible to differentiate
these mechanisms in some individual cases,
it is impossible to do this in the majority.

- Death certificates are unreliable; many
deaths certified as being caused by
coronary heart disease, particularly in the
elderly, are in truth unclassifiable.

- About 25% of non-fatal infarctions are
silent and medically unattended.

- These facts must be taken into account for
interpretation of all community and
epidemiological studies, and also for
interpretation of demographic data which
show geographical differences or secular
changes in mortality from coronary heart
disease.

course no attempt at distinction between
infarction and electrical death is possible in
purely epidemiological studies.

Yet another problem in identification of the
natural history of acute myocardial infarction is
that fully 25% of non-fatal infarctions are
silent.[8] Silent infarction can be detected only
when a subject is seen more than once at
annual intervals or longer, and an ECG
performed on the second occasion shows new
pathological Q waves. Most clinicians can
remember such cases, but an estimate of the
incidence can be made only when a cohort of
the population free from coronary heart disease
is followed for a number of years. This
happened in the Framingham study—a unique
and prestigious study which has taught us more
than any other about the changing pattern of
coronary heart disease during the latter half of
the 20th century.[9]

The declining mortality from coronary heart disease

There is no doubt that mortality from coronary
heart disease is falling. Figure 6.4[10] shows that
age specific mortality for males aged 35–44
years during 1997 was about one third, and of
those aged 65–74 years about two thirds of the
figures for 1968 when the coronary epidemic
was at its height. Age groups 45–54 and 55–64
showed intermediate changes and the picture
was similar in women. Data in fig 4 stop at age
75, however. If evidence from death certificates
is to be believed, more than 60% of coronary
deaths occur in people aged > 75 years.[10]
Death is being postponed, not prevented; it has
been estimated that the global burden of
coronary heart disease will continue to increase
up to the year 2020.[11] Although the incidence
of new events is falling, the prevalence of
coronary heart disease in the community is
increasing.[10]

How does the decline in mortality shown by
the demographers relate to the natural history

of acute myocardial infarction? Of course only
acute events rather than infarctions can be
monitored. However, the most recent evidence
from the MONICA study suggests that over a
10 year period in populations where mortality
decreased, reduction in coronary event rates
accounted for about two thirds of the decrease
while reduced case fatality accounted for about
one third.[12]

Acute myocardial infarction in hospital

For the hospital clinician there is much less
difficulty in the definition of acute myocardial
infarction. Most clinicians will accept that infarction should be diagnosed when at least two
of the following three conditions are present: a
typical or compatible clinical history; sequential electrocardiographic changes; and a rise in
cardiac enzyme activity to at least twice the
upper limit of normal for the hospital laboratory. For patients who die very soon after presentation, a history of prolonged chest pain with
one ECG showing an infarct pattern is
sufficient for the diagnosis. However, even this
seemingly simple definition is open to differing
interpretations. In a recent survey (unpublished) of cases admitted to a district general
hospital we found a substantial overlap between diagnoses based on the above criteria
and those specified by clinical coding using the
International Classification of Diseases, 10th revision (ICD 10) codes. The most common
reason for disagreement was differentiation
between acute myocardial infarction and unstable angina. This of course reflects the
uncertainties described in epidemiological
studies.[6]

Prognosis of hospital treated infarction

Definitions aside, the prognosis of hospital
treated patients has improved considerably
over recent years although the factors determining survival have not changed. More than
30 years ago we constructed a coronary
prognostic index[13] which was based on the age
of patients and the then available methods for
assessment of left ventricular function, namely
the chest radiograph and the systolic blood
pressure on admission to hospital. The index

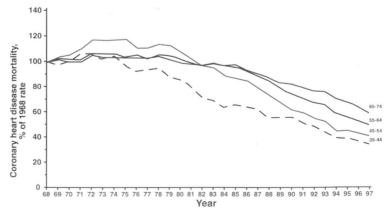

Figure 6.4. Age specific death rates from coronary heart disease in men 1968 to
1997, plotted as a percentage of the rates in 1968. Reproduced from British
Heart Foundation Coronary Heart Disease Statistics 1999, with permission.

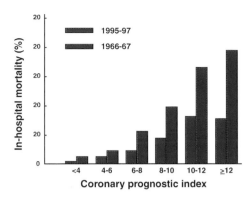

Figure 6.5. Hospital fatality predicted by a coronary prognostic index in patients treated in 1966-67 and 1995-97. Modified and reproduced from Christiansen and Liang[14] with permission of the publisher.

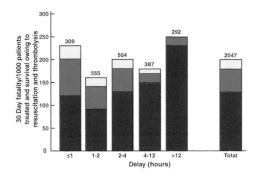

Figure 6.6. Thirty day fatality (red bars), lives saved by resuscitation from cardiac arrest (green bars), and lives estimated to have been saved by thrombolytic treatment (yellow bars) according to delay in presentation to the hospital. Numbers above the bars refer to the numbers of patients in each group. Reproduced from UK heart attack study[17] with permission of BMJ Publishing Group.

has proved to be remarkably robust in predicting relative although not absolute risk. This is shown by a study of 830 patients treated between 1995 and 1997[14] which showed that hospital fatality had fallen by 50% or more compared with 30 years previously (fig 6.5). This decline was most striking in the high risk patients (elderly patients with cardiac failure). Data such as those in fig 6.5 also underline the potential unreliability of crude figures for case fatality as a performance indicator. Both case mix and differences in definition of acute myocardial infarction (see above) can influence hospital fatality rates considerably.

The two major advances in treatment which have changed the natural history of hospital treated infarction over the last 30 years are resuscitation from cardiac arrest and restoration of flow to the infarct related coronary artery by thrombolytic drugs or primary angioplasty. It has been estimated that thrombolysis saves about 30 lives per thousand patients treated,[15] although the benefit may be doubled for those treated within the "golden hour" after the onset of symptoms.[16] Reduction in delay in giving thrombolytic treatment has been a major goal for hospitals in recent years, and various strategies for "fast track" administration either in accident and emergency departments or in coronary care units have been proposed. Pre-hospital treatment on a large scale has so far proved impracticable, and emphasis is placed on reduction in patient delay and use of ambulance paramedics rather than medical practitioners in providing early resuscitation and transport to hospital. Delay is inevitable with this strategy, however; in a recent hospital survey only 2% of patients had thrombolytic treatment started within the "golden hour".[17]

Recent enthusiasm for improving delivery of thrombolytic treatment has to a degree caused clinicians and health administrators to lose sight of the fact that resuscitation from cardiac arrest has done much more than thrombolysis to change the natural history of myocardial infarction for the better. Moreover reduction of delay in coming under care saves more lives by timely defibrillation than by early recanalisation of the infarct related coronary artery. This is shown in fig 6.6[17] which examines the effect of delay on salvage of patients by resuscitation and estimated salvage by thrombolytic treatment, taking delay in its administration into account.[16] Altogether, 80% of the salvage was attributable to resuscitation, and benefit from the "golden hour" was greater for resuscitation than for thrombolysis. Part of the reason for this was, of course, that patients did not receive thrombolytic treatment immediately after coming under care.

Survival after recovery from myocardial infarction

As for early survival, long term survival is most closely related to age and to left ventricular function. Function is traditionally described by ejection fraction which is an arithmetical term derived from the volumes of the ventricle at end diastole and end systole. In a series of patients under 60 years of age studied by left ventriculography before the thrombolytic era, we identified end systolic volume as the major functional determinant of long term survival.[18] For patients with an ejection fraction < 50%, the five year fatality rate was more than twice as great (36%) when end systolic volume was above the median value of 110 ml as when it was below the median (14%). Apart from age and ventricular dilatation, electrical instability as evidenced by occurrence of non-sustained ventricular arrhythmias on Holter monitoring and inducibility on electrophysiologic testing[19] are powerful additional predictors of a poor prognosis.

Conclusion: future prospects for improving the natural history

Many years ago the Framingham investigators concluded that the only road to substantial reduction in premature mortality from coronary heart disease lay in prevention of the disease. Primary prevention in the UK by a population strategy to encourage people to reduce their dietary fat intake has had limited success, although smoking has declined in the coronary age group.[10] Nevertheless, at least some of the decline in mortality must presum-

---

The natural history of acute myocardial infarction

- There are major difficulties in defining the natural history because of:
  - –differentiation from "electrical" death.
  - –difficulties in pathological examination.
  - –unreliability of death certification.
  - –impossibility of recording silent non-fatal infarcts.

- The decline in coronary mortality is occurring among younger people and is caused mainly by reduction in new events.

- The single most promising therapeutic strategy is secondary prevention.

---

ably be the result of primary prevention.[12] Secondary prevention for patients with known coronary disease has great potential for reducing mortality and has the attraction that potential methods for achieving it are soundly evidence based. Recent evidence from the USA[20] suggests that the decline in mortality between 1987 and 1994 may be largely caused by improvements in secondary prevention.[20]

As far as the treatment of myocardial infarction is concerned, it is probably true to say that better application of treatments already known to be effective in the year 2000 have more to offer than the development of new treatments. Reduction of patient delay in calling for help through public education on the symptoms of heart attack and the importance of access to emergency services, and improved response time of ambulances, are of paramount importance. The search for better thrombolytic and antiplatelet agents continues, but is less likely to improve the natural history than is earlier delivery of drugs already known to be effective.

1. **Norris RM, on behalf of the United Kingdom Heart Attack Study Collaborative Group.** Fatality outside hospital from acute coronary events in three British health districts 1994–95. *BMJ* 1998;**316**:1065–70.
- *This is the most recent study of out-of-hospital coronary death to have been performed in the UK.*

2. **de Wood MA, Spores R, Natske LT,** *et al.* Prevalence of total coronary occlusion during the early hours of transmural myocardial infarction. *N Engl J Med* 1980;**303**:897–902.
- *The first study of myocardial infarction by coronary arteriography during the acute stage finally established that coronary thrombosis was the proximate cause of infarction.*

3. **Davies MJ.** Anatomic features in victims of sudden coronary death. *Circulation* 1992;**85**(suppl 1):19–24.
- *Summarises the best available evidence from detailed anatomical studies carried out by an expert pathologist.*

4. **Norris RM.** Sudden cardiac death and acute myocardial infarction in three British health districts: the UK heart attack study. London: British Heart Foundation, 1999:61–4.

5. **Baum RS, Alvarez H, Cobb LA.** Survival after resuscitation from out-of-hospital venticular fibrillation. *Circulation* 1974;**50**:1231–5.
- *The definitive definition between acute myocardial infarction and "electrical" death in survivors from out-of-hospital cardiac arrest.*

6. **Tunstall-Pedoe H, Kuulasmaa K, Amouyel P,** *et al.* Myocardial infarction and coronary deaths in the World Health Organization MONICA registration project: registration procedure, event rates and case fatality rates in 30 populations from 21 countries in 4 continents. *Circulation* 1994;**90**:583–612.
- *This important epidemiological study is quoted to show the difficulties of definition of acute coronary events and consequent uncertainties of geographical comparisons.*

7. **Tunstall-Pedoe H.** Perspectives on trends in mortality and case fatality from coronary heart attacks : the need for a better definition of acute myocardial infarction. *Heart* 1998;**80**:112–3.

8. **Kannel WB, Abbott RD.** Incidence and prognosis of unrecognised myocardial infarction. An update on the Framingham study. *N Engl J Med* 1984;**311**:1144–7.
- *The definitive description of silent infarction from the most prestigious epidemiological study ever performed.*

9. **Kannel WB.** Some lessons in cardiovascular epidemiology from Framingham. *Am J Cardiol* 1976;**37**:269–82.
- *A classic account of coronary risk factors.*

10. **British Heart Foundation.** Coronary heart disease statistics. London: British Heart Foundation, 1999.
- *An invaluable reference source for data on the changing mortality rates and prevalence of risk factors in the UK.*

11. **Murray CJL, Lopez AD.** Alternative projections of mortality and disability by cause 1990—2020; global burden of disease study. *Lancet* 1997;**349**:1498–504.

12. **Tunstall-Pedoe H, Kuulasmaa K, Mahonen M,** *et al.* Contribution of trends in survival and coronary event rates to changes in coronary heart disease mortality: 10-year results from 37 WHO MONICA project populations. *Lancet* 1999;**353**:1547–57.

13. **Norris RM, Brandt PWT, Caughey DE,** *et al.* A new coronary prognostic index. *Lancet* 1969;i:274–8.
- *This article showed by indirect methods that age and impairment of cardiac function are the principal determinants of survival for hospital treated patients.*

14. **Christiansen JP, Liang C-S.** Reappraisal of the Norris score and the prognostic value of left ventricular ejection fraction. Measurement of in-hospital mortality after acute myocardial infarction. *Am J Cardiol* 1999;**83**:589–91.

15. **Fibrinolytic Therapy Trialists (FTT) Collaborative Group.** Indications for fibrinolytic therapy in suspected acute myocardial infarction: collaborative overview of early mortality and major morbidity results from all randomised trials of more than 1000 patients. *Lancet* 1994;**343**:311–22.
- *This comprehensive overview of thrombolytic trials suggested that about 30 lives were saved for every 1000 patients treated.*

16. **Boersma E, Maas ACP, Simoons ML.** Early thrombolytic treatment in acute myocardial infarction: reappraisal of the Golden Hour. *Lancet* 1996;**348**:771–5.

17. **United Kingdom Heart Attack Study (UKHAS) Collaborative Group.** Effect of time from onset to coming under care on fatality of patients with acute myocardial infarction: effect of resuscitation and thrombolytic treatment. *Heart* 1998;**80**:114–20.

18. **Norris RM, White HD, Cross DB,** *et al.* Prognosis after recovery from myocardial infarction: the relative importance of cardiac dilatation and coronary stenoses. *Eur Heart J* 1992;**13**:1611–8.

19. **Richards DAB, Blyth K, Ross DL,** *et al.* What is the best predictor of spontaneous ventricular tachycardia and sudden death after myocardial infarction? *Circulation* 1991;**83**:756–63.

20. **Rosamond WD, Chambless LE, Folsom AR,** *et al.* Trends in the incidence of myocardial infarction and in mortality due to coronary heart disease 1987 to 1994. *N Engl J Med* 1998;**339**:861–7.

7 Management of the post-myocardial infarction patient: rehabilitation and cardiac neurosis

David R Thompson, Robert J P Lewin

Myocardial infarction (MI) is a major cause of mortality and morbidity in the western world. As MI is a life threatening event it is hardly surprising that it often causes distress and impairment of quality of life for patients and their relatives, especially partners. For a substantial minority of families such consequences are profound.

Psychological factors

Most patients are clinically anxious on admission to hospital. This anxiety generally remits over the next couple of days but rises again just before discharge, when many patients may again become clinically anxious. This distress is often deliberately hidden from the staff and other patients. Once home, a reduction in mood—"home coming depression"—is almost universal and patients and partners should be warned that it is likely to happen, otherwise they may worry that their "mind" has been damaged as well as their heart. Patients should be assured that this reaction is not unique to surviving an MI but is common in survivors of any natural disaster. In the majority of patients, unless there are further acute events, anxiety and depression slowly remit over the following weeks. However, about a quarter of patients may remain distressed at one year. It takes only minutes to screen patients using the Hospital Anxiety and Depression Scale, and as many patients come back for an exercise test at 6–12 weeks postdischarge, this may be a good time to identify those likely to have long term adjustment problems and to refer them for appropriate counselling/treatment.

In the first few months of recovery many patients report a fear of resuming sex and, unless this is dealt with, some will never resume it. Partners share the same worries and their fear is often the major factor in reduced sexual activity and enjoyment. There is no evidence that sex is in anyway dangerous, and patients and their partners should be told so in an unequivocal fashion. The exercise involved may even be protective as regular moderate exercise has a very significant protective effect in post-MI patients.

Some patients interpret the normal or explicable feelings of fatigue or minor symptoms of the anxiety they are suffering as relating to the condition of their heart. This often leads to a reduction in social and physical activity (in an effort to protect the heart) and further preoccupation with symptoms. Reduced activity leads to physical deconditioning, often producing more fatigue, more time to dwell on any symptoms or bodily sensations, and therefore generates further anxiety. Other patients become trapped in a downward spiral of increasing disability, and a very small number will succumb to a restricted and fearful lifestyle that has been labelled in many different ways over the years—for example "cardiac neurosis", "neurocirculatory asthenia" or "effort syndrome". These patients are currently described as demonstrating "undue illness behaviour". They demonstrate high levels of anxiety, physical deconditioning, a dependent attitude towards medical care, and often an almost obsessional preoccupation with the details of their medical history.

Health beliefs

Patients' beliefs and perceptions of their illness are critically important in the recovery phase of MI. Patients' beliefs about whether their MI was caused by stress or poor health habits act as a clear starting point for them when deciding to make changes in their personal health behaviours.

MI patients who hold negative models of their illness are less likely to return to work and to have lower levels of functioning regardless of the severity of the MI.

The patients' view of their MI is an important factor in both rehabilitation attendance and in how quickly they return to work.[1] The attributions that patients make for the cause of their MI may also have a major bearing on their recovery. Surveys have shown that the majority of patients blame the MI on "stress", "worry" or "overwork". If a patient believes that his job nearly killed him he may be very reluctant to return. These faulty attributions are often compounded by poor medical communication. Many patients view the heart as "worn out" and fear and avoid activity, thinking that this will further deplete their energy reserves. These damaging beliefs are often reinforced by the media, friends, and family and sometimes by lifestyle advice received from health care professionals.

Practical advice on managing psychological factors

It is important to attend to psychological factors because there is increasing evidence that psychological distress following MI is an independent risk factor for early mortality.[2] There is also more limited evidence that initial distress predicts outcome for return to work and for some other aspects of quality of life outcome,[3] lifestyle changes,[4] and compliance with medical care.[5]

Structured advice and discussion of the factors known to affect recovery is important. Whenever possible it is important to elicit from

40

patients what they think the main cause of the heart attack was. Particular care should be taken to avoid unintentionally reinforcing the common cardiac misconceptions, especially about stress and the value of rest, that many patients have. Advice should be realistic, practical, and concrete (that is, specifying exactly what should be done—for example, "eat five portions of fresh fruit or vegetables every day" instead of "try and eat more fruit"). Advice should take account of social and cultural needs. Every patient should be helped to develop an individualised and concrete plan for recovery to be carried out in the weeks following the MI. The resumption of small amounts of activity should be encouraged from the first full day home. Vague advice such as "listen to your body" or "do what you can manage" is unhelpful. Patients and their families should be warned about the common physical and psychological sequelae. The primary physical problems are unexpected weakness caused by deconditioning, breathlessness on exercise, and angina. Patients are often particularly fearful of exercising to breathlessness and should be advised that this is an important concomitant of increasing cardiovascular fitness.

Common psychological reactions that should be mentioned are:
- low mood;
- tearfulness;
- sleep disturbance;
- irritability;
- anxiety;
- acute awareness of minor somatic sensations or pains;
- poor concentration and memory.

It should be explained that these symptoms are normal, that they are universal, and are part of the natural course of recovery following *any* potentially life threatening event. Partners should be advised to alter the family routines as little as possible except for lifestyle changes, such as smoking or diet, which should begin immediately. They must be tactfully advised against overprotecting the patient or, in a few cases, usually with female patients, from expecting the patient to resume doing all of the housework immediately. The patient's and partner's understanding of the advice should be checked during the course and at the end of each session, by asking them to summarise the advice imparted.

As half of the advice in a five minute consultation is forgotten within a further five minutes, it is helpful if written or tape recorded advice (the interview itself can be taped) is provided. Written information should be produced following the empirically determined guidelines for maximising comprehension and compliance.

Cardiac rehabilitation

Early cardiac rehabilitation programmes centred upon physical restitution of middle aged men who could be returned to work after prolonged bed rest. Modern cardiac rehabilitation

---

Cardiac rehabilitation: general points

- For the majority of patients the best predictors of rehabilitation outcome are psychosocial not physiological.

- Psychological findings about adjustment to MI and lifestyle change must be integrated with routine care.

- Family members, especially the partner, should be included in the rehabilitation process.

- The greater part of any verbal interaction is quickly forgotten, and should be backed up with carefully constructed and empirically evaluated written and taped material.

---

is an activity requiring a range of health skills to bring together medical treatment, education, counselling, exercise training, risk factor modification and secondary prevention, in order to limit the harmful physical and psychological effects of heart disease, reduce the risk of death or recurrence of the cardiac event, and enhance the psychosocial and vocational state of patients.[6]

Cardiac rehabilitation has been defined by the World Health Organization as: " . . .the sum of activities required to influence favourably the underlying cause of the disease, as well as to ensure that patients' best possible physical, mental and social conditions so that they may, by their own efforts, preserve, or resume when lost, as normal a place as possible in the life of the community."[7] The WHO definition is, of course, all embracing but is endorsed by countries in Europe and beyond. In essence, cardiac rehabilitation services are comprehensive programmes involving education, exercise, risk factor modification and counselling, designed to limit the physiological and psychological effects of heart disease, reduce the risk of death or recurrence of the cardiac event, and enhance the psychosocial and vocational state of patients. Thus, cardiac rehabilitation is a multidisciplinary and multifaceted intervention that aims to restore wellbeing and retard disease progression in patients with heart disease.

It has been recommended that every district hospital which treats patients with heart disease should provide a cardiac rehabilitation service, and that individual programmes should evaluate their outcome, and a standard format of audit could be agreed nationally to allow comparison.[6] However, the provision of cardiac rehabilitation is still a neglected topic in some centres and it is likely that there is considerable potential to improve the quality of care and to reduce undesirable variations in service provision. The new National Service Framework for coronary heart disease,[8] developed to improve the quality and consistency of services in terms of prevention and treatment, should be helpful in implementing change.

Early phase of rehabilitation

- Immediately after diagnosis of MI, or as soon as is practical, patients should have their beliefs and knowledge about the MI and their lifestyle assessed and, where necessary, receive counselling.

- Patients should be assessed for psychological problems using validated instruments, such as the Hospital Anxiety and Depression Scale, and if necessary have access to appropriate counselling/treatment and to follow up assessment.

- Counselling should be concrete, with clearly defined and measurable goals, and must take into account the patient's own beliefs about what has happened and what should be done.

- Patients should be prepared for the common physical and emotional sequelae which often only become problematic after discharge from hospital.

Effectiveness

Although there is some scepticism regarding the effectiveness of cardiac rehabilitation, there is strong evidence attesting to its benefits. Most of the evidence pertains to patients who have suffered an MI. Meta-analyses have suggested a significant reduction in total and cardiac mortality of at least 20%. These benefits are likely to be greater for people with more severe disease, and are only seen in trials using a comprehensive individualised approach to lifestyle modification with education and psychological input as well as exercise.

Systematic reviews[9][10] have concluded that there is sufficient evidence available to show substantial benefits, including improvements in exercise tolerance, symptoms, and blood lipid concentrations, psychosocial wellbeing, and reductions in stress and cigarette smoking. Cardiac rehabilitation can promote recovery, enable patients to achieve and maintain better health, and reduce risk of death in people who have heart disease. A combination of exercise, psychological interventions, and education appears to be the most effective form of cardiac rehabilitation. However, important questions remain to be answered as to the optimal mix of components.

Cost and cost-effectiveness

There is an urgent need to assemble information on the cost and cost-effectiveness of cardiac rehabilitation. At present, little is known about the economic aspects of these services.

To date, there has been only one full cost-effectiveness study of cardiac rehabilitation, in the USA.[11] When extrapolated to the UK situation the results suggest a cost per quality adjusted life year (QALY) of £6900, and a cost per life year gained at three years of £15 700.[12] Costs have not been calculated for more than

three years but it is likely that cardiac rehabilitation would be even more cost-effective over longer periods of time. In addition, two trials (one in Sweden and one in the USA) examining the medium to long term implications of cardiac rehabilitation have shown a significant reduction in the costs of readmission to hospital and treatment coupled with savings accruing from an earlier return to work.[12]

Clearly cardiac rehabilitation is not a homogeneous service and there is a range of factors that influence the costs and cost-effectiveness of the process, including the scale of the programme, location, components, intensity of the process, the patient population, and compliance.

Organisation of services

There is a paucity of research regarding the optimal frequency, duration, and mode of delivery of cardiac rehabilitation programmes. Most programmes are organised on an outpatient, hospital basis, usually of 6-12 weeks duration and commencing six weeks after discharge from hospital.

A six week, home based rehabilitation programme, the *Heart Manual*, delivered by a specially trained nurse has been found to be effective in reducing anxiety and depression, visits to the general practitioner and hospital readmissions up to six months after an MI.[13] Other forms of home and community based rehabilitation may be as effective and as safe as hospital based programmes, but more research is needed.

Cardiac rehabilitation involves long term maintenance of changed behaviour. This will take place in the community and patients need access to cardiac support groups and to appropriate cardiac review and follow up.

Access and uptake of services

Only a small proportion of patients with MI is offered or takes up cardiac rehabilitation.[14] Although the overall number of programmes and level have increased notably over the past 15 years, there is wide variation in practice and in the organisation and management of services, and many patients who might benefit do not receive cardiac rehabilitation. Current service provision fails to meet the standard set in national guidelines.[15][16] Most centres tend to restrict access to young, male, white patients who have suffered a (usually first, uncomplicated) MI. Indeed, the majority of cardiac rehabilitation research has been conducted on MI or coronary artery bypass surgery patients. Little is known about the needs and experiences of women, elderly people, and ethnic minorities, who are rarely offered rehabilitation or, when they are, frequently fail to take up services. In addition, very few patients with heart failure or angina are offered rehabilitation, even though they are likely to have a large potential for health gain. More research is required to identify reasons for, and strategies to improve, the current low levels of uptake in these groups.

Process of rehabilitation

National guidelines aim for cardiac rehabilitation to be comprehensive, provide early help for everyone likely to benefit, based on individual assessment of need, and followed by a later menu of options.[15] It should be accompanied by audit and individual monitoring of patient progress.

Ideally, the cardiac rehabilitation process should start at, or even before, the time of hospital admission, continue throughout hospital stay, and hand over seamlessly to the community.

The time course of cardiac rehabilitation can be divided into four phases: in-hospital; early postdischarge; later postdischarge; and long term follow up. Spanning these phases are three essential elements, which are inter-linked and may be overlapping:

- the process of explanation and understanding;
- specific rehabilitation interventions— including where appropriate secondary prevention, exercise training, and psychological support—tailored to the needs of the individual patient;
- the long term process of re-adaptation and re-education.

A flexible approach to the later stages of rehabilitation is essential, with the outcomes (particularly physical activity, smoking cessation, dietary change) being more important than rigid adherence to set procedures.

Involvement of family

Evidence is accumulating that the success of rehabilitation may depend to a large extent upon the involvement of the patient's family, particularly the partner. Arguments for including the partner in the rehabilitation process are both practical and therapeutic. The partner can be incorporated in the programme with little additional effort or cost. It is likely that the partner's attitudes to the patient's MI can affect recovery through, for example, being over concerned and protective. Perhaps as important as the potential health gains for patients are those for partners. As one might expect, partners are often distressed after an MI. Indeed, they often report levels of anxiety and depression that are at least as comparable to, and often higher than, those of patients. Therefore, they may well benefit from the support, information and enhanced feeling of control that they are likely to experience by being included in rehabilitation.

The presence of the partner in rehabilitation can improve confidence and morale in the patient. It is frequently the partner that has the major role in the patient's readjustment during convalescence, and his or her behaviour is an important determinant of the rate and extent of the patient's recovery. Recent studies examining the impact on patients and partners of in-hospital and extended rehabilitation have resulted in less anxiety and depression and more knowledge and satisfaction with care in both patients and partners, with effects enduring up to one year.[17]

Cardiac rehabilitation: early postdischarge

- Support should be continued and need only consist of brief meetings or even telephone calls to go through the goals, reinforce progress, and help the patient solve any practical difficulties that may have arisen.

- Care should be taken to ensure that congruent advice is given by primary care staff.

- Patients should be formally assessed at 6–12 weeks post-MI to ascertain their success in making lifestyle changes and psychological adjustment.

Partners are a valuable resource during the rehabilitation process. They can support patients during the adjustment phase and assist and encourage them in making changes to their lifestyle and promoting healthy behaviours. The routine inclusion of partners in rehabilitation programmes seems warranted.

It is worth acknowledging that the majority of studies on rehabilitation have focused on male patients and female partners and there may be sex related factors that influence partner involvement.

Methodological issues

Some of the methodological problems in trials of rehabilitation have been reviewed.[18] In contrast to the "ideal" placebo controlled evaluation of a single drug or procedure in a homogeneous study group, cardiac rehabilitation research is concerned with the effects of multiple interventions on several outcomes in, by definition, a heterogeneous population. It is important that research on robust and valid ways of evaluating both the totality and components of rehabilitation should continue.

Summary

All MI patients should be offered access to cardiac rehabilitation. This will involve the systematic identification, assessment, treatment, monitoring and evaluation of patients. In order to facilitate this, organisations, facilities and equipment for a comprehensive service need to be developed. This will involve inter-agency collaboration, including hospital, community, voluntary and transport services.

As alluded to in an editorial in *Heart*,[19] the keys to improving cardiac rehabilitation are individual assessment, careful formulation of treatment, effective delivery, and systematic evaluation.

1. **Cooper A, Lloyd G, Weinman J,** *et al*. Why patients do not attend cardiac rehabilitation: role of intentions and illness beliefs. *Heart* 1999;**82**:234–6.

2. **Frasure-Smith N, Lesperance F, Talajic M.** Depression and 18-month prognosis after myocardial infarction. *Circulation* 1995;**91**:999–1005.

3. Petrie KJ, Weinman J, Sharpe N, *et al.* Role of patients' views of their illness in predicting return to work and functioning after myocardial infarction: longitudinal study. *BMJ* 1996;**312**:1191–4.

4. Billing E, Bar-On D, Rehnqvist N. Determinants of lifestyle changes after a first myocardial infarction. *Cardiology* 1997;**88**:29–35.

5. Maeland JG, Havik OE. Use of health services after a myocardial infarction. *Scand J Soc Med* 1989;**17**:93–102.

6. Thompson DR, Bowman GS, de Bono DP, *et al. Cardiac rehabilitation: guidelines and audit standards.* London: Royal College of Physicians, 1997.
• *UK national guidelines for cardiac rehabilitation endorsed by key organisations, including the Royal College of Physicians, the Royal College of Nursing, and the British Cardiac Society.*

7. World Health Organisation. *Needs and action priorities in cardiac rehabilitation and secondary prevention in patients with coronary heart disease.* Copenhagen: WHO, 1993.

8. Department of Health. *National service framework for coronary heart disease.* London: Department of Health, 2000.

9. Wenger NK, Froelicher ES, Smith LK, *et al. Cardiac rehabilitation. Clinical practice guideline No. 17.* Rockville, Maryland: Agency for Health Care Policy and Research and National Heart, Lung and Blood Institute, 1995.
• *A comprehensive and authoritative report based on critical reviews and syntheses of the literature on cardiac rehabilitation.*

10. Dinnes J, Kleijnen J, Leitner M, *et al.* Cardiac rehabilitation. *Quality Health Care* 1999;**8**:65–71.
• *A summary of an Effective Health Care bulletin on cardiac rehabilitation conducted by the NHS Centre for Reviews and Dissemination.*

11. Oldridge N, Furlong W, Feeny D, *et al.* Economic evaluation of cardiac rehabilitation soon after acute myocardial infarction. *Am J Cardiol* 1993;**72**:154–61.

12. Taylor R, Kirby B. The evidence base for the cost-effectiveness of cardiac rehabilitation. *Heart* 1997;**78**:5–6.

13. Lewin B, Robertson IH, Cay EL, *et al.* Effects of self-help post-myocardial infarction rehabilitation on psychological adjustment and use of health services. *Lancet* 1992;**339**:1036–40.

14. Lewin RJ, Ingleton R, Newens AJ, *et al.* Adherence to cardiac rehabilitation guidelines: a survey of cardiac rehabilitation programmes in the United Kingdom. *BMJ* 1998;**316**:1354–5.

15. Thompson DR, Bowman GS, Kitson AL, *et al.* Cardiac rehabilitation in the United Kingdom: guidelines and audit standards. *Heart* 1996;**75**:89–93.

16. American Association of Cardiovascular and Pulmonary Rehabilitation. *Guidelines for cardiac rehabilitation and secondary prevention programs*, 3rd ed. Champaign, Illinois: Human Kinetics, 1999.
• *Expanded and updated US guidelines with a focus on secondary prevention.*

17. Johnston M, Foulkes J, Johnston DW, *et al.* Impact on patients and partners of inpatient and extended cardiac counseling and rehabilitation: a controlled trial. *Psychosom Med* 1999;**61**:225–33.

18. West R. Rehabilitation. In: Pitt B, Julian D, Pocock S, eds. *Clinical trials in cardiology.* London: WB Saunders, 1997:355–78.

19. Thompson DR, de Bono DP. How valuable is cardiac rehabilitation and who should get it? [editorial] *Heart* 1999;**82**:545–6.

8 Intervention in coronary artery disease

Stephan Windecker, Bernhard Meier

Percutaneous transluminal coronary angioplasty (PTCA) was introduced into clinical practice more than 20 years ago.[1] The breathtaking growth of percutaneous coronary interventions (PCI) during the 1990s in Europe (fig 8.1) reflects their widespread acceptance for coronary revascularisation, challenging coronary artery bypass grafting (CABG). This review provides an overview of current coronary interventional techniques with emphasis on adjunctive pharmacologic treatments and indications of PCI in patients with chronic coronary artery disease.

Percutaneous coronary interventions

Balloon angioplasty

The balloon catheter is central not only to balloon angioplasty, but serves also as a complementary instrument for other intracoronary interventions such as delivery of stents or radiation sources. There are three types of balloon catheter (based on the relation between the guidewire and balloon)— fixed wire, over the wire, and Monorail balloon catheters—the latter being the most popular in Europe. There are five possible mechanism by which balloon angioplasty improves coronary haemodynamics[w1]: (1) plaque compression; (2) plaque fracture; (3) stretching of the plaque free wall segment in eccentric lesions; (4) stretching of the vessel wall without plaque compression; and (5) medial dissection (fig 8.2). The most important mechanisms for improved blood flow appears to be the rupture and dehiscence of the atherosclerotic plaque, resulting in numerous fissures and sprouting of blood filled channels. The individual procedural outcome is a combination of different degrees of the above mechanisms, and the final luminal geometry following balloon angioplasty is determined by the ensuing remodelling of the vessel wall.[w2–4]

Despite this crude mechanism of arterial dilatation the initial success rate of balloon angioplasty is > 90% in single lesions.[w5-7] The chief limitations to event free survival following balloon angioplasty have been abrupt vessel closure in the short term and restenosis in the long term.[2 w8] Abrupt vessel closure, defined as the sudden occlusion of the target vessel during or after angioplasty, has been reported in 4–8% of cases.[w9 w10] The pathophysiologic mechanisms underlying abrupt vessel closure are dissection (80% of cases), thrombus formation (20% of cases), and coronary artery spasm.[w11] Abrupt vessel closure becomes apparent in 75% of cases while still in the catheterisation laboratory, the remainder occurring within 24 hours of the procedure. Abrupt vessel closure has been associated with death in 0–8% and myocardial infarction (MI) in 11–54% of cases. In the past > 20% of patients suffering abrupt vessel closure were referred for emergency CABG.[w12] In the meantime coronary artery stents have become the method of choice in treating threatened or abrupt vessel closure, with success rates in excess of 90%.

Restenosis, defined as > 50% diameter stenosis at follow up angiography, has been the most important long term limitation of balloon angioplasty, with an incidence of 30–50% and need for target vessel revascularisation in 20–30% of patients.[w8] Most restenosis occurs during the first four months following balloon angioplasty, and patients who are free of restenosis at six months are considered to be at minimal further risk.

Today's paradigm of PCI is an aggressive approach to initial balloon angioplasty, so called optimal balloon angioplasty, to optimise luminal gain, with provisional stenting as a safety net for suboptimal balloon results (fig 8.2 and 8.3).[3] A stent like balloon angioplasty result, arbitrarily defined in BENESTENT I as a residual stenosis < 30%, resulted in a minimal mean (SD) luminal diameter of 1.84 (0.52) mm (stent group 1.82 (0.64) mm), a binary restenosis rate of 16% (stent group 22%) and a one year event free survival rate of 77% (stent group 77%).[w13] Similarly, patients in the DEBATE study undergoing balloon angioplasty, whose results were assessed physiologically by means of intracoronary Doppler flow velocity measurement, were found to have a favourable restenosis rate (16% v 41%, p = 0.002) and target lesion revascularisation rate (16% v 34%, p = 0.024), as well as freedom from recurrent symptoms or ischaemia (23% v 47%, p = 0.005) at six months follow up, if the coronary flow reserve was > 2.5 and the residual diameter stenosis < 35%.[w14]

A strategy of optimal balloon angioplasty with "provisional" stenting in case of early recoil was compared with coronary artery

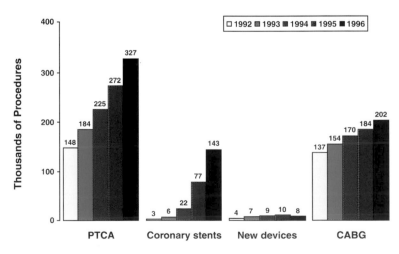

Figure 8.1. Development of cardiac interventions during the 1990s in Europe. Data are obtained from the coronary circulation working group of the European Society of Cardiology and represent more than 30 European countries with a population > 500 million people. Note the steady increase in the number of PTCAs, coronary stent, and CABG procedures, in contrast to new devices.

Percutaneous Coronary Intervention

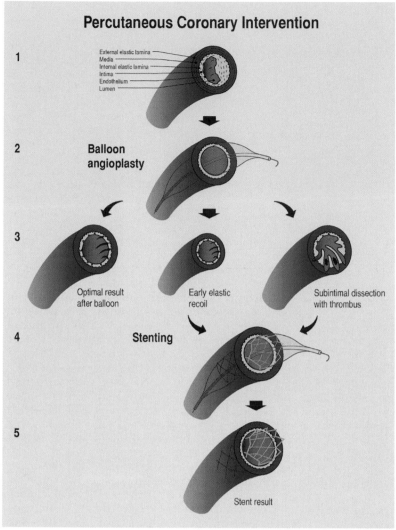

Figure 8.2. Schematic diagram of the primary mechanisms of balloon angioplasty and coronary artery stenting.

stent designs, including bifurcation and side branch stents, covered, coated, and radioactive stents, have been introduced. According to their design, coating, and composition stents differ with respect to radial force, flexibility, profile, trackability, radio-opacity, biocompatibility, thrombogenicity, and risk of in-stent restenosis. However, the basic principle underlying the therapeutic value of stents are independent of their design: increasing the arterial lumen by scoffolding the vessel wall; tagging of the intimal flaps between the stent surface and the vessel wall; and sealing of dissections.

Coronary artery stenting has been shown to be successful in > 95% of patients undergoing elective stent implantation in native vessels (single vessel and multivessel stenting) and saphenous vein grafts, and in > 90% of patients undergoing bailout stenting or stenting in the setting of acute MI.[3] Stenting has proved useful for two applications: (1) as a bailout device, reducing acute ischaemic complications of PTCA; and (2) as an anti-restenosis device reducing the need for reinterventions in the long term. Threatened or abrupt vessel closure is the best indication for coronary artery stenting, with a dramatic reduction in the immediate need for emergency CABG currently to < 1%, and an improved angiographic outcome with less residual stenosis and increased restoration of TIMI III flow. The impact on death and MI during bailout stenting is less well established.

Elective coronary artery stenting has been compared with balloon angioplasty in several randomised trials, and proved efficacious in: (1) prevention of restenosis in native coronary arteries with a diameter > 3.0 mm (BENESTENT I and II, STRESS I and II),[5][6][w19] especially in the case of isolated stenosis of the left anterior descending coronary artery[w20]; (2) treatment of restenosis after initial balloon angioplasty[w21]; (3) de novo lesions in saphenous vein grafts[w22]; (4) acute MI[w23]; and (5) chronic total occlusion.[w24–26] In the BENESTENT I

stenting in 116 patients in the OCBAS trial.[w15] After randomisation to PTCA, 14% of patients crossed over to stenting owing to early luminal loss. Although acute gain was significantly higher in patients implanted with coronary artery stents, there was no difference in net gain at six months between the two groups (1.32 (0.3) mm v 1.24 (0.29) mm for PTCA, p = ns). Furthermore, there was no difference in the angiographic restenosis rate (19% v 16% for PTCA, p = ns) and event free survival (81% v 83% for PTCA, p = ns). The percentage of patients in whom an optimal result can be achieved with balloon angioplasty alone is not known from controlled studies, but probably is around 30–50%.

Coronary artery stents

Coronary artery stents have become an important adjunct to conventional balloon angioplasty owing to their dual function of reducing acute complications and the long term risk of restenosis.[4][w16–18] Various classification schemes of coronary artery stents have been put forward, including: type of delivery system (self expanding, balloon expandable); type of basic structure (mesh, slotted tube, coil, ring, and multidesign); and composition (stainless steel, tantalum, nitinol). More recently additional

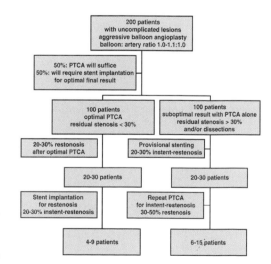

Figure 8.3. Flow diagram illustrating the concept of provisional stenting with random patient numbers. The use of coronary artery stents on a provisional basis is associated with an excellent long term outcome and a low restenosis rate at minimised cost.

Table 8.1 Coronary artery stents as antirestenosis devices—evidence from randomised trials and improved clinical outcome with changes in antithrombotic adjunctive treatment

End points	STRESS Stent (n=205)	PTCA (n=202)	BENESTENT I Stent (n=259)	PTCA (n=257)	BENESTENT II Stent + heparin coating (n=413)	PTCA (n=410)	EPISTENT Stent + abciximab (n=794)	Stent + placebo (n=809)
					% of patients			
Early events (< 30 days)								
Success	99.5	96.5*	–	–	96	95	–	–
Stent thrombosis	3.5	2.7	3.4	1.5	0.2	1.7	0	0.7
Death	0	1.5	0	0	0	0.2	0.3	0.6
MI	5.4	5.0	3.5	3.1	2.7	3.2	4.4	9.4
CABG	2.4	4.0	3.1	1.5	0.7	0.5	0.8	1.2
Vascular access site complications	7.3	4.0	13.5	3.1*	1.2	1.0	1.5†	2.2†
Hospital stay	5.8	2.8*	8.5	3.1*	2.8	2.3	–	–
Events up to 6 months								
Death	1.5	1.5	0.4	0.8	0.2	0.5	0.5	1.2
MI	6.3	6.9	4.3	4.7	3.2	3.6	5.2	10.3*
CABG	4.9	8.4	6.2	4.3	1.5	1.5	4.6	4.3
PCI	11.2	12.4	13.5	23.3*	8	13.7	7.5	9.3
Restenosis	31.6	42.1*	22	32*	16	31*	–	–
TVR	10.2	15.4	13.5	23*	9.2	13.8	8.7	10.6
Events up to 1 year								
Death	–	–	1.2	0.8	1.0	1.0	2.4	1.0*
MI	–	–	5.4	5.1	3.4	4.4	–	–
CABG	–	–	8.1	5.8	1.9	1.5	–	–
PCI	–	–	17.8	26.8*	9.4	15.6*	–	–

*p < 0.05; †defined as major bleeding (minor bleeding episodes were 2.9% for stent + abciximab and 1.7 for stent + placebo).

and STRESS I and II trials patients with discrete de novo lesions in vessels > 3.0 mm diameter were randomised to undergo balloon angioplasty or stent implantation using the Palmaz-Schatz stent. Both studies showed that stents resulted in: (1) higher clinical success rate (STRESS 99% *v* 96% for PTCA, p = 0.04); (2) reduced angiographic restenosis rate at six months (STRESS 30% *v* 46% for PTCA, p < 0.01; BENESTENT 22% *v* 32% for PTCA, p = 0.02); (3) reduced target lesion revascularisation rate (STRESS 10% *v* 15% for PTCA, p = 0.06; BENESTENT 14% *v* 23% for PTCA, p < 0.01); and (4) reduced clinical event rate at one year (BENESTENT 23% *v* 32% for PTCA, p = 0.04; STRESS 18% *v* 27% for PTCA, p < 0.01).[5 6]

Since its introduction stent implantation posed a risk for subacute stent thrombosis with its associated sequelae of MI and death. Two recent modifications have substantially reduced the incidence of subacute stent thrombosis: optimised stent deployment and full stent expansion with circumferential apposition to the vessel wall using routine high pressure (> 10–14 atm) stent inflation;[w27] and dual antiplatelet treatment with aspirin and ticlopidine or clopidogrel.[w28] Intravascular ultrasound assessment of coronary stent placement has not been conclusively shown to improve outcome and is largely omitted in clinical practice. Adoption of these principles led to current subacute stent thrombosis rates of < 2% under elective conditions (table 8.1), and a decrease in bleeding and vascular access site complications and length of hospitalisation to the same level as with conventional PTCA.

Although coronary artery stents serve as antirestenosis devices and reduce target vessel revascularisation requirements compared with balloon angioplasty, they can themselves become a source of in-stent restenosis in 20–30% of cases. While stents counteract pathologic arterial shrinkage of the vessel wall,

they may fail to prevent neointimal proliferation, which culminates in in-stent restenosis. Recently, Bauters and colleagues, studying 103 consecutive patients, reported a 98% procedural success rate with repeat PCI (versus 85% for PTCA) for treatment of in-stent restenosis, and 22% angiographic restenosis and 17% target lesion revascularisation rate at six months' follow up.[w29] However, diffuse in-stent restenosis was associated with significantly higher restenosis rates compared with focal in-stent restenosis (42% for diffuse versus 14% for focal, p < 0.006).

In contrast to PTCA or other devices such as atherectomy or laser angioplasty, coronary artery stenting requires deployment of a permanent prosthesis and therefore requires long term evaluation with respect to potential metal fatigue, stent migration, and inflammatory responses.[w30] Serial clinical and angiographic follow up over a three year period in 143 patients implanted with a Palmaz-Schatz stent revealed a favourable outcome with respect to death (9% at three years), MI (6% at

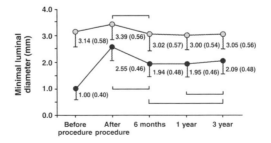

Figure 8.4. Serial changes in mean (SD) minimal luminal diameter of 72 lesions (blue circles) for which sequential studies over a three year period were completed, compared with a reference diameter (red circles). Note the significant improvement in mean minimal luminal diameter during the period from one year to three years after implantation of the stent; p < 0.001 for the comparison between the points linked by brackets. Reproduced from Kimura T et al[15] with permission of the Massachusetts Medical Society.

three years), and target lesion revascularisation (17% at three years).[7] Beside the expected initial loss of gain at six months of follow up owing to intimal proliferation, a late improvement in luminal diameter of the stented coronary artery segments at three years was observed, suggesting that restenosis was in fact prevented and not simply delayed after coronary stenting and indicating long term stabilisation of the lesion (fig 8.4).

Directional atherectomy

The principle of directional atherectomy (DCA) is removal of the atherosclerotic plaque by a rotating blade.[2] The DCA catheter consists of a soft tapered nose cone which serves as a waste basket for ablated tissue, a cylindrical metal housing which contains a coaxial rotating cup shaped blade, and a long flexible shaft for delivery. The metal housing has a window measuring between 9–16 mm on one side and a non-compliant balloon on the opposite side. Once the open window is positioned within the stenosis, the eccentrically positioned balloon is inflated at 2–3 atm for protrusion of the plaque into the cutting chamber. The cutter is connected via a drive cable to a motor outside the patient and rotates at approximately 2000 rpm. By advancing the cutter the plaque material is shaved off and deposited within the nose cone. The balloon is then deflated and the window of the metal housing reoriented by slight rotation; the cutting process is repeated several times to achieve circumferential tissue ablation. Many patients require adjunctive balloon angioplasty for a satisfactory angiographic result.

Complications associated with DCA are side branch occlusion (1–8%), perforation (1%), coronary vasospasm (2%), abrupt vessel closure (1–8%), and distal embolisation (0–13%). DCA has been compared with PTCA in four multicentre randomised trials in native vessels (CCAT, CAVEAT-I, BOAT)[w31–33] as well as saphenous vein grafts (CAVEAT II),[w34] and resulted in better immediate luminal gain and higher procedural success at similar major complication rates. However, the immediate angiographic success failed to translate into improved clinical outcome. While the BOAT trial was the only study to demonstrate a significant reduction in angiographic restenosis rate,[w33] the need for target lesion revascularisation and event free survival at six months and one year were similar between DCA and PTCA in all studies. Disconcertingly, patients in the CAVEAT trial treated by DCA were found to have higher rates of release of creatinine kinase CK-MB after the procedure (19% v 8% for PTCA), a higher one year mortality rate (2.2% v 0.6% for PTCA, p < 0.05), and a higher incidence of MI (7.6% v 4.4% for PTCA; p < 0.01).[w32] Developed initially to reduce restenosis and to treat high grade lesions in the proximal coronary artery tree, DCA has been superceded by the more effective and easier to use coronary artery stent. Owing to DCA's unique feature of actually removing plaque material, its only indication may be the complex bifurcation lesion with plaque shifting not suited for stent implantation.

Rotational atherectomy

Rotational atherectomy is based on the concept of debulking an atherosclerotic plaque by drilling.[2] The rotablator catheter consists of an elliptical burr coated with 20–50 μm diamond microparticles welded to a metal drive shaft which tracks along a central coaxial 0.009 inch guidewire. The drive shaft is connected to an air turbine which generates between 160 000 and 200 000 rpm. The operator controls the speed of rotation and advancement through the atherosclerotic plaque. Multiple passes of the rotablator are typically done with an initial burr-to-artery ratio of 0.5–0.6:1.0 followed by a second larger burr with a 0.75–0.8:1.0 burr-to-artery ratio. Since typically the burr size is only 80% of the vessel reference diameter the residual stenosis is usually treated with adjunctive PTCA. Rotational atherectomy by means of its high speed spinning burr features differential cutting. While the healthy, elastic arterial wall deflects beneath the spinning burr, hard, calcified and non-elastic atherosclerotic plaque should be selectively ablated. The size of the microparticles generated during rotational atherectomy is usually < 5 μm and the amount of microparticles is too small to result in impairment of blood flow.[w35] Complications intrinsic to the rotablator are a potential for heat injury, "slow or no reflow" owing to embolisation of large microparticles or microcavitation bubbles (1.8–6.1%),[w36] [w37] large dissections (10–13%),[w38] and perforation (0–1.5%).

Acute procedural success has been high (90–99%) even in high risk lesions. Rotablation proved superior to PTCA (procedural success 89% v 80% for PTCA, p < 0.05; MACE 3.2% v 3.1%, p = ns) in the ERBAC trial,[8] a randomised comparison of rotablation and PTCA in complex lesions (American Heart Association/American College of Cardiology type B and C). However, rotablation failed to improve six month angiographic restenosis rates (57% v 47% for PTCA, p = 0.14), and both target lesion revascularisation (42% v 32% for PTCA, p = 0.013) and ischaemic

Table 8.2 Results of the ERBAC trial, a randomised comparison between balloon angioplasty, rotational atherectomy, and excimer laser angioplasty

	PTCA	ELCA	PTRA
Early complications (%)	n=222	n=232	n=231
Death	0.9	0.9	0.9
CABG	0.5	2.2	0.9
MI	3.5	3.9	3.5
Q wave MI	1.8	1.3	1.3
Non-Q wave MI	1.7	2.6	2.2
Bailout stenting	3.6	3.0	1.7
Non-surgical reintervention	3.6	3.0	1.7
Results at one year follow up (%)	n=191	n=211	n=205
Death	3.7	1.9	2.4
Q wave MI	2.6	2.4	2.4
CABG	6.3	7.1	7.3
Non-surgical reintervention	27.2	40.3*	36.6*
Target vessel revascularisation	31.9	46.0*	42.4*
Any event	36.6	47.9*	45.9*

ELCA, excimer laser coronary angioplasty; PTRA, percutaneous transluminal rotational atherectomy *p < 0.05

complications (46% *v* 37% for PTCA, p = 0.04) were more frequent in patients undergoing rotablation (table 8.2). Rotational atherectomy may still be of value in the treatment of heavily calcified, non-dilatable lesions. However, in long, calcified lesions the advantage of rotational atherectomy levels off and comes at a price of increased complications.

Contraindications for the use of rotational atherectomy are thrombus containing lesions, degenerated saphenous vein grafts, and lesions $\geqslant$ 25 mm.

Laser angioplasty

Excimer laser coronary angioplasty (ELCA) is the most thoroughly investigated laser technology applied to coronary interventions. It uses a high intensity, short duration (100–200 ns) pulsed wave ultraviolet light (308 nm) generated in a xenon chloride medium with a penetration depth of 100 μm.[w39] The ultraviolet light is transmitted via a fibreoptic bundle arranged around the central lumen of a polyethylene catheter which is available as an over the wire or Monorail system. The laser catheter is advanced over the coronary guidewire to the lesion, and laser energy is applied as the catheter is advanced through the plaque. Excimer laser energy ablates tissue by a combination of three mechanisms[w40]: (1) photomechanical energy resulting in acoustic shockwaves as the principal modus of luminal gain [w41–43]; (2) photothermal energy which vapourises tissue[w44 w45]; and (3) photochemical energy which is able to break directly the intramolecular bonds.[w46] To achieve an optimal final result adjunctive balloon angioplasty is required in almost all cases (> 95%).

ELCA has been compared with PTCA in the ERBAC trial.[8] There was no difference between PTCA and laser angioplasty with respect to procedural success (77% *v* 80% for PTCA, p = ns) and major in-hospital complications (4.3% *v* 3.1% for PTCA, p = ns). However, at six months' follow up the angiographic restenosis rate (59% *v* 47% for PTCA, p = 0.04), target lesion revascularisation rate (46% *v* 32% for PTCA, p = 0.01), and late ischaemic events (48% *v* 37% for PTCA, p = 0.02) were significantly more frequent in patients treated with laser angioplasty (table 2).

Complications associated with excimer laser angioplasty are perforations (1–3%) and a high incidence of dissections (13–21%) caused by the formation of intravascular vapour bubbles. The only indication where laser angioplasty may prove of some value is for revascularisation of chronic total occlusions with a laser guidewire. In the randomised TOTAL trial the excimer laser wire increased the initial success rate from around 50% to 60%.[w47] However, this effect was largely confined to crossover cases, and conventional guidewires but not specific recanalisation systems or newer generation hydrophilic wires were assessed.

Adjunctive pharmacologic treatment

The therapeutic effect of arterial vessel enlargement through PCI is accompanied by various degrees of arterial injury with exposure of thrombogenic components. Depending on the degree of activation of the coagulation cascade, as well as platelet adhesion and aggregation, this may result in intracoronary thrombus formation and subsequent ischaemic sequelae. Therefore, inhibition of platelets and the coagulation system has always been central to interventional investigations.

Anticoagulants during PCI
Heparin

Unfractionated heparin is a glycosaminoglycan mixture composed of variable length polysaccharides with molecular weights ranging from 3000 to 50 000 daltons.[w48] Heparin exerts its anticoagulant effect by formation of the heparin-antithrombin III complex, which inhibits thrombin and activated factors IX, X, XI, and XII. Although there is general agreement that patients undergoing PCI should receive heparin before the intervention, controversy surrounds the issue of optimal heparin dosage and the need for prolonged heparin infusion following PCI. Narins and colleagues observed an inverse relation between the level of anticoagulation (measured by activated clotting time (ACT)) and the occurrence of acute ischaemic complications,[w49] and the recommended adequate threshold for anticoagulation is arbitrarily set at an ACT of > 300 seconds. This contrasts with several randomised and open prospective studies which established data on the safety and efficacy of routine low dose heparin (5000 IE) in patients undergoing PCI independent of the level of ACT,[w50–52] and failed to demonstrate an additional benefit of continuous heparin infusion after PCI in low risk patients.[w51 w53] Without increasing the risk for ischaemic complications, the approach of routine low dose heparin during PCI offers the advantages of a lower incidence of bleeding complications, faster sheath removal, and shorter hospitalisation. In addition it does not preclude the administration of unplanned, adjunctive glycoprotein IIb/IIIa receptor inhibitors, which would be preferable in case of ischaemic complications.

Low molecular weight heparins, obtained by chemical or enzymatic depolymerisation of the polysaccharide chains of unfractionated heparin, have a better bioavailability, result in more reproducible anticoagulation without need of monitoring, and induce less platelet activation compared with unfractionated heparins.[w54] The REDUCE trial, a restenosis study, randomly compared intravenous administration of the low molecular weight heparin reviparin with unfractionated heparin during PCI and revealed a significant reduction in early major ischaemic events (first three days) in favour of reviparin (reviparin 4% *v* heparin 8%, p = 0.03), but no long term clinical or angiographic benefit at six months of follow

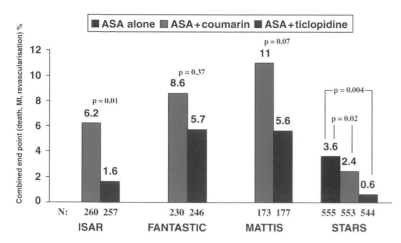

Figure 8.5. Summary of results of four randomised coronary artery stent thromboprophylaxis trials. Dual antiplatelet treatment with aspirin and ticlopidine was superior to oral anticoagulation and aspirin treatment in the prevention of major adverse cardiac events in all trials. In the STARS trial dual antiplatelet treatment was superior to aspirin alone.

up.[w55] The role of low molecular weight heparins in the prevention of bleeding and ischaemic complications during PTCA and coronary stenting is currently under investigation, and these agents may replace unfractionated heparin as they have for other indications.

Direct thrombin inhibitors
In contrast to heparin direct thrombin inhibitors such as hirudin, hirulog, argatroban, and others do not require antithrombin III as a cofactor, and inhibit both circulating and clot bound thrombin. Three randomised trials with over 6700 patients compared the efficacy of unfractionated heparin with hirudin (HELVETICA, GUSTO IIb)[w56 w57] and hirulog (Hirulog angioplasty study)[w58] during PCI. Patients receiving direct thrombin inhibitors had a lower incidence of bleeding complications; however, the therapeutic benefit was modest at best with a reduction in ischaemic complications limited to subgroups and acute events only. In light of these results and the availability of more potent glycoprotein IIb/IIIa receptor antagonists, the role of direct thrombin inhibitors will probably be reserved for patients with adverse reactions to heparin, for example, heparin induced thrombocytopenia.

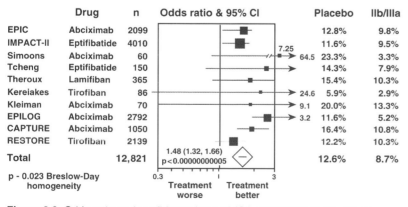

Figure 8.6. Odds ratio and confidence interval (CI) concerning death, MI, or additional coronary revascularisation at 30 days with glycoprotein IIb/IIIa receptor antagonists compared with placebo. Reproduced with permission from Meier B. Balloon angioplasty. In: Topol EJ, ed. Comprehensive cardiovascular medicine. Philadelphia: Lippincott-Raven, 1998:2251–84.

Vitamin K antagonists
Coumarin derivatives were administered in conjunction with full dose heparin, aspirin, and dipyridamole as thromboprophylaxis early in the coronary stent era. However, subsequent clinical trials established the superiority of a dual antiplatelet treatment over oral anticoagulants in preventing both cardiac events and bleeding complications after coronary artery stenting.[9 w28 w59 w60] This clinical benefit, coupled with the salutary effects of shorter hospitalisation time, reduced cost, and simplification of the pharmacological regimen, no longer support the use of oral anticoagulants after stent implantation.

Antiplatelet agents during PCI
Aspirin
The beneficial effect of aspirin during PCI has been shown in the Montreal heart study, in which treatment with aspirin and dipyridamole was superior to placebo in the prevention of periprocedural Q wave MI (aspirin and dipyridamole 2% v placebo 7%, p = 0.01).[w61] Dipyridamole has not been found to provide an additional benefit over aspirin alone in subsequent studies.[w62] Low dose aspirin (75–325 mg per day) is recommended in patients undergoing PCI, ideally administered at least one day before the procedure and continued indefinitely thereafter.

Thienopyridines
Ticlopidine and clopidogrel are thienopyridine derivatives which inhibit platelet function independent of aspirin by interference with the platelet ADP receptor.[w63] The interest in dual antiplatelet treatment with aspirin and ticlopidine in patients undergoing coronary stent implantation stemmed from the pathophysiological understanding that stent thrombosis was predominantly mediated by platelets rather than abnormalities of coagulation activation.[w64] Furthermore, intensive anticoagulation after stent placement was complicated by excessive vascular access site problems, prolonged hospitalisation, and increased cost, seriously limiting the benefits of coronary artery stents. Several randomised clinical trials assessed the efficacy of dual antiplatelet treatment with aspirin and ticlopidine compared with aspirin alone and aspirin-anticoagulant treatment after coronary stent implantation in low (STARS),[9] intermediate (ISAR, FANTASTIC),[w60 w65] and high risk (MATTIS)[w59] patient populations (fig 8.5). These trials showed that: (1) dual antiplatelet treatment with aspirin and ticlopidine is superior to both aspirin monotherapy and a combination of aspirin and oral anticoagulation in the prevention of stent thrombosis; (2) rates of bleeding and vascular complications are less frequent; and (3) hospitalisation duration is shorter with antiplatetet compared with anticoagulant treatment.

Moussa and colleagues[w66] recently compared the safety and efficacy of ticlopidine with clopidogrel in a longitudinal uncontrolled study, and found no difference in rates of stent thrombosis or major adverse cardiac events at one month follow up. In the CLASSICS trial clopidogrel with and without a loading dose was compared with ticlopidine in patients undergoing coronary stenting. The findings of the study at 28 days of follow up were: (1) a superior safety profile of clopidogrel with a significantly reduced combined end point of major bleeding complications, neutropenia, and thrombocytopenia (ticlopidine 9% v clopidogrel 5%, p = 0.005); (2) a well tolerated loading dose of clopidogrel without increased bleeding complications; and (3) a comparable efficacy with respect to major adverse cardiac events. Therefore, it is anticipated that clopidogrel will replace ticlopidine as the thienopyridine of choice.

Glycoprotein IIb/IIIa inhibitors

While platelets may be activated by numerous agonists, platelet aggregation, the prerequisite for thrombus formation, has one final common pathway mediated by the platelet glycoprotein IIb/IIIa receptor, a member of the integrin family. Therefore, inhibition of the glycoprotein IIb/IIIa receptor appealed as the therapeutic target in the prevention of largely platelet mediated ischaemic complications during PCI. Several randomised trials have assessed the role of glycoprotein IIb/IIIa receptor antagonists during coronary interventions, including the monoclonal antibody abciximab (EPIC, EPILOG, EPISTENT, CAPTURE, RAPPORT),[10] [w67-70] the peptide molecule eptifibatide (IMPACT II),[w71] and the non-peptide molecule tirofiban (RESTORE)[w72] in over 15 000 patients with clinical presentations ranging from stable coronary artery disease to unstable angina pectoris and acute MI. All trials consistently demonstrated benefits in the reduction of early death, non-fatal MI, and urgent revascularisation (fig 8.6).[11] While this effect was maintained in patients receiving abciximab during long term follow up, the benefits have not been durable with tirofiban and eptifibatide. Specifically, abciximab is the only glycoprotein IIb/IIIa receptor antagonist reported to reduce mortality significantly in a subgroup of patients in the EPIC trial admitted with an acute coronary syndrome (three year mortality reduction 60%, p = 0.01),[w73] and more recently in the EPISTENT trial (one year mortality reduction of 50%, p = 0.04).[12] In summary glycoprotein IIb/IIIa receptor antagonists administered during PCI appear to: (1) reduce the incidence of death or non-fatal MI complicating PCI (in case of abciximab); (2) reduce the need for bailout stenting during PCI; (3) provide benefit in all patient subgroups, and (4) do not result in excessive bleeding complications if weight adjusted lower doses of heparin are adhered to.

Indications for PCI in chronic coronary artery disease

The indications for PCI have expanded during the past two decades, and no absolute contraindications remain (table 8.3). Single vessel coronary artery disease (CAD) remains the principal indication for PCI, with over 80%[w74] of procedures performed in Europe and over 90% in the USA. This exponential growth of PCI has been largely at the expense of medical treatment rather than surgical revascularisation. Beside clinical and angiographic factors, operator volume has been recognised as a major determinant of outcome in several recent studies.[w75-78] There is no upper patient age limit to the applicability of PCI; however, the threshold is shifted in favour of PCI compared with CABG in the very elderly owing to the higher perioperative morbidity and mortality in this patient population. Initial concerns of a sex difference in the outcome of PCI with women,

Table 8.3   *Indications and contraindications for PCI*

Clinical indications	Angiographic indications

Angina pectoris
  –de novo angina pectoris
  –stable angina pectoris
  –unstable angina pectoris
  –recurrent angina pectoris
  –after PCI (restenosis)
  –after CABG (graft attrition)
	1–4 lesions amenable to PCI
	  –not immediately life threatening
	  –vessel diameter ≥2.5 mm
	  –lesion(s) subtending function, viable,
	    or collateral dependent myocardium

Angina equivalent
  –arrhythmias, sudden death survivors
  –dyspnoea
  –dizziness
	Angiographic contraindications (relative)
	Left main stenosis (exceptions: protected
	  by graft or collaterals, ideal lesion,
	  inoperable patient\)

Myocardial infarction
  –acute myocardial infarction (primary PCI)
  –postinfarct angina pectoris
  –rescue PTCA (failed thrombolysis, cardiogenic
    shock)
	Left main equivalent stenoses
	  (exceptions: staged procedure, ideal
	  lesions, inoperable patient)

Objective signs of reversible ischaemia
  –resting ECG
  –exercise induced ischaemia
	Lesion characteristics
	  Chronic total occlusion
	    –no collaterals to distal artery
	    –long and old
	    –no stump
	    –extensive bridging collaterals

Clinical contraindications
  –rapidly terminal cardiac or other systemic
    disease
	Thrombotic stenosis with
	  non-significant underlying lesions
	Diffusely diseased, small calibre native
	  coronary artery
	Diffusely diseased old venous vein graft

Table 8.4   *Randomised comparison of medical treatment with PCI in patients with stable CAD*

End points	ACME (6 months follow up)		RITA-2 (32 months follow up)		AVERT (18 months follow up)	
	Medical treatment (antianginals) (n=107)	PCI (PTCA) (n=105)	Medical treatment (antianginals) (n=514)	PCI (PTCA) (n=504)	Medical treatment (atorvastatin) (n=164)	PCI (PTCA, stent) (n=177)
			% of patients			
Death	0.9	0	1.4	2.2	0.6	0.6
MI	2.8	4.8	1.9	4.1	2.4	2.8
Death or MI	3.7	4.8	3.3	6.3†	3.0	3.4
Angina						
Free	53.9	36.5**	–	–	–	–
Improved	–	–	–	–‡	41	54*
CABG	0	7**	5.8	7.9	1.2	5.1
PTCA	9	16	17.1	11.1	11.0	11.9
Repeat hospitalisation	–	–	–	–	6.7	14.1

*p < 0.05; †p < 0.02; **p < 0.01; ‡17% excess of grade 2+ angina in the medical group 3 months after randomisation.

Table 8.5   Randomised comparison of CABG with PCI

End points	Lausanne (proximal LAD, follow up 5 years)		SIMA (proximal LAD, follow up 2.4 years)		BARI (multivessel CAD follow up 5 years)		ARTS (multivessel CAD follow up 1 year)	
	CABG (n=66)	PTCA (n=68)	CABG (n=54)	Stent (n=67)	CABG (n=914)	PTCA (n=915)	CABG (n=605)	Stent (n=600)
				% of patients				
Death	3	9	–	–	10.7	13.7	2.8	2.5
Q wave MI	6	3	–	–	–	–	4.0	5.3
Death or MI	9	12	7	7	19.6	22.3	6.8	7.8
CABG	0	5	–	–	1	31	0.5	4.7
PCI	9	33	–	–	7	23	3	12.2
CABG or PTCA	9	38*	0	21.0*	8.0	54.0*	3.5*	17.0*

*p < 0.05.
There are no differences in death or myocardial infarction between patients undergoing PCI compared with CABG. Patients undergoing PCI have to undergo significantly more often a second revascularisation procedure than their surgical counterparts. Note the decrease in repeat revascularisation between patients undergoing only PTCA (Lausanne study, BARI) compared with coronary artery stenting (SIMA, ARTS) by approximately one half.

felt to be at higher risk for acute ischaemic complications, did not find confirmation in more recent registries and clinical trials. While acute thrombotic coronary occlusion, even of the left main stem, represents no major hurdle for performing PCI, chronic total occlusion is the single most important reason not to attempt PCI. The following comparison of PCI with alternative treatments is limited to patients with chronic coronary artery disease.

PCI versus medical treatment

PCI has been compared with medical treatment in patients with CAD in several randomised clinical trials (table 8.4). In the ACME trial[13] involving patients with symptomatic single vessel CAD, the group allocated to PTCA had earlier and more complete relief of angina and better exercise performance during follow up. However, patients undergoing PTCA had an increased risk of undergoing emergency CABG because of procedural complications, although there were no differences with respect to death and infarction. Similar findings were reported in the RITA-2 trial[14] comparing PTCA with medical treatment in symptomatic patients with single and double

vessel disease. Patients undergoing PTCA featured greater relief of angina and better exercise performance at an increased risk of death and MI (6% PTCA group *v* 3% medically treated group, p = 0.02), largely because of enzyme elevations at the time of the procedure.

In the recently reported AVERT trial a strategy of aggressive lipid lowering treatment with atorvastatin was compared with PCI in minimally symptomatic (Canadian Cardiovascular Society class I–II), mostly single vessel CAD patients.[w79] There was a non-significant trend towards a reduction in the composite end point of death, MI, revascularisation, and worsening angina in patients allocated to atorvastatin (13% atorvastatin group *v* 21% PCI group, p = ns), but the differences in favour of atorvastatin treatment were exclusively limited to a decreased revascularisation and rehospitalisation rate. As in previous trials patients undergoing PCI in AVERT had significantly improved symptoms compared with medically treated patients, and one wonders why the interventionally treated patients had adequate cholesterol control withheld despite established evidence of their beneficial effect in secondary prevention. All the above studies comparing PCI with medical treatment do not reflect current practice of interventional cardiology with widespread utilisation of coronary stents and glycoprotein IIb/IIIa inhibitors, which contributed significantly to a decrease in major adverse cardiac events and target vessel revascularisation. In summary, PTCA effectively relieves symptoms and improves exercise performance at the cost of a small incidence of MI and a need for reinterventions because of restenosis in patients with single vessel CAD.

PCI versus bypass surgery

PTCA has been compared with left internal mammary artery (LIMA) grafting in 134 patients with isolated proximal left anterior descending artery (LAD) stenosis in the randomised Lausanne study (table 8.5).[w80] At five years of follow up there were no differences between patients allocated to PTCA and LIMA grafting with respect to death, Q wave MI, functional status, and antianginal drug treatment. However, patients allocated to PTCA had more frequent non-Q wave infarction related to abrupt closure or unstable angina related to restenosis, and required addi-

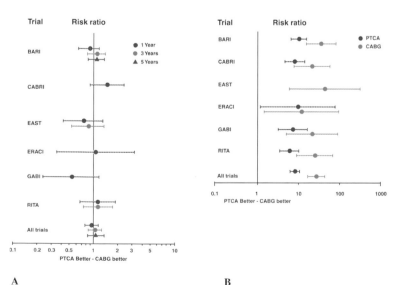

A   **B**

Figure 8.7. (A) Risk ratio and 95% confidence intervals for death or MI after CABG or PTCA for multivessel CAD at one, three, and five years in six randomised trials. (B) Risk ratio and 95% confidence intervals for reintervention after an initial strategy of CABG or PTCA for multivessel CAD at one year of follow up in six randomised trials. Reproduced with permission from Meier B. Balloon angioplasty. In: Topol EJ, ed. Comprehensive cardiovascular medicine. Philadelphia: Lippincott-Raven, 1998:2251–84.

tional revascularisation procedures more often compared with surgically revascularised patients. The same investigators initiated a randomised trial in 123 patients with isolated proximal LAD stenosis comparing coronary stenting with LIMA grafting. There were no differences in the incidence of in-hospital death and MI, with low rates in both groups. During follow up the combined end point of death and MI was equal; however, 21% of stented patients required additional revascularisation compared with no patients in the surgical group.

Several randomised trials compared PTCA with CABG in patients with multivessel CAD.[15 16 w81-85] The results of these trials have been remarkably consistent (fig 8.7) and revealed that an initial strategy of PTCA and CABG in selected patients with multivessel CAD results in: (1) similar survival and freedom from MI 1–7 years after the procedure; (2) a better relief of angina in CABG patients at least during the first year after the intervention; (3) an increased need for further coronary interventions in patients allocated to PTCA mostly during the first year after the intervention; and (4) similar long term costs during a follow up period of 5–8 years. An important issue raised in the BARI trial[56] was that the subgroup of treated diabetic patients had significantly better survival rates with CABG (66% PTCA v 81% CABG, p = 0.003).

The advent of coronary stents has significantly reduced the need for target lesion revascularisation and therefore trials have been initiated comparing stent supported PTCA with CABG in patients with multivessel CAD (ARTS, SOS, ERACI-II). The one year follow up results of ARTS have recently been reported (P Serruys, European Society of Cardiology, Barcelona, 1999) and revealed: (1) a similar incidence of death, MI and stroke; (2) an increased need for additional revascularisation procedures in patients initially treated by coronary stenting, and (3) a cost saving of 4278 Euros during the initial hospitalisation and of 2965 Euros at one year follow up in favour of coronary stenting. The most important finding of ARTS is the reduction by more than half in the need for additional revascularisation procedures in patients undergoing coronary stenting (17%) as compared with the previous PTCA/CABG trials featuring revascularisation rates of 30–40% at one year follow up, confirming the hypothesis that stents improve long term outcome (table 8.5). An even further improvement of PCI can be predicted by the addition of glycoprotein IIb/IIIa inhibitors to coronary stenting as indicated by the complementary benefit of abciximab and coronary stenting in the EPISTENT trial[12] (table 8.1). Compared with coronary stenting alone, the addition of abciximab resulted in improved survival at one year follow up (2.4% stent alone v 1.0% stent plus abciximab, p = 0.04) and an 18% reduction in target vessel revascularisation (10.6% stent alone v 8.7% stent plus abciximab, p = 0.2), which became significant in diabetic

patients (16.6% stent alone v 8.1% stent plus abciximab, p = 0.02).

In summary, since there are no major differences in prognosis between the two treatment modalities, in non-diabetic patients with multivessel disease and maintained left ventricular function amenable to both PCI and CABG, the choice of revascularisation method rests on weighing the more invasive nature of CABG against the increased need of additional revascularisation after PCI.

1. **Grüntzig AR, Senning Å, Siegenthaler WE.** Nonoperative dilatation of coronary-artery stenosis. Percutaneous transluminal coronary angioplasty. *N Engl J Med* 1979;**301**:61–8.
• *Original paper by Andreas Grüntzig introducing balloon angioplasty into clinical practice.*

2. **Bittl JA.** Advances in coronary angioplasty. *N Engl J Med* 1996;**335**:1290–302
• *Recent comprehensive review about percutaneous coronary interventions, adjunctive pharmacologic treatment and comparison with medical and surgical treatment in patients with coronary artery disease.*

Trial acronyms

ACME: Angioplasty Compared with Medicine

ARTS: Arterial Revascularisation Therapy Study

AVERT: Atorvastatin Versus Revascularization Treatment Investigators

BARI: Bypass Angioplasty Revascularization Investigation

BENESTENT: Belgium-Netherlands Stent Study

BOAT: Balloon versus Optimal Atherectomy Trial

CAPTURE: Chimeric 7E3 Anti-Platelet in Unstable Angina Refractory to Standard Treatment Trial

CAVEAT: Coronary Angioplasty Versus Excisional Atherectomy Trial

CLASSICS: CLopidogrel plus Aspirin Stent International Cooperative Study

DEBATE: Doppler Endpoints Balloon Angioplasty Trial Europe

EPIC: Evaluation of IIb/IIIa platelet receptor antagonist 7E3 in Preventing Ischemic Complications trial

EPILOG: Evaluation of PTCA to Improve Long-term Outcome by c7E3 GP IIb/IIIa receptor blockade trial

EPISTENT: Evaluation of Platelet GP IIb/IIIa Inhibitor for Stenting

ERBAC: Excimer laser, Rotational atherectomy, and Balloon Angioplasty Comparison Study

FANTASTIC: Full Anticoagulation Versus Ticlopidine plus Aspirin After Stent Implantation Trial

GUSTO: Global Use of Strategies To Open Occluded Coronary Arteries

HELVETICA: Hirudin in a European Trial Versus Heparin in the Prevention of Restenosis After PTCA

IMPACT: Integrilin to Manage Platelet Aggregation to Combat Thrombosis Trial

ISAR: Intracoronary Stenting and Antithrombotic Regimen Trial

MATTIS: Multicenter Aspirin and Ticlopidine After Intracoronary Stenting Trial

OCBAS: Optimal Coronary Balloon Angioplasty with Provisional Stenting versus Stent Trial

RAPPORT: Reo Pro and Primary PTCA Organisation and Randomized Trial

REDUCE: Reduction of Restenosis After PTCA, Early Administration of Reviparin in a Double-blind, Unfractionated Heparin and Placebo Controlled Evaluation

RESTORE: Randomised Efficacy Study of Tirofiban for Outcomes and Restenosis Trial

RITA: Randomised Intervention Treatment of Angina Trial

SOS: Stent Or Surgery trial

STARS: Stent Anticoagulation Regimen Study

STRESS: Stent Restenosis Study

3. **Narins CR, Holmes DR Jr, Topol EJ.** A call for provisional stenting: the balloon is back! *Circulation* 1998;**97**:1298–305.
  • *Excellent summary of the state of contemporary percutaneous coronary interventions and description of the concept of provisional stenting.*

4. **Goy JJ, Eeckhout E.** Intracoronary stenting. *Lancet* 1998;**351**:1943–9.
  • *Recent review of the coronary artery stents with focus on established evidence from clinical trials.*

5. **Serruys PW, De Jaegere P, Kiemeneij F,** *et al.* A comparison of balloon-expandable-stent implantation with balloon angioplasty in patients with coronary artery disease. *N Engl J Med* 1994;**331**:489–95.

6. **Fischman DL, Leon MB, Baim DS,** *et al.* A randomized comparison of coronary-stent placement and balloon angioplasty in the treatment of coronary artery disease. *N Engl J Med* 1994;**331**:496–501.

7. **Kimura T, Yokoi H, Nakagawa Y,** *et al.* Three-year follow-up after implantation of metallic coronary-artery stents. *N Engl J Med* 1996;**334**:561–6.

8. **Reifart N, Vandormael M, Krajcar M,** *et al.* Randomized comparison of angioplasty of complex coronary lesions at a single center. Excimer laser, rotational atherectomy, and balloon angioplasty comparison (ERBAC) study. *Circulation* 1997;**96**:91–8.

9. **Leon MB, Baim DS, Popma JJ,** *et al.* A clinical trial comparing three antithrombotic-drug regimens after coronary-artery stenting. Stent anticoagulation restenosis study investigators. *N Engl J Med* 1998;**339**:1665–71.

10. **EPILOG Investigators.** Platelet glycoprotein IIb/IIIa receptor blockade and low-dose heparin during percutaneous coronary revascularization. The EPILOG investigators. *N Engl J Med* 1997;**336**:1689–96.

11. **Topol EJ, Serruys PW.** Frontiers in interventional cardiology. *Circulation* 1998;**98**:1802–20
  • *Review article dealing with PCI and special emphasis on coronary artery stents, adjunctive pharmacologic therapy and future perspectives.*

12. **Lincoff AM, Califf RM, Moliterno DJ,** *et al.* Complementary clinical benefits of coronary-artery stenting and blockade of platelet glycoprotein IIb/IIIa receptors. Evaluation of platelet IIb/IIIa inhibition in stenting investigators. *N Engl J Med* 1999;**341**:319–27.

13. **Parisi AF, Folland ED, Hartigan P.** A comparison of angioplasty with medical therapy in the treatment of single-vessel coronary artery disease. *N Engl J Med* 1992;**326**:10–16.

14. **RITA-2 Trial Participants.** Coronary angioplasty versus medical therapy for angina: the second randomised intervention treatment of angina (RITA-2) trial. RITA-2 trial participants. *Lancet* 1997;**350**:461–8.

15. **Pocock SJ, Henderson RA, Rickards AF,** *et al.* Meta-analysis of randomised trials comparing coronary angioplasty with bypass surgery. *Lancet* 1995;**346**:1184–9.

16. **BARI Investigators.** Comparison of coronary bypass surgery with angioplasty in patients with multivessel disease. The bypass angioplasty revascularization investigation (BARI) investigators. *N Engl J Med* 1996;**335**:217–25.

53

website
extra

Additional references appear on the Heart website

www.heartjnl.com

SECTION II: HEART FAILURE

9 Epidemiology, aetiology, and prognosis of heart failure

John J McMurray, Simon Stewart

Heart failure is now recognised as a major and escalating public health problem in industrialised countries with ageing populations. Any attempt to describe the epidemiology, aetiology, and prognosis of heart failure, however, must take account of the difficulty in defining exactly what heart failure is. Though the focus of this article is the symptomatic syndrome it must be remembered that as many patients again may have asymptomatic disease that might be legitimately labelled "heart failure"—for example, asymptomatic left ventricular systolic dysfunction. More comprehensive reviews of the epidemiology and associated burden of heart failure have been published by McMurray and colleagues[1] and more recently by Cowie and colleagues.[2]

Data relating to the aetiology, epidemiology and prognostic implications of heart failure are principally available from five types of studies:

- Cross sectional and longitudinal follow up surveys of well defined populations. These have almost exclusively focused on those individuals with clinical signs and symptoms indicative of chronic heart failure.
- Cross sectional surveys of individuals who have been medically treated for signs and symptoms of heart failure within a well defined region.
- Echocardiographic surveys of individuals within a well defined population to determine the presence of left ventricular systolic dysfunction.
- Nation wide studies of annual trends in heart failure related hospitalisation identified on the basis of diagnostic coding at discharge.
- Comprehensive clinical registries collected in conjunction with clinical trials. These include a large proportion of individuals who were identified on the basis of having both impaired left ventricular systolic dysfunction and signs and symptoms of heart failure.

Within the context of the specific limitations of the type of data available from these studies, the current understanding of the aetiology, epidemiology, and prognostic implications of chronic heart failure are discussed here.

Epidemiology of heart failure

Prevalence

Table 9.1 summarises the reported prevalence of heart failure according to whether this was estimated from a survey of individuals requiring medical treatment from a general practitioner or from population screening. Despite the wide variation in the reported prevalence of heart failure (undoubtedly caused by differing research methods, in addition to inherent differences in the sociodemographic and risk factor profiles of study cohorts), overall these data demonstrate that the prevalence of clinically overt heart failure increases considerably with age. These data also suggest that the prevalence of heart failure has increased over the past few decades.

Studies of patients visiting a general practitioner
There have been several large studies examining the number of patients being treated for signs and symptoms of chronic heart failure by a general practitioner, undertaken in the UK over the past 40 years. Only some of the more recent of these can be reviewed here. For example, Paramshwar and colleagues[w1] examined the clinical records of diuretic treated patients in three general practices in northwest London in 1992 to identify possible cases of heart failure. From a total of 30 204 patients, a clinical diagnosis of heart failure was made in 117 cases (46 male and 71 female), giving an overall prevalence of 3.9 cases/1000. Prevalence of heart failure increased considerably with age—in those aged under 65 years the prevalence rate was 0.6 cases/1000 compared

Table 9.1 Reported prevalence of heart failure[1] [2]

Study	Location	Overall prevalence rate	Prevalence rate in older age group
Surveys of treated patients			
RCGP (1958)	UK national data	3/1000	–
Gibson et al (1966)	Rural cohort, USA	9–10/1000	65/1000 (>65 years)
RCGP (1986)	UK national data	11/1000	–
Parameshwar et al (1992)	London, UK	4/1000	28/1000 (> 65 years)
Rodeheffer (1993)	Rochester, UK	3/1000 (< 75 years)	–
Mair et al (1994)	Liverpool, UK	15/1000	80/1000 (> 65 years)
RCGP (1995)	UK national data	9/1000	74/1000 (65–74 years)
Clarke et al (1995)	Nottinghamshire, UK	8–16/1000	40–60/1000 (> 70 years)
Population screening			
Droller and Pemberton (1953)	Sheffield, UK	–	30–50/1000 (> 62 years)
Garrison et al (1966)	Georgia, USA	21/1000 (45–74 years)	35/1000 (65–74 years)
Framingham (1971)	Framingham, USA	3/1000 (< 63 years)	23/1000 (60–79 years)
Landahl et al (1984)	Sweden (males only)	3/1000 (< 75 years)	80–170/1000 (> 67 years)
Eriksson et al (1989)	Gothenburg, Sweden	–	130/1000 (> 67 years)
NHANES (1992)	USA national data	20/1000	80/1000 (> 65 years)
Cardiovascular health study (1993)	USA national data	20/1000	80/1000 (> 65 years)
RCGP (1995)	UK national data	9/1000 (25–74 years)	74/1000 (65–74 years)

to 28 cases/1000 in those aged over 65 years. However, objective investigation of left ventricular function had been undertaken in less than one third of these patients. Using similar methods, Mair and colleagues[w2] identified a total of 266 cases of heart failure from 17 400 patients within two general practices in Liverpool. Undertaken in 1994, the overall prevalence rate was 15 cases/1000 patients with 80 cases/1000 in those aged $\geq$ 65 years.

More recently, Clarke and colleagues[w3] reported an even larger survey of heart failure based on similar methods and including analysis of prescription of loop diuretics for all residents of the English county of Nottinghamshire. They estimated that between 13 017 and 26 214 patients had been prescribed frusemide (furosemide) in this region of central England. Case note review of a random sample of those patients receiving such treatment found that 56% were being treated for heart failure. On this basis they calculated an overall prevalence rate of 8–16 cases/1000. Once again, heart failure prevalence increased with advancing age with the rate increasing to between 40–60 cases/1000 among those aged $\geq$ 70 years.

Population studies based on clinical criteria.
There are now many population studies of heart failure and only some can be reviewed here. At entry into the Framingham study, 17 of 5209 persons (3 cases/1000) screened for heart failure on the basis of clinical criteria were thought to have heart failure; all were less that 63 years of age.[w4] After 34 years follow up, prevalence rates increased as the cohort aged. The estimated prevalence of heart failure in the age groups 50–59, 60–69, 70–79, and $\geq$ 80 years was 8, 23, 49, and 91 cases/1000 persons respectively.[3] NHANES-1 (national health and nutrition examination survey) reported the heart failure prevalence rate within the US population. Based on self reporting, and a clinical scoring system, this study screened 14 407 persons of both sexes, aged 25–47 years, between 1971 and 1975, with detailed evaluation of only 6913 subjects and reported a prevalence rate of 20 cases/1000.[w5] The study of men born in 1913 examined the prevalence of heart failure in a cohort of 855 Swedish men at ages 50, 54, 57, and 67 years.[w6] The prevalence rate of "manifest" heart failure rose dramatically from 21 cases/1000 at age 50 years to 130 cases/1000 at age 67 years.

Prevalence of left ventricular systolic dysfunction
In only a few of the two types of prevalence study described above was objective evidence of cardiac dysfunction obtained. Consequently, it is unclear whether all patients really had heart failure and, if they did, what the cause of heart failure was. There have, however, been four recent estimates of the population prevalence of left ventricular systolic dysfunction as determined by echocardiography emanating from Scotland,[4] the Netherlands, England, and Finland.

The Scottish study targeted a representative cohort of 2000 persons aged 25–74 years living north of the River Clyde in Glasgow. Of those

selected 1640 (83%) underwent a detailed assessment of their cardiovascular status and underwent echocardiography. Left ventricular systolic dysfunction was defined as a left ventricular ejection fraction (LVEF) $\leq$ 30%. The overall prevalence of left ventricular systolic dysfunction using this criterion was 2.9%. Concurrent symptoms of heart failure were found in 1.5% of the cohort, while the remaining 1.4% were asymptomatic. Prevalence was both greater in men and increased with age: in men aged 65–74 years it was 6.4% and in age matched women 4.9%.

The Rotterdam study in the Netherlands, though examining individuals aged 55–74 years, reported similar findings. Overall the prevalence of left ventricular systolic dysfunction, defined in this case as fractional shortening of $\leq$ 25%, was 5.5% in men and 2.2% in women.[w7]

The Helsinki ageing study describes clinical and echocardiographic findings in 501 subjects (367 female) aged 75-86 years.[w8] The prevalence of heart failure, based on clinical criteria, was 8.2% overall (41 of 501) and 6.8%, 10%, and 8.1% in those aged 75, 80, and 85 years, respectively. These individuals had a high prevalence of moderate or severe mitral or aortic valve disease (51%), ischaemic heart disease (54%), and hypertension (54%). However, of the 41 subjects with "heart failure" only 11 (28%) had significant left ventricular systolic dysfunction (diagnosed by the combined presence of fractional shortening < 25% and left ventricular dilation), and in 20 cases no echocardiographic abnormality was identified. Of the 460 without symptoms of heart failure 43 (9%) also had left ventricular systolic dysfunction. The overall prevalence of left ventricular systolic dysfunction was therefore 10.8% (95% confidence interval (CI) 8.2% to 13.8%).

More recently, Morgan and colleagues[w9] studied 817 individuals aged 70–84 years selected from two general practices in Southampton, England. Left ventricular function was assessed qualitatively as normal, mild, moderate or severe systolic dysfunction. The overall prevalence of all grades of dysfunction was 7.5% (95% CI 5.8% to 9.5%). Prevalence of left ventricular dysfunction doubled between the ages of 70–74 years and > 80 years.

Preserved left ventricular systolic function
One of the most controversial issues pertaining to the subject of heart failure at present is the occurrence of the syndrome in patients with preserved left ventricular systolic function (and no other obvious cause, such as valve disease). A full discussion of this topic is beyond the scope of this article. There are, however, two recent studies of this type of heart failure. The Olmsted county study, Minnesota, found that 43% of patients with chronic heart failure had an LVEF $\geq$ 50%.[5] Similarly, the Framingham investigators found that 51% of their cohort with heart failure had an LVEF of $\geq$ 50% (see also Helsinki ageing study above).[6]

Table 9.2   Reported incidence of heart failure.[1][2]

Study	Location	Incidence rate (whole population)	Incidence rate in older age groups
Eriksson et al (1989)	Sweden (men born in 1913)	–	10/1000 (61–67 years)
Remes et al (1992)	Eastern Finland	1–4/1000 (45–74 years)	8/1000 (> 65 years)
Ho et al (1993)	Framingham, USA	2/1000	–
Rodeheffer et al (1993)	Rochester, USA	1/1000 (< 75 years)	16/1000 (> 65 years)
Cowie et al (1999)	London, UK	1/1000	12/1000 (> 85 years)

Incidence

There is much less known about the incidence than the prevalence of heart failure. Table 9.2 shows reported incidence rates from the largest population based studies. The most detailed incidence data emanate from the Framingham heart study.[3] Like other population based prevalence studies heart failure was defined according to a clinical scoring system. The only "cardiac" investigation was chest radiography. At 34 years follow up, the incidence of heart failure was approximately 2 new cases/1000 in persons aged 45–54 years, increasing to 40 new cases/1000 in men aged 85–94 years. Using similar criteria, the study of men born in 1913 reported incidence rates of "manifest" heart failure of 1.5, 4.3, and 10.2 new cases/1000 in men aged 50–54, 55–60, and 61–67 years, respectively.[w6] The Rochester epidemiology project also reported the incidence of heart failure in a US population during 1981 in persons aged 0–74 years.[w10] The annual incidence was 1.1 new cases/1000. Once again incidence was higher in men compared to women (1.57 v 0.71 cases/1000, respectively). It also increased with age, the rate of new cases increasing from 0.76/1000 in men aged 45–49 years to 1.6/1000 in men aged 65–69 years.

The most recent incidence study was reported by Cowie and colleagues from the Hillingdon district of London with a population of approximately 150 000.[7] In a 15 month period, 122 patients were referred to a special heart failure clinic. This represented an annual referral rate of 6.5/1000 population. Using a broad definition of heart failure, only 29% of these patients were clearly diagnosed as having heart failure (annual incidence 1.85/1000 population).

Heart failure admissions

A different type of epidemiological information comes from reports of heart failure related hospital admissions on a country to country basis; however, these also need to be interpreted with some caution because of their retrospective nature and variations in coding practices and changing admission thresholds over time. Figure 9.1 shows the reported hospitalisation rates from Scotland,[8] Spain, the USA, Sweden, New Zealand, and the Netherlands for the period 1978 to 1993. As such, hospitalisation for heart failure appears to be a growing problem on a global scale. For example, studies undertaken in the UK suggest that in the early 1990s 0.2% of the population were hospitalised for heart failure per annum and that such admissions accounted for more than 5% of adult general medicine and geriatric hospital admissions—outnumbering those associated with acute myocardial infarction.[8] In the USA heart failure continues to be the most common cause of hospitalisation in people over the age of 65 years.[9]

An admission for heart failure is frequently prolonged and in many cases followed by readmission within a short period of time. For example, in the UK the mean length of stay for a heart failure related admission in 1990 was 11.4 days on acute medical wards and 28.5 days on acute geriatric wards. Within the UK about one third of patients are readmitted within 12 months of discharge, while the same proportion are reportedly readmitted within six months in the USA.[8][9] Such readmission rates are usually higher than the other major causes of hospitalisation, including stroke, hip fracture, and respiratory disease. Moreover, although there is evidence to suggest that an increasing number of heart failure patients are surviving a heart failure related hospital admission, there is a parallel decrease in the number of patients who are discharged on an independent basis to their own homes. On a sex specific basis, men tend to be younger than women when admitted for the first time with heart failure, but because of greater female longevity, the number of male and female admissions are roughly equal.

Cost of heart failure

In any health care system, hospital admissions represent a disproportionate component of total health care expenditure. Not surprisingly, considering the high rates of hospitalisation for heart failure and the ongoing treatment and care it requires, the overall management of heart failure requires a significant amount of health care expenditure in industrialised nations. Figure 9.2 shows that heart failure is reported to consume 1–2% of health care expenditure in a number of industrialised countries.[1] Moreover, considering the increasing rates of hospitalisation it is likely that these reported estimates fall short of the current burden of heart failure.

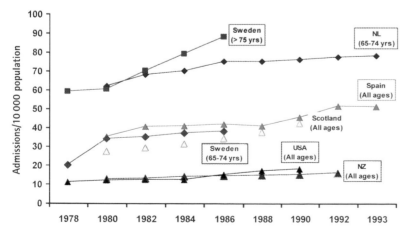

Figure 9.1. Comparison of heart failure admissions rates per annum (recorded hospital admissions/10 000 population at risk) in western developed countries 1978 to 1993. Adapted from data in McMurray et al.[1]

Aetiology of heart failure

In western developed countries, coronary artery disease, either alone or in combination with hypertension, seems to be the most common cause of heart failure. It is, however, very difficult to be certain what is the primary aetiology of heart failure in a patient with multiple potential causes (for example, coronary artery disease, hypertension, diabetes mellitus, atrial fibrillation, etc). Furthermore, even the absence of overt hypertension in a patient presenting with heart failure does not rule out an important aetiological role in the past, with normalisation of blood pressure as the patient develops pump failure. Even in those with suspected coronary artery disease the diagnosis is not always correct and in the absence of coronary angiography must remain presumed rather than confirmed. In this context, even coronary angiography has its limitations in identifying atherosclerotic disease.

The initial cohort of the Framingham heart study was monitored until 1965; hypertension appeared to be the most common cause of heart failure, being identified as the primary cause in 30% of men and 20% of women and a cofactor in a further 33% and 25%, respectively. Moreover, electrocardiographic evidence of left ventricular hypertrophy in the presence of hypertension carried an approximate 15 fold increased risk of developing heart failure. In the subsequent years of follow up, however, coronary heart disease became increasingly prevalent before the development of heart failure and, as the identified cause of new cases of heart failure, increased from 22% in the 1950s to almost 70% in the 1970s.[w11] During this period, the relative contribution of hypertension and valvar heart disease declined dramatically. Figure 9.3 is a summary of the changing association of coronary artery disease, hypertension, diabetes, and valvar heart disease with the sub-

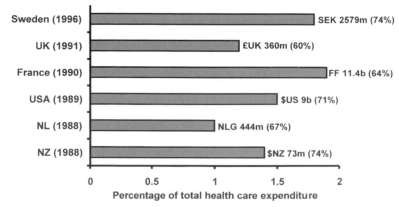

Figure 9.2. Cost of chronic heart failure compared with the total health expenditure in Sweden, the UK, France, the USA, the Netherlands, and New Zealand. The figures represent the component of hospital costs contributing to total expenditure quoted in the local currency and (in parentheses) as a proportion of total health care expenditure for that country. Adapted from data in McMurray et al.[1]

sequent development of heart failure over the period 1950 to 1987.[10] As such there was an approximate 5% and 30% decline in the prevalence per decade of hypertension during this period among men and women, respectively. The declining contribution of hypertension most probably reflects the introduction of anti-hypertensive treatment; the parallel decline in the prevalence of left ventricular hypertrophy supports this supposition. It is also probable that during this same period, progressively greater accuracy in determining the presence of coronary heart disease contributed to its increasing importance in this regard.

As noted above, however, any interpretation of the Framingham data has to consider the fact that heart failure was identified on clinical criteria alone and undoubtedly included individuals without associated left ventricular systolic dysfunction. Conversely, the large scale clinical trials have largely recruited patients who have reduced left ventricular ejection fractions and applied an extensive list of exclusion criteria. Table 9.3 is a summary of the most commonly attributed causes and associates of heart failure in a number of clinical trials and registries.[11-17] As such it demonstrates that coronary artery disease appears to be the most common underlying cause of heart failure, consistent with the more recent Framingham experience.

Common precursors of chronic heart failure

- Coronary artery disease (for example, consequent upon acute myocardial infarction)

- Chronic hypertension

- Cardiomyopathy (for example, dilated, hypertrophic, alcoholic, and idiopathic)

- Valve dysfunction (for example, diseases of the aortic and mitral valve)

- Cardiac arrhythmias/conduction disturbance (for example, heart block and atrial fibrillation)

- Pericardial disease (for example, constrictive pericarditis)

- Infection (for example, rheumatic fever, Chagas disease, viral myocarditis, and HIV)

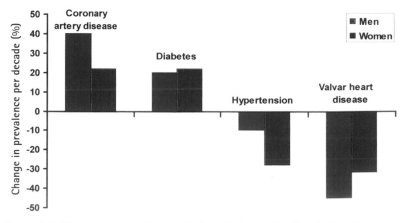

Figure 9.3. Change in causal factors for heart failure in the Framingham heart study during the period 1950 to 1987. Adapted from data reported by Kannel WB et al.[10]

Table 9.3   Aetiology of heart failure in clinical trials and registers.[11-17]

	Clinical trials					Registers	
	SOLVD 1991	DIG Study 1997	MERIT-HF 1999	ATLAS 1999	RALES 1999	SOLVD 1992	SPICE 1999
Size of cohort	2569	6800	3991	3192	1663	6273	9580
Mean age	61	64	64	64	65	62	66
Male (%)	80	78	78	79	73	74	74
Aetiology of heart failure							
Ischaemic	71%	70%	66%	64%	54%	69%	63%
Non-ischaemic	–	29%	34%	35%	46%	31%	–
Hypertensive	–	(9%)	–	(20%)	–	7%	4%
IDCM	18%	(15%)	–	(28%)	–	13%	17%
Valvar	–	–	–	(6%)	–	–	5%
Other	–	6%	–	–	–	11%	–
Unknown	–	–	–		–	–	6%
Comorbidity							
Hypertension	42%	–	44%	46%	–	43%	27%
Diabetes	26%	–	25%	29%	–	23%	–
Atrial fibrillation	10%	–	17%	–	–	14%	–
Current angina	37%	–	–	27%	–	–	–
Respiratory disease	26%	–	–	–	–	15%	–

In the study of left ventricular function in North Glasgow,[4] 95% v 71% of symptomatic and asymptomatic individuals with definite left ventricular systolic dysfunction had evidence of coronary artery disease (p = 0.04). Those individuals with symptomatic heart failure were also more likely to have a past myocardial infarction (50% v 14%; p = 0.01) and concurrent angina (62% v 43%; p = 0.02). Hypertension (80%) and valvar heart disease (25%) were also more prevalent in those individuals with both clinical and echocardiographically determined heart failure compared to the remainder of the cohort, including those with asymptomatic left ventricular dysfunction (67% and 0%, respectively).[4] One recent study, however, reports an unknown aetiology for heart failure in a disturbingly high proportion of cases.[7]

Therefore, the aetiological importance of many of the associated causes of heart failure will depend on both the age cohorts examined and the type of criteria used to determine the presence of heart failure.

Prognosis

Heart failure, irrespective of whether it has been detected on the basis of being actively treated (for example, during a hospital admission) or in otherwise asymptomatic individuals, is a lethal condition.

There are some data to suggest that heart failure related mortality is comparable to that of cancer. For example, in the original and subsequent Framingham cohort, the probability of someone with a diagnosis of heart failure dying within five years was 62% and 75% in men and 38% and 42% in women, respectively.[18] In comparison, five year survival for all cancers among men and women in the US during the same period was approximately 50%. The general applicability of these data is, however, limited by the few events recorded overall, the relative homogeneity of the Framingham population, and the exclusion of older individuals. The Rochester

epidemiology project has also described the prognosis in 107 patients presenting to associated hospitals with new onset heart failure in 1981, and 141 patients presenting in 1991. The median follow up in these cohorts was 1061 and 1233 days, respectively. The mean age of the 1981 patients was 75 years rising to 77 years in 1991. The one year and five year mortality was, respectively, 28% and 66% in the 1981 cohort and 23% and 67% in the 1991 cohort.[w12] In other words, though the same diagnostic criteria used in the Framingham study were used in the Rochester project, the prognosis was somewhat better in the latter.

The only other large, representative, epidemiological study reporting long term outcome in patients with heart failure is the NHANES-I.[w5] The initial programme evaluated 14 407 adults aged 25 and 74 years in the USA between 1971 and 1975. Follow up studies were carried out in 1982-84 and again in 1986 (for those aged > 55 years and alive during the 1982-84 review). The estimated 10 year mortality in subjects aged 25–74 years with self reported heart failure was 42.8% (49.8% in men and 36% in women). Mortality in those aged 65–74 years was 65.4% (71.8% and 59.5% in men and women, respectively). These mortality rates are considerably lower than those observed in Framingham. The patients in NHANES-I were non-institutionalised and their heart failure was self reported. Follow up was incomplete. NHANES-I was also carried out in a more recent time period than Framingham when prognosis in heart failure patients may have improved. Framingham investigators in 1993 looked at patients developing heart failure in the period 1948 to 1988 and the Rochester investigators in the period 1981 to 1991. In both of these studies no temporal change in prognosis was identified.

All three of these studies describe a mixed population of patients, some of whom had systolic left ventricular dysfunction and others who did not. The true contribution of heart failure to overall mortality or coronary artery disease related mortality is almost certainly underestimated. Although heart failure is highly prevalent among the elderly, representing the terminal manifestation of a number of cardiovascular disease states, and has been shown to be associated with extremely poor survival rates, official statistics continue to attribute only a small proportion of deaths to this syndrome. This reflects a common policy of coding the cause of death as the underlying aetiology (for example, coronary artery disease rather than heart failure itself).

Future burden of heart failure

Despite a decline in age adjusted mortality from coronary heart disease (CHD) in developed countries overall, the number of patients with chronic CHD is increasing. This is principally the result of two separate trends. Firstly, the proportion of elderly in the population is increasing rapidly and these subjects have the highest incidence of CHD and hypertension. Secondly, survival in those with coronary artery disease is improving. In particular, it has been shown that survival after acute myocardial infarction has increased notably over the past decade, at least in part because of better medical treatment.[19] As coronary artery disease is the most powerful risk factor for heart failure (and its most important precursor) it is likely that the aforementioned trends will lead to an increase its future prevalence. Chronic heart failure may, therefore, become a more common manifestation of chronic heart disease and contribute to many more deaths. Two formal projections of the future burden of heart failure have been undertaken in respect to the Netherlands[20] and Australia.[w13] For example, an analysis of demographic trends in the Netherlands has predicted that the prevalence of heart failure caused by coronary heart disease will rise by approximately 70% from 1985 to 2010.

Summary

- Heart failure represents a major and escalating public health problem.

- The overall prevalence of clinically identified heart failure is estimated to be 3–20 cases/1000 population, but rises to > 100 cases/1000 population in those aged ≥65 years.

- Prevalence of confirmed left ventricular systolic dysfunction also increases with age and is more common in men. However, these rates are far less than reported for the syndrome of heart failure.

- The overall annual incidence of clinically overt heart failure in middle aged men and women is approximately 0.1–0.2%. However, with each additional decade of life there is an approximate doubling of this rate and the incidence of heart failure in those aged > 85 years is approximately 2–3%.

- Although reported incidence rates are higher in men than women, greater longevity in women tends to balance overall prevalence rates on a sex specific basis.

- Heart failure admission rates appear to be steadily increasing in all industrialised countries, especially among older individuals. Overall, annual admission rates for 1990 ranged from 10–40 admissions/10 000 population and increased to > 75 admissions/10 000 population in those aged > 65 years.

- The cost of managing heart failure in the early 1990s was estimated to be 1–2% of total health care expenditure. Because hospital care consumes a significant proportion of this expenditure, and rates of heart failure related hospitalisation have probably risen, this may be an underestimate of the current cost of heart failure.

- Heart failure is associated with an approximately 60% mortality rate within five years of diagnosis.

- The combination of increasing survival post acute myocardial infarction and increased longevity in western developed nations is likely to lead to an increase in the overall prevalence of heart failure.

1. **McMurray JJ, Petrie MC, Murdoch DR,** et al. Clinical epidemiology of heart failure: public and private health burden. Eur Heart J 1998;**19**:P9–16.

2. **Cowie MR.** Annotated references in epidemiology. Eur J Heart Failure 1999;**1**:101–7.
   - An update of a comprehensive overview of the epidemiology of heart failure published by the same author in 1997.

3. **Ho KK, Pinsky JL, Kannel WB,** et al. The epidemiology of heart failure: The Framingham study. J Am Coll Cardiol 1993;**22**:6A-13A.
   - A follow up report of the classic incidence and natural history study conducted in a community in northeastern USA, starting in 1946 and continuing to this day. It describes the long term follow up of a sizeable cohort of individuals with chronic heart failure.

4. **McDonagh TA, Morrison CE, Lawrence A,** et al. Symptomatic and asymptomatic left-ventricular systolic dysfunction in an urban population. Lancet 1997;**350**:829–33.
   - The first population survey of men and women to report the prevalence estimates of left ventricular systolic dysfunction using echocardiography. It was carried out in north Glasgow, which has a very high prevalence of coronary artery disease and hypertension.

5. **Senni M, Tribouilloy CM, Rodeheffer RJ.** Congestive heart failure in the community: a study of all incident cases in Olmsted County, Minnesota, in 1991. Circulation 1998;**98**:2282–9.

6. **Vasan RS, Larson MG, Benjamin EJ,** et al. Congestive heart failure in subjects with normal versus reduced left ventricular ejection fraction: prevalence and mortality in a population-based cohort. J Am Coll Cardiol 1999;**33**:1948–55.

7. **Cowie MR, Wood DA, Coats AJ,** et al. Incidence and aetiology of heart failure; a population-based study. Eur Heart J 1999;**20**:421–8.
   - A contemporary, London based, population survey of the incidence and new cases of chronic heart failure in men and women.

8. **McMurray J, McDonagh T, Morrison CE,** et al. Trends in hospitalization for heart failure in Scotland 1980–1990. Eur Heart J 1993;**14**:1158–62.
   - A survey of heart failure related hospitalisations in Scotland during the period 1980 to 1990. It represents the first European report of its kind.

9. Haldeman GA, Croft JB, Giles WH, *et al.* Hospitalization of patients with heart failure: national hospital discharge survey 1985–1995. *Am Heart J* 1999;**137**:352–60.
● *A survey of heart failure related hospitalisations in the USA during the period 1985 to 1995. It represents the most up to date report from an industrialised nation.*

10. Kannel WB, Ho KK, Thom T. Changing epidemiological features of cardiac failure. *Eur Heart J* 1994;**72**:S3–9.
● *Using data from the long term surveillance of the Framingham cohorts, an important overview of the changing epidemiology and aetiology of heart failure.*

11. The SOLVD Investigators. Effect of enalapril on survival in patients with reduced left ventricular ejection fractions and congestive heart failure. *N Engl J Med* 1991;**325**:293–302.

12. Pitt B, Zannad F, Remme WJ, *et al.* The effect of spironolactone on morbidity and mortality in patients with severe heart failure. Randomized aldactone evaluation study investigators. *N Engl J Med* 1999;**341**:709–17.

13. The Digitalis Investigation Group. The effect of digoxin on mortality and morbidity in patients with heart failure. *N Engl J Med* 1997;**336**:525–33.

14. MERIT Investigators. Effect of metoprolol CR/XL in chronic heart failure: metoprolol CR/XL randomised intervention trial in congestive heart failure (Merit-HF). *Lancet* 1999;**353**:2001–7.

15. Packer M, Poole-Wilson PA, Armstrong PW, *et al.* Comparative effects of low and high doses of the angiotensin converting enzyme inhibitor, lisinopril, on morbidity and mortality in chronic heart failure. *Circulation* 1999;**100**:2312–18.

16. SOLVD Investigators. Natural history and patterns of current practice in heart failure. *J Am Coll Cardiol* 1993;**4A**:14A-19A.

17. Bart BA, Ertl G, Held P, *et al.* Contemporary management of patients with left ventricular systolic dysfunction. Results from the study of patients intolerant of converting enzyme inhibitors (SPICE) registry. *Eur Heart J* 1999;**20**:1182–90.
● *A clinical trial based registry that contains data from 105 study centres in eight countries in North America and Europe.*

18. Ho KKL, Anderson KM, Karmel WB, *et al.* Survival after the onset of congestive heart failure in the Framingham heart study subjects. *Circulation* 1993;**88**:107–15.
● *Another follow up report of the Framingham study describing extremely poor survival rates in those individuals diagnosed with chronic heart failure.*

19. Rosamund WD, Chambless LE, Folsom AR, *et al.* Trends in the incidence of myocardial infarction and in mortality due to coronary artery disease. *N Engl J Med* 1998;**339**:861–7.

20. Bonneux L, Barendregt JJ, Meeter K, *et al.* Estimating clinical morbidity due to ischaemic heart disease and congestive heart failure: the future rise of heart failure. *Am J Public Health* 1994;**84**:20–8.
● *The first population based modelling exercise of its kind, this study estimated the future prevalence and associated burden of chronic heart failure in the Netherlands.*

website
extra

Additional references appear on the Heart website

www.heartjnl.com

10 The diagnosis of heart failure

Allan D Struthers

Heart failure is a difficult disease to define. It is easy to recognise heart failure in its moderate/severe version where the patient has pronounced symptoms and signs accompanied by echocardiographic evidence of left ventricular (LV) systolic dysfunction.[1] However, the problem of defining heart failure arises in its milder forms where patients may complain of dyspnoea but do not have echocardiographic evidence of LV systolic dysfunction. The complexities of what represents heart failure are illustrated in fig 10.1 but space precludes a detailed discussion of the definition of heart failure.

To overcome the various difficulties in defining heart failure, the European Society of Cardiology (ESC) has developed guidelines for the diagnosis of heart failure.[2] However, like all statements which are meant to define the undefinable, there is a certain deliberate vagueness about them. For example, they do not specify what they mean by cardiac dysfunction. Does an elderly lady whose echocardiogram meets criteria for "diastolic dysfunction" and who has swollen ankles have heart failure, even if she has no breathlessness or fatigue? Despite this caveat, the ESC guidelines have clarified the situation, even if one can still point to isolated patients who remain ambiguous with the ESC definition.

At a more pragmatic level, the clinician who is faced with a patient with suspected heart failure should try to answer two major questions:
1. Are the patient's symptoms cardiac in origin?

2. If so, what kind of cardiac disease is producing these symptoms?

In order to answer these questions, the clinician goes through the standard process of assessing the patient's symptoms, then the patient's signs, and finally arranging appropriate investigations. Obtaining the answer to the above questions is much more complex than it is with some other disease. For example, absolute levels of blood glucose make or break the diagnosis of diabetes mellitus. Similarly, absolute levels of blood pressure decide whether a patient has hypertension or not (even if the cutoff values for blood pressure and blood glucose do change repeatedly). Heart failure is much more difficult because it is not definable by an absolute level of any one parameter. Even if one could define a set of echocardiographic criteria to make the diagnosis, experts would never agree on the cutoff values and, even if they did, echocardiography is much more subject to interobserver bias than is a blood glucose. In order to set the scene, it is also worth saying how poor clinicians are at diagnosing mild heart failure using purely symptoms and signs. This information comes from the many open access echo services which have been set up throughout the country. In these, general practitioners are asked to send up all patients whom they suspect may have heart failure. To the surprise of many, it was found that only 25% of those sent up had LV systolic dysfunction on their echocardiogram—that is, 75% had normal LV systolic function.[3 4] This is not to criticise doctor's skills. Rather this says how non-specific are the symptoms and signs which classically lead us to suspect heart failure (table 10.1).[5]

Clinical history

The most classic symptom of heart failure is exertional dyspnoea. Unfortunately, exertional dyspnoea is also a common symptom in the general population. Indeed, with sufficient exercise, normal individuals will experience dyspnoea. Furthermore, in the general population, an individual patients' level of "fitness" will determine at what stage during exercise he or she experiences dyspnoea. Another problem is that there are a whole host of other non-cardiac diseases which also produce dyspnoea. Obvious examples are respiratory dis-

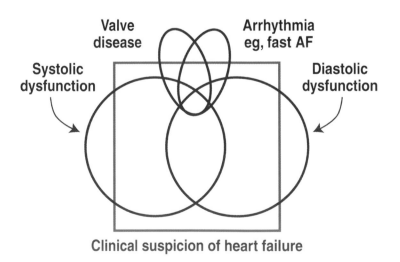

Figure 10.1. The various subcategories of heart failure.

Table 10.1 *Predictive values of clinical features*[5]

	Sensitivity (%)	Specificity (%)	PPV (%)	NPV (%)
Past history of myocardial infarction	59	86	44	92
Ingesting diuretic	73	41	19	89
Dyspnoea on exertion	100	17	18	100
Orthopnoea	22	74	14	83
Paroxysmal nocturnal dyspnoea	39	80	27	87
Oedema in history	49	47	15	83
Jugular venous pressure distension	17	98	64	86
Crackles	29	77	19	85
Gallop rhythm	24	99	77	87
Oedema on examination	20	86	21	85

PPV, positive predictive value; NPV, negative predictive value.

eases, anaemia, and simple obesity. All these factors make exertional dyspnoea a very non-specific symptom.

There are more extreme versions of dyspnoea which are more useful diagnostically. Orthopnoea is certainly more specific since it does not occur in normal individuals and probably not in respiratory disease. However, heart failure patients have to be quite severe before orthopnoea occurs, and diuretics are usually instituted long before orthopnoea becomes a problem. Indeed, if orthopnoea occurs, it is likely that premonitory symptoms have been ignored (either by the patient or the doctor). Thus, orthopnoea is a specific symptom but it has low sensitivity. Another extreme version of dyspnoea is paroxysmal nocturnal dyspnoea (PND). This results from nocturnal fluid redistribution which causes an increased LV filling pressure. Like orthopnoea, PND is a specific but insensitive symptom because again it signifies fairly severe heart failure which should have been noted and treated beforehand. Another small practical point is that in some patients, a very careful history is required to differentiate the PND of heart failure from the nocturnal dyspnoea and wheezing of asthma.

Fatigue and lethargy are common problems in heart failure, but they are probably even harder to define and assess than dyspnoea. Fatigue is an intermittent symptom in normal individuals as well as being a recognised symptom of nearly every disease that exists. Fatigue is therefore so unspecific as a symptom as to render it virtually worthless in guiding you to a diagnosis of heart failure or not.

A history of ankle oedema is another common presenting feature, but there are many alternative causes for it. Cor pulmonale (right heart failure caused by lung disease) also causes ankle oedema although the lung disease is usually so extreme as to be clinically obvious. Ankle oedema is much more helpful in diagnosing heart failure in men than in women. Elderly ladies commonly have ankle oedema which is not caused by heart failure: its precise cause is unknown although venous insufficiency accompanied by pelvic obstruction to venous blood flow are commonly blamed. In fact, it is elderly ladies with swollen ankles who most commonly cause the "false positives" which are seen in open access echo referrals.

Perhaps the best clue from the history is not a symptom which the patient complains of, but

a past history of a previous myocardial infarction. Less useful but also worth noting is a past history of hypertension. It should be noted, however, that many elderly patients experience clinically "silent" myocardial infarctions. Other useful features in the history are excessive alcohol intake, a past history of rheumatic fever making valve disease possible, and the use of a drug such as a non-steroidal anti-inflammatory (NSAID) which might precipitate heart failure.

Physical signs

As with the symptoms, the physical signs fall into two categories. Firstly, there are physical signs which occur in so many other diseases that they are non-specific and hence of low predictive value. These are tachycardia, pulmonary crepitations, and peripheral oedema. On the other hand, there are physical signs which are relatively specific to heart failure but they are also insensitive because they only occur once heart failure has become quite severe. These latter physical signs are elevation of the jugular venous pressure, gallop rhythm, and displacement of the apex beat. There is a further problem with these latter physical signs in that the ability of doctors to detect these more specific signs is variable.

Thus, it can be seen that few symptoms or signs are valuable on their own. However, clinical medicine is not about using single parameters to make diagnoses. As a clinician, one assesses the overall probability of a diagnosis based on the whole history and examination. When one does that, it becomes clear that heart failure is not as hard to diagnose correctly as the above discussion would imply. For example, a man with a past history of a myocardial infarction who now develops ankle oedema is very likely to have heart failure. On the other hand, heart failure is unlikely in a patient who complains of fatigue with no relevant past history and no other symptoms/signs of heart failure.

Investigations

The main purpose of investigations is to confirm or refute the diagnosis of heart failure *and* to define the precise underlying cardiac cause. The latter is especially important as treatment is based on the underlying cause and not simply on the existence of heart failure. For example, heart failure can be caused by valve disease, where the correct treatment may be surgery, or by LV systolic dysfunction, where the correct treatment will be diuretics, angiotensin converting enzyme (ACE) inhibitors, β blockers, and spironolactone.

Blood analysis
It goes without saying that all patients with suspected heart failure should have blood sent for haematological and biochemical analysis (including thyroid function and cholesterol). These

65

tests will not only exclude anaemia and hypothyroidism but will also detect other entities which might need treatment, such as cholesterol.

Chest *x* ray

The chest *x* ray is routinely performed and can produce useful information. Cardiac enlargement (cardiothoracic ratio > 50%) implies cardiomegaly and if this is present it is a good guide to heart failure. However, many heart failure patients will not exhibit cardiomegaly so that it tends to be a specific but insensitive test which identifies severe heart failure only. The other helpful findings at chest *x* ray are pulmonary oedema (bat's wing appearance), upper lobe diversion, fluid in the horizontal fissures, and Kerley B lines in the costophrenic angles. In extreme cases, pleural effusions may be present although clearly there are alternative explanations for pleural effusions such as bronchial carcinoma, pneumonia or pulmonary emboli. Clearly the chest *x* ray can also reveal other clues as to non-cardiac disease which might cause the dyspnoea. A lung tumour might be obvious, and emphysema might also be present. Nevertheless, the chest *x* ray should be seen as a whole—for example, the finding of cardiomegaly plus bilateral pleural effusions with no other parenchymal lung disease makes heart failure extremely likely (although it should still be confirmed by echocardiography).

Electrocardiogram

The 12 lead ECG should be routinely performed. The situation with the ECG is very different for heart failure than it is for angina—that is, a completely normal resting ECG does not by any means exclude the diagnosis of angina whereas it does virtually exclude the presence of heart failure. Put another way, LV systolic dysfunction is rare in the presence of a completely normal 12 lead ECG. In practice, what this means is that if a patient has dyspnoea and a completely normal ECG, then the doctor should first consider alternative diagnoses for the patient's dyspnoea, rather than heart failure. On the other hand, an abnormal resting ECG will often occur in the absence of LV systolic dysfunction.[6] Overall therefore, an abnormal resting ECG is sensitive (94%) with excellent negative predictive value (98%) but it is much less specific (61%) and has poor positive predictive value (35%). Although most studies support this finding, in general, there are contrary data including one paper where 27% of cases were missed with this approach.[7] Therefore, if in a certain area the availability of echocardiography is limited, then a possible strategy is to limit echocardiography to those with abnormal ECGs as well as those with cardiac murmurs.

Echocardiography

The real gold standard investigation in suspected heart failure is echocardiography. It is clearly the most valuable single investigation. A qualitative assessment can be made to decide whether LV systolic function is normal or impaired (hypokinetic). This may well be all

Ability of a normal ECG to exclude LV systolic dysfunction?[6]

● Sensitivity	94%
● Specificity	61%
● Positive predictive value	35%
● Negative predictive value	98%

that is necessary in routine clinical use. However, it can be quantified by measuring various parameters—for example, fractional shortening, LV ejection fraction (LVEF) or wall motion index. Fractional shortening is the quickest and, for clinical purposes, is usually sufficient. When it comes to research, more accurate quantification is preferable which is why the LVEF or the wall motion index are more usually used in research studies. Another useful measure is whether the left ventricle is dilated or not. Again, this can be described qualitatively or quantitatively by LV diameters or LV volume indices. LV dilatation and LV systolic dysfunction usually accompany each other, but occasionally the left ventricle is dilated even although its systolic function is normal. LV dilatation implies impending LV systolic dysfunction and should probably be treated as such.

In true systolic dysfunction, secondary mitral incompetence is often seen—that is, the mitral ring becomes stretched owing to LV dilatation. It is crucial to distinguish this from primary mitral valve disease, where surgery is the treatment of choice. In secondary mitral incompetence caused by LV systolic dysfunction, surgery used not to be indicated since optimised medical treatment reduces the LV dilatation and can hence reduce the secondary mitral incompetence. However, this situation may be changing as mitral valve replacement is now thought to be of benefit in selected cases of secondary mitral incompetence.

Clearly, echocardiography will also be able to assess valve structure and function and identify patients with aortic stenosis, etc, who would benefit from surgery.

Echocardiography will also be able to assess diastolic function although this is a contentious issue. The problem is that the left ventricle (like the aorta) becomes stiffer as it ages and it is difficult to define when this stiff left ventricle constitutes diastolic dysfunction. No echocardiographic criteria are fully accepted as measures of diastolic dysfunction. It should be recognised, however, that there is one extreme version of diastolic dysfunction which can cause severe pulmonary oedema. This is when the left ventricle is so stiff that left atrial pressure increases and leads to fast atrial fibrillation with profound dyspnoea. The short term treatment here is to reverse the abnormal rhythm, but longer term strategies to prevent LV stiffness which leads to atrial fibrillation should be explored. As yet, no established treatment exists for diastolic dysfunction per se.

Value of BNP as a screening tool in two important situations

- Ability of a high BNP concentration to identify heart failure in symptomatic patients in primary care[8]

Sensitivity	97%
Specificity	84%
Positive predictive value	70%
Negative predictive value	98%

- Ability of BNP to identify LV systolic dysfunction in a cross section of the community[9]

Sensitivity	76%
Specificity	87%
Positive predictive value	16%
Negative predictive value	98%

In a small proportion of patients, echocardiographic windows are poor and in that situation radionuclide ventriculography is often used instead to assess LV systolic function. Although it does so very reliably, unfortunately it does not give useful structural information about valves or LV mass.

Open access echocardiography

Because of the key role of echocardiography in assessing such patients, the concept of direct access or open access echocardiography has arisen. Francis and colleagues showed the true value of such a service.[4] Among the referred patients who were already being treated for heart failure, only 36% of men and 18% of women had definitely impaired LV systolic function. In fact, the echo result led to a change in treatment for 70% of those patients who were already taking diuretics for suspected heart failure—this change was often the cessation of unnecessary treatment. However, open access echocardiography is not without its problems. These problems relate to guidelines on whom to refer, interpretation of the results, and on the maintenance of echocardiographic standards. General practitioners should ideally receive guidelines on whom to refer. In addition, echocardiography can be difficult to interpret in some cases without a fuller assessment of the individual patient. The main difficulty here is that many symptomatic patients will not have systolic dysfunction but may have "diastolic dysfunction". Whether such diastolic dysfunction seen on an echocardiogram is the cause of the patient's symptoms or not is often a difficult judgement even for an experienced cardiologist. Hence the lack of systolic dysfunction in an open access echo service could be falsely reassuring to the general practitioner. In fact it may be better referring this kind of difficult patient to a hospital consultant who can then assess the echo result as part of the whole clinical picture.

Despite this important caveat, open access echo services continue to flourish and expand. Dialogue between referring general practitioners and consultants should help to iron out dif-

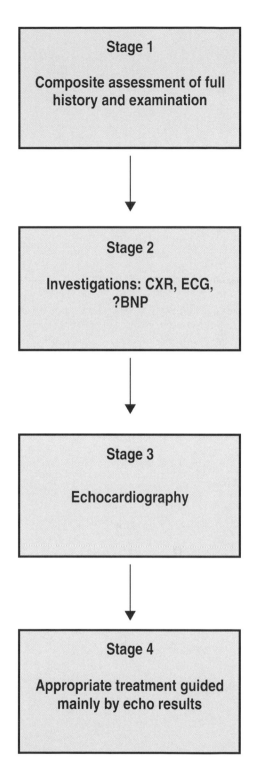

Figure 10.2. Diagnosing heart failure in practice. CXR, chest x ray; BNP, B-type natriuretic peptide.

ficulties and to identify two separate groups: those patients who only need a factual echo report, and those who require further interpretation of the echo with knowledge of the whole clinical picture.

Natriuretic peptides for prescreening patients for echocardiography

General practitioners would still like more guidance as to whom to refer for echocardiography, especially since they are aware that only

25% of those referred for echo turn out to have LV systolic dysfunction. They are aware that a completely normal ECG can be used to select patients for echocardiography, although this does miss some cases of LV systolic dysfunction. In addition, general practitioners are unsure about their ability to differentiate between ECGs with minor abnormalities and totally normal ECGs. Therefore, there arose the idea that plasma concentrations of natriuretic peptides could help identify who to refer for echocardiography. The best measures are B-type natriuretic peptide (BNP) or N-terminal BNP (N-BNP). Although many papers have addressed this question, most of them were based on hospital patients and suffer from the weakness that the blood was taken from patients already on diuretics, which distort the relation between BNP and LV function since they reduce the BNP concentration but do not alter the echo. In one study set in general practice, BNP was 97% sensitive and 84% specific at identifying heart failure.[8] In another study set in the community, BNP was 76% sensitive and 87% specific in identifying LV systolic dysfunction.[9]

Despite most of the data being very positive, the use of BNP or N-BNP has not yet entered routine clinical practice. The reasons for this are that there are virtually no studies yet of general practitioners using BNP/N-BNP in routine practice and before diuretic treatment or referral; in addition, the cost-effectiveness of such a strategy still needs to be established. Future studies should clarify these important issues which may lead to general practitioners using BNP/N-BNP to preselect symptomatic patients for echocardiography.

Conclusions

The diagnosis of heart failure has three stages (fig 10.2). Firstly, the clinical history and examination have many pointers, none of which should be used in isolation, but when put together lead to a relatively accurate assessment of the likelihood of the patient having heart failure. The next stages are the preliminary investigations of chest x ray, ECG, and in the future perhaps BNP.[10] This second stage is mainly to preselect patients for the next stage which is the gold standard investigation of echocardiography—that is, if the second stage excludes heart failure then echocardiography would then become unnecessary and alternatively diagnosis should be considered. The third stage is the definitive investigation of echocardiography which would not only confirm heart failure definitely but even more importantly classify the cause of the heart failure into systolic dysfunction, diastolic dysfunction or valve disease. This differentiation is essential since the treatment is very different for each subcategory of heart failure.

Summary

- Symptoms which suggest heart failure tend to be either sensitive (for example, dyspnoea) or specific (PND, orthopnoea), but no symptom is both.

- Physical signs which suggest heart failure tend to be specific (raised jugular venous pressure, gallop rhythm), but none of them are sensitive.

- Echocardiography is essential to diagnose heart failure in suspected cases. Open access echo services seem popular.

- The ECG can be used as a prescreen to select patients for echocardiography, but some cases of LV systolic dysfunction (2–27% in different reports) are missed by this approach.

- Measurement of natriuretic peptides (BNP and N-BNP) might become an alternative way to prescreen suspected patients for echocardiography, but more work is required to establish feasibility and accuracy.

1. **Dargie HJ, McMurray J.** Diagnosis and management of heart failure. *BMJ* 1994;**308**:321–8.
- *An excellent summary of how to diagnose heart failure.*

2. **Task Force on Heart Failure of the European Society of Cardiology.** Guidelines for the diagnosis of heart failure. The task force on heart failure of the European Society of Cardiology. *Eur Heart J* 1995;**16**:741–51.
- *The definitive guidelines and definition on how to diagnose heart failure.*

3. **Wheeldon NM, MacDonald TM, Flucker CJ**, et al. Echocardiography in chronic heart failure in the community. *QJM* 1993;**86**:17–23.
- *The first paper to show that only a minority of patients on diuretic treatment in the community have LV systolic dysfunction.*

4. **Francis CM, Caruena L, Kearney P**, et al. Open access echocardiography in management of heart failure in the community. *BMJ* 1995;**310**:634–6.
- *The first description of how an open access echo service worked in the UK.*

5. **Davie AP, Francis CM, Caruana L**, et al. Assessing diagnosis of heart failure: which features are any use. *QJM* 1997;**90**:335–9.
- *A large assessment of the accuracy of various symptoms and signs in diagnosing LV systolic dysfunction.*

6. **Davie AP, Francis CM, Love MP**, et al. Value of the ECG in identifying heart failure due to LV systolic dysfunction. *BMJ* 1996;**312**:222.
- *The first report that a normal ECG virtually excludes LV systolic dysfunction.*

7. **Sandler DA, Steed RP, Hadfield JW.** Opening access to echocardiography for GPs in North Derbyshire. *Br J Cardiol* 2000;**7**:94–100.

8. **Cowie M, Struthers AD, Wood DA**, et al. The value of natriuretic peptides in assessment of patients with possible new heart failure in primary care. *Lancet* 1997;**350**:1349–53.
- *A formal assessment of how valuable BNP concentrations are in patients referred with suspected heart failure.*

9. **McDonagh T, Robb SD, Murdoch DR**, et al. Biochemical detection of LV systolic dysfunction. *Lancet* 1998;**351**:9–13.
- *A formal assessment of how good natriuretic peptide concentrations are in screening for LV systolic dysfunction in the community.*

10. **Davies MK, Gibbs CR, Lip GYM.** ABC of heart failure: investigation. *BMJ* 2000;**320**:297–300.
- *An excellent up to date review of heart failure investigations.*

website extra

Additional references appear on the Heart website

www.heartjnl.com

11 Non-transplant surgery for heart failure

Stephen Westaby

Thrombolysis and PTCA save lives during acute myocardial infarction, but incomplete or delayed reperfusion results in akinesia or dyskinesia. If more than 20% of the left ventricular circumference is dyskinetic, the remaining contractile cavity dilates to increase stroke volume. When more than 50% of the myocardium is impaired, increased wall tension (LaPlace's law) triggers progressive left ventricular failure with regression to myocyte fetal genetics and apoptosis.[1][2] In Britain, most heart failure is caused by coronary artery disease, particularly in patients over 60 years old. There are now hundreds of thousands of patients with debilitating symptoms despite maximal medical treatment. Less than 300 cardiac transplants per year are undertaken in a labour intensive way by 10 separate units. In a short time, more palliated young patients with congenital heart disease will require these organs. Consequently, the treatment of older patients with coronary disease and idiopathic dilated cardiomyopathy requires a radical rethink.

Table 11.1 Relation between infarct size and mortality[3]

	Three year mortality (%)	p Value
Myocardial infarction or scar $\geq$ 23%	43	0.014
Myocardial infarction or scar < 23%	5	
EF $\leq$ 43%	38	0.029
EF > 43%	6	
EF $\leq$ 43% without viable myocardium	63	0.059
EF $\leq$ 43% with viable myocardium*	13	

*For all patients with viable myocardium the three year mortality rate was 8% (80% had CABG). For patients with only fixed scar > 23% mortality rate was 50% (p = 0.018). Only 40% had CABG with no difference in mortality with or without CABG. EF, ejection fraction.

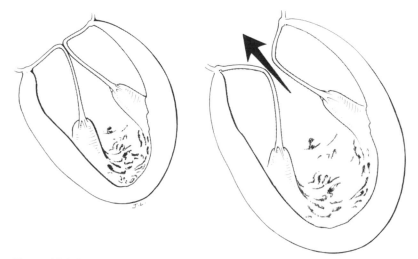

Figure 11.1. Progressive left ventricular dilatation causes mitral regurgitation and volume overload.

The following account of current and emerging surgical strategies for heart failure concentrates on those patients with left ventricular ejection fraction (LVEF) < 30%, mean pulmonary artery pressure > 25 mm Hg, left ventricular circumferential akinesia or dyskinesia > 60%, and left ventricular end diastolic volume (LVEDV) > 250 ml (LVEDV index (LVEDVI) > 140 ml). Most of these patients are New York Heart Association (NYHA) functional class III or IV with medical treatment. In coronary disease the relation between infarct size and mortality has been well defined (table 11.1).[3] From the coronary artery surgery study registry, five year survival for patients with LVEF < 25% was 41% with medical treatment and 62% with surgery.[4] For patients with dilated cardiomyopathy, mortality untreated is directly related to the severity of systolic dysfunction. Increased chamber sphericity and the presence of mitral regurgitation are markers of worse prognosis (one year mortality 54–70%). In the failing heart, mitral regurgitation occurs secondary to annular dilatation, altered left ventricular geometry or papillary muscle dysfunction (fig 11.1). Volume overload causes progressive left ventricular and annular dilatation, worsened mitral regurgitation, and decreased survival.

Coronary revascularisation in heart failure patients

High risk coronary bypass is the most frequent conventional operation in heart failure patients. Incomplete myocardial infarction leaves viable but ischaemic myocardium within involved segments (flow/metabolism mismatch). Hibernating myocardium is an unstable substrate for postinfarction dysrhythmic events and mortality, independent of age or LVEF (event rate 43% v 8% for scar).[5] Hibernating myocardium will recover contractile performance with reduced risk of dysrhythmia after coronary revascularisation, but for global improvement in left ventricular function, sufficient reversibly ischaemic territory must be present. Differentiation between reversible ischaemia and infarction is made on clinical grounds (angina which responds to sublingual nitrates) and objectively by positron emission tomography (PET) scan or dobutamine stress echocardiography.[6] Heart failure patients without reversible ischaemia do not have an improved outlook with coronary bypass, and LVEF alone is a poor predictor of surgical

- Cardiac transplantation is a very rare commodity.

- All transplant candidates with coronary disease should be assessed for hibernating myocardium then revascularisation.

- Those candidates with dilated cardiomyopathy should be considered for mitral repair.

- Left anterior descending coronary occlusion causes muscle loss in the apex, septum and anterolateral free wall.

- In 20% of patients cardiac failure occurs within 15 months when the normal elliptical left ventricle loses its apex and becomes spherical.

- The non-infarcted myocardium progressively dilates and further impairs function.

- When more than 50% of the circumference is asynergic surgical left ventricle restoration reduces left ventricular end systolic volume index (LVESVI) to < 80 ml/m² and avoids progressive failure.

Table 11.2   Guidelines for coronary bypass versus transplantation in end stage coronary artery disease[10]

CABG	Transplant
Prevailing hibernation	Prevailing scar
Short duration of heart failure	Prolonged heart failure
Low dose diuretics	High dose diuretics
No right ventricular failure	Chronic right ventricular failure
Stable cardiac output	Progressively lower output
Cardia index > 2.0 l/min/m²	Cardiac index < 2.0 l/min/m²
LVEDP < 24 mm Hg	LVEDP > 24 mm Hg
Good target vessels	Poor vessels
First operation	Previous revascularisation

LVEDP, left ventricular end diastolic pressure.

outcome when compared with the extent of reversible ischaemia.[3 7] In fact, survival benefit from coronary bypass increases as LVEF decreases. Other contraindications to high risk coronary surgery are poor target vessels, a pulmonary artery pressure > 60 mm Hg, and significantly impaired right ventricular function.

The ethos for revascularisation of the failing ventricle can be summarised as simplicity, safety, and speed. The intra-aortic balloon pump is employed preoperatively. Only good target vessels to documented reversibly ischaemic myocardium are grafted to keep the cross clamp time short. Moderate and severe mitral regurgitation are corrected and full thickness scar excised where feasible. Those with access to left ventricular assist devices (LVADs) employ these to keep the perioperative mortality below 10–15%.[8] Non-cardiac risk factors for death include great age, female sex, a history of hypertension or chronic obstructive airways disease, and the presence of peripheral vascular disease or renal impairment. In selected patients with hibernating myocardium but poor target vessels to some areas, concomitant transmyocardial laser revascularisation has been shown to improve survival.[9]

Useful data regarding patient selection and outcome for high risk revascularisation have emerged from transplant centres where end stage heart failure patients were selected out for myocardial revascularisation. Hausmann and colleagues in Berlin compared 225 revascularised transplant candidates with 231 others who received a donor organ.[10] The important differences between the groups were the longer duration of symptoms, the presence of right heart failure, and a greater incidence of

previous revascularisation in the heart transplant recipients. Operative risk in the coronary bypass group was significantly higher for those with a greatly increased left ventricular end diastolic pressure (LVEDP) (> 24 mm Hg), a low preoperative cardiac output (< 2.0 l/min/m²), and for patients in NYHA class IV. Hospital mortality was 7.1% for the coronary artery bypass graft (CABG) patients versus 18.2% in the transplant group. There was no significant difference in hospital mortality in patients with LVEF between 10–20% versus those between 20–30%. Survival for the CABG group was 78.9% after six years versus 68.9% in the transplant group. Reinvestigation of CABG patients showed a significant decrease in mean (SD) pulmonary artery pressure from 28.2 (4.7) mm Hg to 21.2 (3.9) mm Hg (p < 0.01). Pulmonary capillary wedge pressure fell from 19.2 (4.3) mm Hg to 13.1 (2.8) mm Hg (p < 0.01). Left ventricular ejection fraction improved from a mean of 0.24 (0.03) to 0.39 (0.06) (p < 0.0001). Others have reported similar findings.[11 12] Table 11.2 provides guidelines suggesting coronary bypass in preference to cardiac transplantation for patients with end stage coronary disease. Table 11.3 summarises the surgical treatment options in end stage ischaemic heart disease.

Left ventricular restoration

Patients with large left ventricular aneurysms gain symptomatic relief from simple linear aneurysmectomy. So called "ventricular restoration" has recently extended from scarred paradoxical segments to akinetic areas which were not previously thought suitable for surgery.[13] The goal of surgical reversal of remodelling is to exclude the infarcted septum and free wall and reshape the left ventricle from globular to elliptical without critically reducing

- High risk (5–15% mortality) revascularisation is the treatment of choice for patients with ejection fraction < 20%, reversible ischaemic cardiomyopathy and graftable target vessels.

- Contraindications to coronary bypass are pulmonary artery pressure > 60 mm Hg, right heart failure, and poor target vessels.

Table 11.3   Decision making in the surgery of end stage ischaemic heart disease

Condition	Intervention
Reversible ischaemia LVESVI < 60ml/m²	CABG alone
Full thickness scar and left ventricular aneurysm	Linear resection ± CABG
Akinetic/dyskinetic left ventricle LVESVI > 60 ml/m² Reversible ischaemia	Surgical remodelling ± CABG
Class III/IV mitral regurgitation	Mitral repair ± CABG
No reversible ischaemia LVESVI > 100 ml/m² Pulmonary hypertension (PAP > 70 mm Hg) Right ventricular failure	Left ventricular assist device or transplantation (no conservative option)

LVESVI, left lentricular end systolic volume index (normal is < 30 ml/m²); CABG, coronary artery bypass grafting; PAP, pulmonary artery pressure.

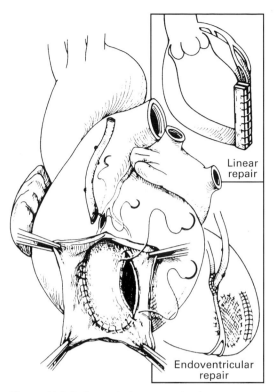

Figure 11.2. Left ventricular restoration by endoventricular patch repair (the Dor procedure) as opposed to simple linear aneurysmectomy.

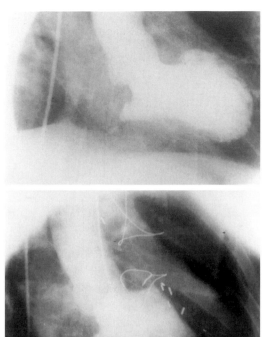

Figure 11.3. The Dor procedure restores an elliptical shape from the globular failing left ventricle (courtesy of Dr Vincent Dor).

cavity volume. This improves global function and arrests progression of left ventricular failure. Ventricular dysrhythmias and mitral regurgitation are addressed during the same procedure.

In the Dor procedure, or the Buckberg modification, the left ventricle is opened through scar and subtotal endocardectomy (fig 11.2), performed over the septum and posterior wall.[14] In the event of recurrent ventricular arrhythmias, cryotherapy is applied at the limits of the resection. The boundary between normal endocardium and scar is defined and a circumferential endoventricular (Fontan) circular suture passed between 1–2 cm outside the limit of healthy muscle. This circular constricting suture is tied to reduce the size of the left ventricle around a balloon inflated within the cavity to a diastolic volume of 50–70 ml/m². The residual apical defect is then closed with a Dacron patch cut according to the circumference of the circular suture after removing the balloon. The technique restores an elliptical shape (fig 11.3) with improved function over the globular failing ventricle. Intraoperative echocardiography has shown a decrease in LVEDV from a mean of 194 ml to 128 ml (p = 0.001) and an improvement in LVEF from a mean of 29% to 41% (p = 0.003). The operation can be performed in patients with very low LVEF (< 20%) and pulmonary hypertension with a hospital mortality of 12–18%. This compares with a 3% mortality for those with ejection fraction > 30%. Most patients improve to NYHA I or II, but 10% of survivors are not improved and about 25% have persistently raised pulmonary artery pressure through impaired diastolic compliance.

Linear left ventricular aneurysm resection and the Dor procedure both improve remote myocardial function secondary to a reduction in wall tension. This "LaPlace" concept was expanded by Batista in his partial left ventriculectomy operation.[15] The much hyped procedure was devised to reduce left ventricular volume and wall stress, thereby improving LVEF and symptomatic status.[16] It was widely adopted as an alternative to transplantation without adequate guidelines or convincing information on sustainability or survival. The technique itself consists of a wedge resection of posterolateral left ventricular wall either between or including the papillary muscles. The incision begins at the apex of the ventricle and extends to within 2–3 cm of the mitral annulus (fig 11.4). Full thickness myocardial excision proceeds irrespective of the coronary anatomy and usually removes the obtuse marginal branches in the circumflex territory. The cavity is then reconstituted along its long axis with a continuous suture.

There is surprisingly little information on the amount of myocardium excised. The Cleveland Clinic group weighed the resected specimen, which ranged from 30–290 g (mean 96 g).[17] The San Paolo group removed a posterolateral segment measuring 10.9 (2) cm × 5 (0.8) cm, equivalent to about 20% of the left ventricular circumference.[18] When the resection includes the base of one or both papillary muscles (88% of cases), the valve is either replaced with a prosthesis or the papillary muscles are reimplanted with transfixion sutures at the margins of the ventriculotomy (fig 11.5). If the mitral subvalvar apparatus is preserved, the free margins of the anterior and posterior leaflets are sewn together to produce

- The goal of left ventricular restoration surgery (Dor procedure) is to reshape (from globular to elliptical) and reorganise the ventricle, not to reduce the volume. Reversible ischaemia, mitral regurgitation, and dysrhythmias should be addressed at the same time.

- Left ventricular end systolic volume index (LVESVI) is a strong predictor of death in heart failure (LVESVI > 60 ml/m² carries a one year mortality of 33%).

- Patients with a good outcome from the Dor operation have an LVESVI > 40 ml/².

- Coronary bypass alone improves ejection fraction only if the preoperative LVESVI is < 100 ml/m².

- Linear left ventricular remodelling (the Batista operation) is unpredictable with an unacceptable early failure rate and late mortality.

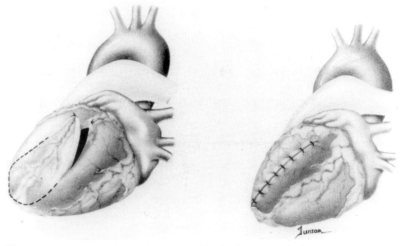

Figure 11.4. Partial left ventriculectomy (the Batista operation).

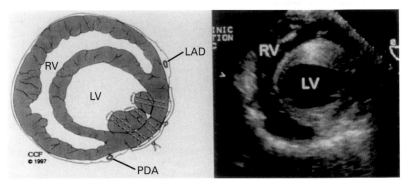

Figure 11.5. Diagrammatic and echocardiographic illustration of the partial left ventriculectomy operation. The mitral subvalvar apparatus is preserved by reimplanting the papillary muscles at the margins of the ventriculotomy.

a double channelled mitral valve (Alfieri method)[19] (fig 11.6). Even published hospital mortality has been prohibitive, ranging from 1.9–27% with an average of 17.4%.[20] Low hospital mortality has been achieved only with the aid of long term LVAD support (20% of patients), and cardiac transplantation.

In survivors, there is a significant decrease in both end diastolic and end systolic volume indices. While LVEF initially improves, restudy at 12 months fails to show significant differences between preoperative LVEF (17.7 (4.6)) and late LVEF (23.7 (6)) in matched patients. The suggested mechanism for improvement in LVEF is reduction of systolic wall stress rather than a change in contractility. There is an inverse relation between the decrease of circumferential end systolic stress and increase in LVEF. In McCarthy's series, mean LVEF improved from 13% to 21% and peak oxygen consumption from 11 ml/kg/min to 16 ml/kg/min at 12 months.[17] Twelve month survival at the Cleveland Clinic was 80% though LVADs were required for bridge to transplantation in 16% of patients. However, freedom from heart failure of any cause (relisting for transplant, death or class IV symptoms) was only 50% by 12 months and 38% at two years.

Though the reduced ventricular geometric dimensions may be sustained up to 12 months (fig 11.7), pump function begins to deteriorate after six months. The first sign is a rise in left atrial pressure. The discrepancy between geometry and sustainability of mechanical function is attributed to the fact that mass reduction causes changes in diastolic compliance.

Though late data are scarce, we defined a 16% mortality from all reported series through progressive heart failure (38%), sudden or arrhythmic death (38%), stroke, transplant heart failure, sepsis or hepatic failure.[20] The procedure has been abandoned in ischaemic cardiomyopathy through a prohibitive incidence of fatal dysrhythmias caused by stretch-

ing of the scar tissue.[21] In reality, most centres who enthusiastically embraced partial left ventriculectomy have now radically cut back operating only on highly selected dilated cardiomyopathy patients. With emerging alternatives the Batista operation is destined to join skeletal muscle cardiomyoplasty in the dustbin of heart failure operations.

Management of mitral regurgitation in heart failure patients

As the failing left ventricle dilates the papillary muscles are displaced, the coaptation of the mitral valve leaflets is decreased, and a central jet of mitral regurgitation appears (fig 11.1). Mitral regurgitation leads to more volume

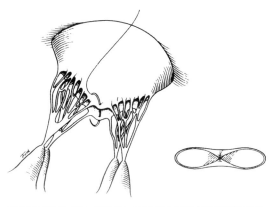

Figure 11.6. The Alfieri suture for mitral regurgitation. This creates a double channel mitral orifice.

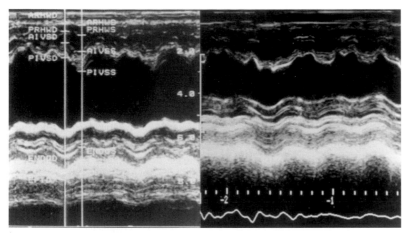

Figure 11.7. One dimensional (M mode) echocardiography showing dramatically improved left ventricular function in an infant six months after partial left ventriculectomy for ischaemic cardiomyopathy in anomalous left coronary artery from the pulmonary artery.

Table 11.4 Mitral valve repair in dilated cardiomyopathy. Left ventricular function and flow before and after annuloplasty

Variable	Preoperatively	Postoperatively	% change*	p Value
End diastolic volume (ml)	335 (107)	307 (103)	18 (9)	0.06
End systolic volume (ml)	227 (101)	237 (98)	−15 (14)	0.03
Stroke volume (ml)	58 (13)	70 (21)	+12 (10)	0.02
Ejection fraction (%)	18 (5)	24 (10)	+31 (24)	0.03
Mitral inflow (l/mm)	12.4 (5.3)	5.4 (0.5)	−49 (22)	0.02
Forward cardiac output (l/min)	3.2 (1.0)	4.7 (0.9)	+52 (38)	0.01
Regurgitant volume (l/min)	9.2 (5.4)	0.8 (0.6)	88.6 (10.1)	0.01
Regurgitant fraction (%)	70 (14)	15 (11)	−79 (15)	<0.001

Values are mean (SD). *Percentage change from preoperative study at 4–6 months postoperatively.
NYHA class fell significantly from 3.9 (0.4) to 1.8 (0.5) (p < 0.001).
Reproduced from Bolling *et al. J Thorac Cardiovasc Surg* 1998;**115**: 381-8. with permission of the publisher.

overload of the already dilated left ventricle. Reports of prohibitive operative mortality for mitral valve replacement in dilated cardiomyopathy patients in the early 1980s suggested that the failing ventricle deteriorates further, if the "blow off" into the left atrium is removed. However, new information shows that mitral valve repair (or replacement) with preservation of the subvalvar apparatus carries low perioperative mortality, good medium term survival, and symptomatic relief through improvement in cardiac index.[22]

There are now a number of clinical situations where mitral valve repair with or without revascularisation improves outlook for the heart failure patient.

These include:
- Ischaemia manifest by angina and variable mitral regurgitation which becomes significantly worse during an acute ischemic episode, causing dyspnoea at rest or left ventricular failure with pulmonary oedema.
- Acute myocardial ischaemia or infarction located inferobasally (right coronary or dominant circumflex distribution) which causes sudden posteromedial papillary muscle dysfunction and mitral regurgitation.
- Acute catastrophic pulmonary oedema caused by papillary muscle rupture (inferobasal in 75% of cases) several days after acute myocardial infarction.
- Chronic progressive dyspnoea (NYHA III or IV) associated with previous myocardial infarction, an enlarged dysfunctional left

ventricle, and varying degrees of pulmonary hypertension. This comprises the largest group.
- Patients with idiopathic dilated cardiomyopathy and annular dilatation producing moderate to severe mitral regurgitation through inadequate leaflet coaptation.

The recommended threshold for mitral repair in ischaemic regurgitation is a left ventricular end systolic volume index > 80 ml/m^2 or a calculated regurgitant fraction > 50% of the forward LVEF. Patients with angina, good target vessels, mild to moderate mitral regurgitation, and reversible ischaemia posterolaterally on the PET scan can be treated by revascularisation alone. Should valve replacement prove necessary, as much of the subvalvar apparatus as possible should be conserved to maintain left ventricular geometry and function. Division of all chordae tendonae is accompanied by a 47% reduction in LVE$_{max}$.

Ischaemic mitral regurgitation is a functional problem of unsuccessful coordination of the entire mitral apparatus rather than simple failure of a single papillary muscle. Two techniques have provided symptomatic improvement in this condition. Firstly, mitral annuloplasty with significant undersizing of the valve ring greatly increases leaflet coaptation.[23] Systolic anterior motion (SAM) is avoided because of widening of the aortomitral angle and increased left ventricular size. The undersized valve ring acutely remodels the base of the myopathic heart, helping to re-establish an ellipsoid shape to the left ventricle. Second, and simpler, is the Alfieri stitch. This can be performed either centrally (fig 11.6) or towards the side of the ischaemic papillary muscle.

Bolling has shown the important effect of mitral repair in patients with end stage dilated cardiomyopathy.[22] All had severe left ventricular systolic dysfunction with preoperative LVEF ranging from 8–25% (mean 16 (3)%). The average duration of cardiomyopathy was 4 (6) years (range 0–16). All patients underwent remodelling ring annuloplasty with an undersized flexible ring. Half had tricuspid annuloplasty. Hospital mortality was < 2% while 12 and 24 month survival were 82% and 72%. All patients were restored to NYHA class I or II with mean postoperative LVEF of 26%. Peak exercise Vo$_2$ max rose from a mean of 14.5 to 18.6 ml/kg/min. Echocardiography at two years showed a pronounced reduction in sphericity, regurgitant volume, and regurgitant fraction. LVEF, end diastolic and end systolic volumes were all improved (table 11.4).

Mechanical blood pumps

Ideal treatment for chronic refractory heart failure should be reliable, cost effective, easy to implement, and capable of providing a physiological level of circulatory support. Existing cardiac support devices such as the pacemaker and implantable defibrillator are already widely accepted for patients of all ages. Within the

74

next 10 years a user friendly miniaturised LVAD is destined to become the treatment of choice to relieve symptoms and prolong life in older heart failure patients.

Total heart replacement became virtually redundant when it was clear that more than 90% of patients could be sustained with left ventricular support alone. Only those with advanced right ventricular pathology or fixed pulmonary hypertension require biventricular support. Those LVADs currently used for bridge to transplantation have their origins in the 1970s and can be regarded as first generation blood pumps. The Novacor (Baxter Health Care, California, USA) and Thermo-Cardio Systems (Woburn, Massachusetts, USA) LVADs consist of a blood sac in series with the native left ventricle and compressed by a pusherplate mechanism, either electrically or pneumatically driven.[24 25] Bioprosthetic heart valves dictate the direction of flow. This mechanism mimics the native left ventricle by providing pulsatile stroke volume with either variable or fixed pump rate. The patients own left ventricle is completely offloaded so that the aortic valve does not open. While large external pneumatic consoles have been replaced by implantable electric systems with portable control and power source, the serious problem of LVAD size, noise, driveline infection, and thromboembolism persist. These devices are unsuitably large for most female patients or children. Nevertheless, some bridge to transplant patients have survived with acceptable quality of life for up to four years.[26]

The new axial flow impeller pumps are the next generation of artificial hearts.[27] In animal studies these compact, silent, non-pulsatile blood pumps provide up to 6 litres flow per minute, without significant haemolysis or thromboembolism. The thumb sized Jarvik 2000 heart fits within the apex of the failing left ventricle and pumps blood to the descending thoracic aorta (fig 11.8).[28] The impeller supported by blood immersed microceramic bearings revolves at up to 18 000 rpm accelerating blood so rapidly through a narrow channel that the cellular components remain undamaged. The controller and batteries are the size of a portable telephone and fit easily onto a normal belt. While transcutaneous power induction is under development, we have devised an infection resistant skull mounted percutaneous titanium pedestal for the first human implants.[29] The extracardiac NASA/de Bakey axial flow pump has already been tested for bridge to transplantation in humans with mixed results owing to mechanical problems.

Other ingenious blood pumps with magnetically suspended rotors (without bearings) are under development. These next generation, fully implantable miniature artificial hearts greatly increase the future scope of circulatory support, but mechanical reliability and freedom from complications remains to be established. We must also define the effects of chronic non-pulsatile blood flow, though the recovering native heart will transmit a pulse through the device. We anticipate that the cost of a blood pump will be less than that of multi-

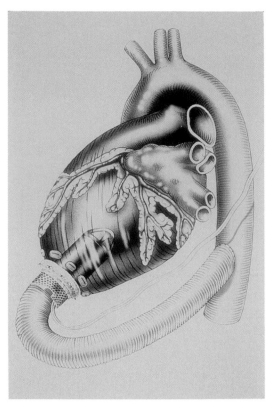

Figure 11.8. The intraventricular "Jarvik 2000 Heart", an axial flow impeller pump which rotates at between 8000 and 18 000 rpm without damaging the blood.

- A realistic blood pump for long term circulatory support must be unobtrusive, silent, mechanically reliable with economic energy consumption, non-thrombogenic, free from constant infection risk and able to provide between 3–10 litres flow per minute without haemolysis. Such devices are now available for human implant.

- In the next 10 years blood pumps will be used for heart failure in the same way that pacemakers and implantable defibrillators are used for dysrhythmia.

ple hospital admissions for stabilisation during the last year of the patient's life. The device will replace most drug treatment and require only a maintenance dose of warfarin.

Reversal of remodelling with an LVAD

One of the revelations of the past five years is the effect of chronic left ventricular offloading on the remodelled left ventricle.[30] Reduction in cardiac workload by strict prolonged bed rest is known to result in functional and symptomatic improvement, though the benefits are limited by the adverse effects of inactivity on the skeletal muscles, vascular tone, and autonomic nervous system. However, when myocardial rest is accompanied by whole body exercise training the combined benefits become apparent. These are the conditions achieved during long term bridge to transplantation with the Thermocardio Systems and Novacor LVADs. The improved systemic blood flow reverses multisystem organ failure and enables resumed physical activity, while the left ventricle is completely offloaded. Renal and hepatic failure improve whereas serum aldosterone concentrations, plasmin renin activity, atrial natriuretic peptide, and norepinephrine concentrations revert to normal.[31] In dilated cardiomyopathy patients bridged to transplantation, left ventricular size regresses with normalisation of pressure volume relations, resolution of left ventricular hypertrophy, and decreased myocytolysis, fibrosis, and apoptosis.[32] Comparison of myocardial biopsies taken at the time of LVAD implantation, then later during transplantation, show regression of myocyte hypertrophy with normalisation of calcium, phospholipid, and fatty acid metabolism. Realisation that recovering hearts were being discarded by transplantation, together with the incontrovertible shortage of organ donors, led to the concept of bridge to myocardial recovery.[33]

Although the scope for bridge to recovery is obvious, there are certain requirements before this strategy has a chance for success. The first is a user friendly LVAD for patients of all sizes. This must be simple to implant and remove without the risk of driveline infection and easy for the patient to control. The axial flow pumps with a skull mounted percutaneous pedestal or transcutaneous power induction are promising in this respect. Second, the LVAD should be employed before diffuse fibrosis renders reversal of ventricular remodelling unachievable.[34] Strategies to promote myocardial recovery with drugs, growth factors, gene therapy, and inhibitors of apoptosis are under investigation and markers for sustainability of recovery explored.[35] In this respect, the Berlin group has used the disappearance from the serum of the autoantibody against the β_2 adrenergic receptor, suggesting that this reflects abatement of the immune process causing functional impairment.[36]

Clinical reports of bridge to recovery demonstrates the importance of myocardial pathology. Patients with acute myocarditis who are in terminal decline can be supported with an LVAD or BIVAD until resolution of the inflammatory process. Even those who require external cardiac massage and conventional cardiopulmonary bypass to sustain life during LVAD implantation can be restored to near normal cardiac function.

In a study of weaning of dilated cardiomyopathy patients from chronic left ventricular support, Muller compared factors which distinguished those with well sustained recovery from others who slipped back into heart failure.[35] Patients with long lasting recovery were younger, had a shorter history of heart failure, had a more rapid improvement in cardiac performance, and needed a shorter duration of LVAD support before cardiac indices justified device removal. The duration over which the autoantibodies disappeared from the serum was shorter (8.8 (2.3) weeks v 9.7 (3.3) weeks, p = 0.0027) in patients with sustainable recovery. Not different were mean age (41.5 (9.9) years v 50.3 (11.2)), mean LVED diameter at the time of device placement (75.2

(7.9) mm v 78.7 (4.8) mm), LVEF (14.8 (2.9)% v 17.0 (2.3)%), and mean LVED diameter two months after LVAD placement (53.7 (6.2) mm v 55.6 (7.2) mm). The Berlin group concluded that an LVAD offloading period of between 8–10 weeks was optimum in patients destined for sustainable recovery, and that longer support could lead to myocyte atrophy. Others have reservations about this limited duration and report success for much longer periods.[1]

Summary

The scope of heart failure surgery is developing rapidly but relies increasingly upon expensive diagnostic techniques and mechanical circulatory support. The major issues are not ethical but economic. New miniature axial flow and centrifugal blood pumps are emerging from bioengineering laboratories and will eventually be used as frequently for heart failure as is the pacemaker for rhythm problems. In the future, new drugs, gene therapy, and autogenous myocyte culture will promote left ventricular repair during circulatory support, thereby freeing the limited number of donor organs for younger complex congenital hearts.

1. **Klein M, Herman M, Gorlin R.** A haemodynamic study of left ventricular aneurysm. *Circulation* 1967;**35**:614–30.

2. **Olivetti G, Abbi R, Quaina F,** *et al.* Apoptosis in the failing human heart. *N Engl J Med* 1997;**336**:1131–41.

3. **Yoshida F, Gould KL.** Quantitative relation of myocardial infarct size and myocardial viability by positron emission tomography to left ventricular ejection fraction and 3 year mortality with and without revascularisation. *J Am Coll Cardiol* 1993;**22**:984–97.

4. **Emond M, Mock MB, Davis KB,** *et al.* Long-term survival of medically treated patients in the coronary artery surgery study (CASS). *Circulation* 1994,**90**:2645–57.

5. **Lee KS, Marwick TH, Cook SA,** *et al.* Prognosis of patients with left ventricular dysfunction, with and without viable myocardium after myocardial infarction. Relative efficacy of medical therapy and revascularisation. *Circulation* 1994;**90**:2687–94.
   • *After myocardial infarction, residual viable but ischaemic myocardium is an unstable substrate for further events. This study shows surgical revascularisation reduces the risk of these events, though age and the severity of left ventricular function remain the best predictor of death.*

6. **Williams MJ, Odabashiar J, Lauer MS,** *et al.* Prognostic value of dobutamine echocardiography in patients with left ventricular dysfunction. *J Am Coll Cardiol* 1996;**27**:132–9.

7. **Di Carli MF, Davidson M, Little R,** *et al.* Value of metabolic imaging with positron emission tomography for evaluating prognosis in patients with coronary artery disease and left ventricular dysfunction. *Am J Cardiol* 1994;**73**:527–33.

8. **Louie HW, Laks H, Milgalter E,** *et al.* Ischemic cardiomyopathy. Criteria for myocardial revascularisation and cardiac transplantation. *Circulation* 1991;**84**:(suppl III):III290–5.

9. **Allen KB, Delrossi EJ, Realyvasquez F,** *et al.* Transmyocardial revascularisation combined with coronary artery bypass grafting versus bypass grafting alone: a prospective randomized multi-centre trial. *J Thorac Cardiovasc Surg* In press.

10. **Hausmann H, Topp H, Siniawski H,** *et al.* Decision making in end stage coronary artery disease: revascularisation or heart transplantation. *Ann Thorac Surg* 1997;**64**:1296–1302.
   • *This paper reviews the outcomes of patients subject to high risk coronary revascularisation or transplantation in a pool of end stage heart failure patients referred for transplantation. Patients with hibernating myocardium treated by coronary bypass had a better long term outlook than those transplanted. The article outlines which patients should undergo coronary bypass in preference to transplantation.*

11 **Kaul TK, Agnihotri AK, Fields BL,** *et al.* Coronary artery bypass grafting in patients with an ejection fraction of twenty per cent or less. *J Thorac Cardiovasc Surg* 1996;**111**:1001–12.

12. **Mickleborough LL, Maruyama H, Yasushi T,** *et al.* Results of revascularisation in patients with severe left ventricular dysfunction. *Circulation* 1995;**92**:(suppl 2):73–9.

13. **Buckberg GD.** Defining the relationship between akinesia and dyskinesia and the cause of left ventricular failure after anterior infarction and reversal of remodelling to restoration. *J Thorac Cardiovas Surg* 1998;**116**:47–9.

14. **Dor V, Sabatier M, DiDonato M,** *et al.* Efficacy of endoventricular patch plasty in large post infarction akinetic scar and severe left ventricular dysfunction: comparison with a series of large dyskinetic scars. *J Thorac Cardiovasc Surg* 1998;**116**:50–9.
• *The Dor procedure remodels the globular failing left ventricle back to an elliptical shape with improved function. This paper describes the functional improvement and outlook for those patients with ischaemic cardiomyopathy.*

15. **Batista RJV, Nery P, Bocchino L,** *et al.* Partial left ventriculectomy to treat end stage heart disease. *Ann Thorac Surg* 1997;**64**:634–8.

16. **Dickstein ML, Spotnitz HM, Rose EA,** *et al.* Heart reduction surgery: An analysis of the impact on cardiac function. *J Thorac Cardiovasc Surg* 1977;**113**:1032–40.

17. **McCarthy PM, Starling RC, Wong J,** *et al.* Early results with partial left ventriculectomy. *J Thorac Cardiovasc Surg* 1997;**114**:755–65.

18. **Moreira LFP, Stolf NAG, Bocchi EA,** *et al.* Partial left ventriculectomy with mitral valve preservation in the treatment of patients with dilated cardiomyopathy. *J Thorac Cardiovasc Surg* 1998;**115**:800–7.

19. **Fucci L, Sandrelli L, Pardini A,** *et al.* Improved results with mitral valve repair using new surgical techniques. *Eur J Cardiothorac Surg* 1995;**9**:621–7.

20. **Katsumata T, Westaby S.** An objective appraisal of partial left ventriculectomy for heart failure. *Journal of Congestive Heart Failure and Circulatory Support* 1999;**1**:97–106.

21. **Bach DS, Bolling SF.** Early improvement in congestive heart failure after correction of secondary mitral regurgitation in end-stage cardiomyopathy. *Am Heart J* 1995;**129**:1165–70.

22. **David TE.** Techniques and results of mitral valve repair for ischemic mitral regurgitation. *J Cardiac Surg* 1994;**9**(suppl):274–7.

23. **McCarthy PM, Portner PM, Tobler HG,** *et al.* Clinical experience with the Novacor ventricular assist system. *J Thorac Cardiovasc Surg* 1991;**102**:573–81.

24. **Frazier OH, Rose EA, MacMannus Q,** *et al.* Multicentre clinical evaluation of the Heartmate 1000 IP left ventricular assist device. *Ann Thorac Surg* 1992;**53**:1080–90.

25. **Frazier OH, Rose EA, McCarthy P,** *et al.* Improved mortality and rehabilitation of transplant candidates treated with a long term implantable left ventricular assist system. *Ann Thorac Surg* 1995;**222**:327–38.

26. **Belland S, Jeevanandam V, Eiser H.** Reduced myocardial matrix metaloproteinase expression as a result of sustained mechanical support with left ventricular assist devices in patients with severe dilated cardiomyopathy [abstract]. *J Heart Lung Transplant* 1998;**17**:84.

27. **Westaby S, Katsumata T, Houel R,** *et al.* Jarvik 2000 Heart—potential for bridge to myocyte recovery. *Circulation* 1998;**98**:1568–74.

28. **Jarvik RK, Westaby S, Katsumata T,** *et al.* LVAD power delivery. A new percutaneous approach to avoid infection. *Ann Thorac Surg* 1998;**65**:470–3.
• *Power line infection is one of the restricting elements which must be overcome before LVADs can be used with widespread efficacy. This short paper describes an innovative method to avoid drive line infection pending the development of transcutaneous power induction.*

29. **Levin HR, Oz MC, Cherr JM,** *et al.* Reversal of chronic ventricular dilation in patients with end stage cardiomyopathy by prolonged mechanical offloading. *Circulation* 1995;**91**:2717–20.

30. **James KB, McCarthy PM, Thomas JD,** *et al.* Effect of the implantable left ventricular assist device on neuroendocrine activation in heart failure. *Circulation* 1995;**92**(suppl II):191–5.

31. **Frazier OH, Benedict CR, Radovancevic B,** *et al.* Improved left ventricular function after chronic left ventricular unloading. *Ann Thorac Surg* 1996;**62**:675–82.

32. **Mann DL, Willerson MD.** Left ventricular assist devices and the failing heart. A bridge to recovery, a permanent assist device or a bridge to far? *Circulation* 1998;**98**:2367–9.

33. **Mancini DM, Beniaminovitz A, Levin H,** *et al.* Low incidence of myocardial recovery after left ventricular assist device implantation in patients with chronic heart failure. *Circulation* 1998;**98**:2383–9.

34. **Kirshenbaum LA, de Moissac D.** The bcl-2 gene product prevents programmed cell death of ventricular myocytes. *Circulation* 1997;**96**:158–5.

35. **Muller J, Wallukat G, Weng Y,** *et al.* Weaning from mechanical support in patients with dilated cardiomyopathy. *Circulation* 1997;**96**:542–9.

36. **Hetzer R, Loebe M, Potapov EV,** *et al.* Circulatory support with pneumatic paracorporeal ventricular assist device in infants and children. *Ann Thorac Surg* 1998;**66**:1498–506.
• *This paper from the Berlin Heart Institute describes their experience of mechanical circulatory support in infants and young children. The very important finding was that infants with myocarditis and terminal circulatory shock could be resuscitated, supported for 2–3 weeks, and eventually have normal hearts after removal of the device.*

SECTION III: CARDIOMYOPATHY

12 The cardiomyopathies: an overview

Michael J Davies

The recent revision (table 12.1) of the definition of a cardiomyopathy by the World Health Organization[1] recognises that ventricular dysfunction can result from a failure to correct volume or pressure overload in valve disease or to control hypertension. Loss of myocardium caused by coronary artery disease also leads to severe ventricular dysfunction. All of these end stage conditions are categorised as specific cardiomyopathies. The second form of cardiomyopathy is caused by intrinsic disorders of the myocardium itself and is subdivided on the basis of the pathophysiology. Such a functional rather than an aetiological classification has drawbacks but reflects our current state of knowledge. The different functional abnormalities produce characteristic changes in ventricular shape easily recognised in short axis echocardiographic planes and by pathologists (fig 12.1).

Table 12.1 *The cardiomyopathies, as defined by the World Health Organization[1]*

Specific (secondary to external processes)	Intrinsic to myocardium
Hypertensive cardiomyopathy	Dilated cardiomyopathy (DCM)
Valvar cardiomyopathy	Hypertrophic cardiomyopathy (HCM)
Ischaemic cardiomyopathy	Arrhythmogenic right ventricular dysplasia
Cardiomyopathy secondary to systemic disease	(ARVD)
Inflammatory cardiomyopathy	Obliterative cardiomyopathy (OCM)

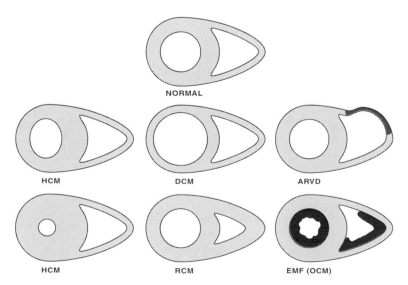

Figure 12.1. The morphological expression of the intrinsic cardiomyopathies as seen in short axis cuts across the right and left ventricle at mid septal level. Hypertrophic cardiomyopathy may be symmetric or asymmetric. HCM, hypertrophic cardiomyopathy; DCM, dilated cardiomyopathy; RCM, restrictive cardiomyopathy; ARVD, arrhythmogenic right ventricular dysplasia; EMF, endomyocardial fibrosis; OCM, obliterative cardiomyopathy,

Structural changes in dilated cardiomyopathy

- Increased left ventricular mass

- Normal or reduced left ventricular wall thickness

- Increased left ventricular cavity size

- Histology
  - myocyte nuclear size increase
  - myofibrillary loss within myocyte
  - focal myocyte death
  - increase in interstitial T lymphocytes/macrophages
  - interstitial fibrosis

Dilated cardiomyopathy

The pathophysiological entity dilated cardiomyopathy (DCM) is heterogeneous with regard both to its pathogenesis and its morphology. Common to the whole group is a poorly contracting dilated left ventricle with a normal or reduced left ventricular wall thickness. The lack of an increase in left ventricular wall thickness tends to mask a significant increase in left ventricular mass. In the terminal stages thrombus may develop in the apices of both ventricles. The histological changes within the myocardium are listed above. The individual myocytes are increased in length rather than in width and lose the normal number of intracellular contractile myofibrils, and thus appear empty and vacuolated on histology (fig 12.2). The degree of this histological change closely correlates with declining left ventricular function. The myocyte nuclei increase in size because of the synthesis of DNA and become polyploid. Death of individual myocytes occurs both by apoptosis and necrosis. Fibrosis characteristically is interstitial and begins to surround and isolate individual myocytes. The number of macrophages and T lymphocytes in the interstitial spaces is often increased compared with normal hearts. All of these histological changes vary widely in degree and type from case to case and give no information on causation.

Pathogenesis of dilated cardiomyopathy

In most cases of DCM no definite cause is identifiable. Some known causes, and some hypotheses, exist. The most prevalent toxic cause of DCM is alcohol. A wide range of structural abnormalities in the myocardium has been associated with high alcohol intake, and it is difficult to define the exact point at which these abnormalities can be called DCM. There is an excess of sudden death in alcoholics with large fatty livers even when the heart appears structurally normal. The spectrum continues through an isolated increase in left

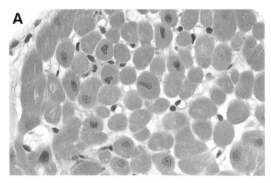
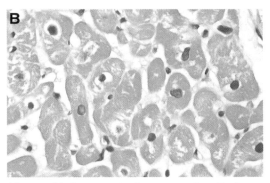

Figure 12.2. Dilated cardiomyopathy. (A) Normal cardiac biopsy, with the myocytes in cross section. Each myocyte has a uniform pink cytoplasm owing to the majority of the cell being filled by myofibrils. (B) Biopsy from a case of DCM. The myocytes have lost myofibrils and empty spaces have appeared within the cytoplasm.

ventricular mass, followed by left ventricular hypertrophy with interstitial fibrosis and fatty change or myofibrillary loss in myocytes, and culminating in fully developed DCM. There are no specific morphological features indicating alcohol as a cause of DCM; the best evidence may come from the results of totally withdrawing alcohol.

Single gene mutations in either the structural proteins of the myocyte, such as dystrophin, metavinculin, and lamin, or of mitochondrial DNA are recognised causes of DCM.[2] The majority of the skeletal muscle dystrophies, including the Duchene and Becker types, may have cardiac involvement. In some families cardiac involvement may be dominant and present first.[3] Knowledge of the genes capable of causing DCM is far less well established than in hypertrophic cardiomyopathy (HCM), but the frequency of familial DCM is increasingly recognised as being far higher than initially realised. As many as 30% of index cases of DCM will have other family members with evidence of left ventricular dysfunction or enlargement on echocardiography.[4]

One view gaining ground is that DCM can be split into groups—one has histological evidence of chronic myocarditis while another group has evidence of viral persistence by polymerase chain reaction (PCR) analysis of myocardial tissue myocardium. Yet another group has neither myocarditis nor viral carriage. The definition of chronic myocarditis[5] is based on an increase in the number of activated chronic inflammatory cells in the interstitial tissues. The cells have to be positively identified by immunohistochemistry as T cells or activated macrophages. More than 14 per square millimetre of myocardium is regarded as positive, particularly when associated with increased expression of class II major histocompatibility complex (MHC) antigens on endothelial and other cells. The hypothesis, as yet unproven by trials, is that each subgroup of DCM needs tailored treatment—that is, interferon, immunosuppression, etc—to improve prognosis. The differentiation of the four possible permutations—viral presence or absence, myocarditis presence or absence—takes sophisticated technology by the laboratory and would not be feasible to carry out in centres taking an occasional cardiac biopsy.

Hand in hand with the concept of chronic myocarditis is the idea that there is evidence of enhanced immune damage in some cases of DCM. Many cases show increased expression of class II antigens in the myocardium, and circulating autoantibodies to a wide range of components of the myocyte are present. Given that in DCM myocyte loss is occurring, the unanswered question is whether these antibodies are the cause of myocyte death or are nothing more than a secondary phenomenon.

Some forms of cardiomyopathy which are difficult to classify may also belong in the DCM group. Patients may present with very mild symptoms and a left ventricle which is dilated. These cases may be early forms of DCM and their frequency is increased in asymptomatic family members of index DCM cases. Myocardial fibrosis may occur without any clear cause, such as coronary disease, and be associated with ventricular arrhythmias rather than left ventricular dilatation and heart failure. Such cases have been equated in the past with healed myocarditis but are increasingly being recognised as familial, although the genes are not identified.

Hypertrophic cardiomyopathy

The heart of a patient with archetypal HCM has an asymmetric or a symmetric increase in left ventricular wall thickness (fig 12.1) with a left ventricular cavity which is reduced in size. A high proportion of cases are now recognised to be caused by mutations in genes coding for myofibrillary proteins. At least nine individual genes coding for different myofibrillary proteins have been identified.[6] Affected individuals are heterozygous and produce a mixture of the normal (known by geneticists as the wild form) protein and abnormal (mutant) protein. The abnormal protein interferes with the organisation or function of the myofibrils within the myocyte producing the histological feature of myocyte disarray (fig 12.3). The unexplained feature is that while some cases appear to have the whole of the left ventricle involved, in others it is confined to a specific region, the most common being anteroseptal close to the left ventricular outflow tract. Other distributions include the posteroseptal region, lateral region,

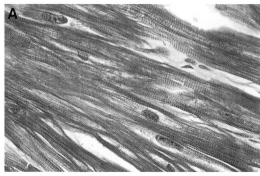

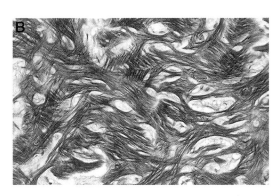

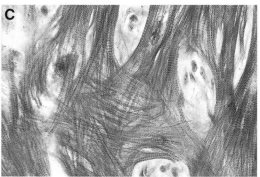

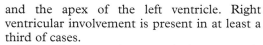

Figure 12.3. Hypertrophic cardiomyopathy. In sections stained to show the myofibrillary structure blue (PTAH stain) in the normal myocardium (A), the myocytes are arranged in parallel, and within the myocyte myofibrils are parallel in the long axis of the cell. Regular cross striations are seen. (B) Myocyte disarray in a case of HCM, with the cells arranged in whorls around foci of connective tissue. (C) Higher power magnification shows the myofibrils within the cell also criss cross and have lost their normal parallel arrangement.

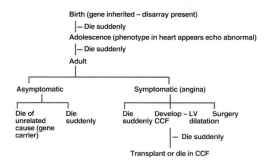

Figure 12.4. The range of natural histories encountered in subjects with HCM caused by myofibrillary gene mutations. CCF, chronic cardiac failure; LV, left ventricular.

and the apex of the left ventricle. Right ventricular involvement is present in at least a third of cases.

Where the upper interventricular septum is involved encroachment of myocardial muscle on the left ventricular outflow tract occurs; this, combined with systolic anterior movement of the mitral valve, leads to contact between the septal endocardium and the anterior cusp. Endocardial thickening develops on the septum as a mirror image of the anterior cusp. This band of severe endocardial thickening, which may be up to 1 cm thick, is removed in subaortic surgical resections. The anterior cusp of the mitral valve develops fibrosis caused by mechanical trauma and incurs a risk of bacterial endocarditis. The genes which cause HCM can be associated with dysplastic changes in the small intramyocardial arteries, significantly reducing the lumen size. These changes may play a role in causing angina and are associated with increasing fibrosis which, over the years, may alter the ventricular shape from HCM to become more like DCM.

An unexplained feature of HCM is the variation in the appearances of the heart (phenotype), even within a family in which all the members have the same gene mutation. The exact mutation does cause some variation in the phenotype. Of the genes so far identified as being responsible for HCM, left ventricular outflow obstruction is a feature of β heavy chain myosin gene mutations while symmetric, rather modest left ventricular wall thickening is found in troponin T mutations. Onset in late adult life is characteristic of myosin binding protein C mutations. The rapid expansion of knowledge concerning the phenotype of the myofibrillary genes creates semantic problems. In troponin T families the left ventricular mass may not be raised and the left ventricular wall thickness may be normal, yet there is myocyte disarray and a risk of sudden death. Thus there is HCM without hypertrophy.

The potential natural history (fig 12.4) of HCM caused by the myofibrillary genes is well known, but it is not easy to predict which path an individual will follow or indeed the frequency of each path in the general community.

HCM is compatible with long life but there is a constant risk of sudden death. Sudden deaths in HCM can occur at any age, from childhood to over 90 years, in subjects who have been asymptomatic all their life. The characteristic morphological changes in ventricular shape in HCM do not develop until early adolescence, making it impossible to identify gene carriers with certainty by echocardiography alone in children.

It is now recognised that cases exist in which there is an increase in left ventricular mass, with striking symmetric or asymmetric left ventricular wall thickening, yet disarray is absent and mutations in the myofibrillary genes are not found. These cases indicate that other genes outside the sarcomeric complex can produce thick walled left ventricles. Mitochondrial gene disorders, glycogen storage disease, and Fabry's disease are among the known causes of the phenomenon.

Restrictive cardiomyopathy

Restrictive cardiomyopathy (RCM), in which the left ventricle is nearly normal in shape but there is a failure of the myocardium to relax in diastole, is one form of cardiomyopathy where cardiac biopsy may help. The most common form is myocardial amyloid. It is usually easy to recognise amyloid on histology by its characteristic green colour under polarised light after staining with Sirius red dye. Amyloid is not, however, evenly distributed in the ventricle and false negatives occur. Some cases develop a florid myocardial fibrotic response masking the amyloid. For these reasons electron microscopy studies of the biopsy may improve the sensitivity. Other causes of restriction include diffuse perimyocyte fibrosis. This pattern of fibrosis is seen to a degree in many cases of DCM, but when in a uniform distribution it appears to cause predominant restriction. The pathogenesis of this form is unknown. Another form of RCM is familial and associated with myocyte disarray on biopsy, but without other clinical or morphological features of HCM. The gene(s) responsible have not yet been identified.

Arrhythmogenic right ventricular dysplasia

First recognised in young subjects with normal exercise tolerance who died suddenly, arrhythmogenic right ventricular dysplasia (ARVD) is characterised by areas in the right ventricle where there is transmural replacement of the myocytes largely by adipose tissue, but with some fibrosis leading to focal areas of aneurysmal dilatation. The first cases recognised were at the extreme end of the spectrum, but family studies[7] and wider clinical studies using magnetic resonance imaging in subjects with unexplained ventricular tachycardia revealed that the areas of abnormality may be small—no more than 1–2 cm across. About a third of cases have concomitant left ventricular involvement with fibrofatty replacement of myocytes, often subpericardial and maximal on the posterior wall. In most but not all cases the myocardial involvement, while acting as a substrate for arrhythmias, does not significantly reduce right or left ventricular contractile function.

In patients with a known family history or with clear ECG and echocardiographic changes suggesting ARVD, cardiac biopsy is a useful confirmatory investigation but is rarely diagnostic in its own right. The focal nature of the disease means false negatives are common, while simple adipose infiltration into the right ventricular myocardium without replacement of myocytes or fibrosis is a common finding in normal subjects, particular women. Biopsy findings of fat in the right ventricular wall can be overinterpreted and lead to false positives. The diagnosis of ARVD has to be based on the concordance of clinical and pathological features.

ARVD is genetic and several sites of candidate genes have been identified on different chromosomes. At present what these genes control or produce is unknown. The histological changes are different from those in DCM because although myocytes are being lost in both conditions, in ARVD there is a predominant replacement by adipose tissue. One suggestion is that in ARVD myocytes are being lost by apoptosis which does not invoke replacement fibrosis. In many cases of ARVD there is an inflammatory cell infiltrate in the abnormal areas of myocardium. This has been interpreted as a myocarditic component but could be a secondary rather than a primary change. Once the candidate genes are identified it may become clear how the phenotype is produced.

The frequency of ARVD is impossible to establish accurately at present because the less striking cases are underdiagnosed both in life and after death. It appears to be a major cause of sudden death in young people in northern Italy, while in the UK HCM remains numerically more important as a cause of sudden death.

Obliterative cardiomyopathy

In this condition thrombus develops on the endocardium of the apex and inflow segments of one or both ventricles. The ventricular cavity begins to be obliterated and the tricuspid and mitral valves are involved. The thrombus undergoes conversion to fibrous tissue as the disease progresses. The ultimate expression is of a small ventricular cavity with massive endocardial thickening by fibrosis leading to the condition known as endomyocardial fibrosis. In temperate climates the disease is caused by endocardial damage resulting from the release of cationic proteins from activated eosinophils in the circulation.[8] In many cases the thrombus is infiltrated by eosinophils but this is not a prerequisite for the condition. Any cause of systemic hypereosinophilia, including eosinophilic leukaemia, Churg Strauss syndrome, Bechet's syndrome, and idiopathic hypereosinophilia, can cause endomyocardial fibrosis. While hypereosinophilia persists and degranulated eosinophils are present in the circulation the deposition of thrombus continues. Cases in which the eosinophilia occurred in a single episode in the past may present at the end stage of the disease, with massive endocardial fibrosis restricting both ventricular contraction and cavity volume. Recognition of the cause can only be made by a history of previous disease likely to be associated with increased eosinophil activation. Decortication of the thick layer of fibrous tissue, with replacement of the mitral or tricuspid valves, may be needed. In tropical countries in Asia, Africa, and South America an identical end stage cardiac disease occurs, but the link to previous hypereosinophilia is less well established, and other factors such as nutritional deficiency or ingestion of unknown toxins are widely debated as causes.

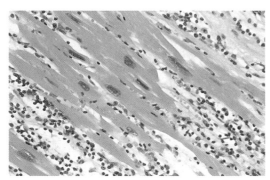

Figure 12.5. Acute myocarditis. There is a heavy but focal increase of lymphocytic cells in the interstitial tissues of the myocardium.

Inflammatory cardiomyopathy (myocarditis)

The clinical picture of acute myocarditis is characterised by the rapid onset of cardiac failure or arrhythmias, or both, with fever, malaise, myalgia, and sometimes pericarditis; it has a morphological counterpart (Dallas criteria)[9] of myocyte necrosis, usually in a multifocal but sometimes regional distribution, with a heavy interstitial infiltrate of T lymphocytes (fig 12.5). In practice the characteristic morphology occurs only in fatal and severe cases, and biopsy of the myocardium often shows no evidence of the typical tissue changes despite a confident clinical diagnosis of acute myocarditis. The reported positivity rate varies from centre to centre but is usually no more than 10%. In biopsy positive cases of myocarditis there is no clear evidence that immunosuppression is beneficial with regard to outcome. The biopsy negative but clinically positive cases create a diagnostic challenge and are likely to be heterogeneous in origin. Some may be genuine cases of myocarditis, but the biopsy is taken after the T lymphocyte infiltrate has cleared. Other cases may reflect the limitations of cardiac biopsy because with a focal disease the sample taken may come from an area of normal myocardium.

A significant number of cases of clinically suspected myocarditis prove to have interstitial fibrosis and therefore represent longstanding disease. A factor such as viral infection may have precipitated non-specifically the onset of symptoms as the first presentation of DCM. In the absence of any current evidence that treatment other than supportive therapy for cardiac failure will improve prognosis, it is not clear whether myocardial biopsy will give any data of value for treating individual subjects. Centres carrying out large numbers of cardiac biopsies to elucidate the mechanisms of cardiac disease for the future have more justification for biopsy.

Viral infection and acute myocarditis

The major cause of acute myocarditis is perceived to be viral, involving in particular the coxsackie group of viruses. This is based on very well established links between viruses and acute myocarditis in animals such as mice (coxsackie) and dogs (parvovirus). What occurs in other animals is likely to occur in man. Coxsackie genomic material is found in about a third of human cases of acute myocarditis using PCR technology on myocardial tissue. The younger the subject the more likely is virus to be found. One facet of viral myocarditis in experimental animals is that viral replication ceases before the myocyte damage occurs. It is therefore rarely possible to culture replicating virus from the heart. The same is true of human acute myocarditis, and diagnosis has to be based on PCR on cardiac tissue and rising titres in sequential serology.

It is probable that human myocarditis can be caused by viruses other than those from the coxsackie group, and the adeno group is beginning to be seen as potentially cardiotoxic. A very wide range of viruses such as those responsible for chicken pox, measles, rubella, and mumps often cause a minor degree of what is taken to be myocarditis based on ECG changes. A small subgroup of myocarditis may be caused by non-viral organisms, such as the spirochaete *Borrelia burgdorferi* in Lyme disease, toxoplasma, and leptospira, while in South America *Trypanosoma cruzi* is by far the most common cause of the acute myocarditis of Chagas' disease.

Patients with biopsy positive or negative myocarditis may die in the acute phase or recover. Recovery is usually complete although there are a few reported cases of slow progression into DCM. Trials are underway to investigate the possibility that cases in which virus can be detected by PCR on biopsy tissue have a different pattern of behaviour and prognosis, and should be treated with interferon.

The Dallas criteria for acute myocarditis on cardiac biopsy defined the need for severe myocyte damage plus a T lymphocyte interstitial inflammatory cell infiltrate. A form of myocarditis occurs in which myocyte damage is mild or absent but there is a florid interstitial inflammatory cell infiltrate of a more pleomorphic type containing plasma cells and eosinophils. This form of chronic myocarditis may be associated with ventricular arrhythmias rather than cardiac failure. Its pathogenesis is unknown but drug hypersensitivity has been implicated in some cases.

Giant cell myocarditis

Myocardial involvement by sarcoid has a range of patterns.[10] There may be a diffuse distribution of giant cell granulomas or a single regional mass of sarcoid tissue which is initially expanded in volume, but as fibrosis develops the mass shrinks and may develop into a ventricular aneurysm. Cardiac biopsy to diagnose myocardial sarcoid in a subject with chronic arrhythmias can give a specific positive diagnosis but the false negative rate is high.

A different form of idiopathic giant cell myocarditis[11] occurs as an acute onset disease with very severe cardiac failure leading to death within a week unless cardiac transplantation is available. There are irregular areas of myocardial necrosis, at the margins of which are large giant cells but no organised granulomas such as occur in sarcoid. No virus has been implicated. The only known association is with autoimmune disease and thymomas, although the majority of cases occur suddenly in subjects who have no other pre-existing disease. Recurrence of the giant cell myocarditis in donor hearts can occur.

1. **Richardson P.** Report of the WHO/ISFC task force on the definition and classification of cardiomyopathy. *Circulation* 1996;**93**:341–2.
• *For better or worse this is the latest revision of nomenclature in the cardiomyopathy field and legitimises the term when applied to end stage cardiac failure in ischaemic or valve disease. Intrinsic myocardial disease remains classified by pathophysiology not aetiology.*

2. **Graham RM, Owens WA.** Pathogenesis of inherited forms of dilated cardiomyopathy. *N Engl J Med* 1999;**341**:1759–62.
• *A review of the current state of knowledge concerning gene mutations that cause DCM.*

3. **Politano L, Nigro V, Nigro G,** *et al.* Development of cardiomyopathy in female carriers of Duchenne and Becker muscular dystrophies. *JAMA* 1996;**275**:1335–8.

4. **Michels W, Mills P, Miller F,** *et al.* The frequency of familial dilated cardiomyopathy in a series of patients with idiopathic dilated cardiomyopathy. *N Engl J Med* 1992;**326**:77–82.

5. **Kuhl U, Noutsias M, Seeberg B,** *et al.* Immunological evidence for a chronic intramyocardial inflammatory process in dilated cardiomyopathy. *Heart* 1996;**75**:295–300.
• *A review of the myocardial changes in DCM that could indicate there is a chronic myocarditis/autoimmune element to the disease.*

6. **Bonne G, Carrier L, Richard P,** *et al.* Familial hypertrophic cardiomyopathy: from mutations to functional defects. *Circ Res* 1998;**83**:580–93.
• *A review of the mutations in sarcomeric protein genes and the mechanisms by which clinical disease is produced.*

7. **Corrado D, Basso C, Thiene G,** *et al.* Spectrum of clinicopathologic manifestations of arrhythmogenic right ventricular cardiomyopathy/dysplasia: a multicenter study. *J Am Coll Cardiol* 1997;**30**:1512–20.
• *A comprehensive review of the cardiac phenotype of ARVD based on a multicentre study in Europe and showing that left ventricular involvement also occurs.*

8. **Chusid M, Dale D, West B,** *et al.* The hypereosinophilic syndrome: analysis of fourteen cases with review of the literature. *Medicine* 1975;**54**:1–28.

9. **Mason J.** Endomyocardial biopsy—the balance of success and failure. *Circulation* 1985;**71**:185–8.

10. **Silverman K, Hutchins G, Bulkley B.** Cardiac sarcoid: a clinicopathological study of 84 unselected patients with systemic sarcoidosis. *Circulation* 1978;**58**:1204–11.

11. **Cooper LT Jr, Berry GJ, Shabetai R.** Idiopathic giant-cell myocarditis—natural history and treatment. Multicenter giant cell myocarditis study group investigators. *N Engl J Med* 1997;**336**:1860–6.

13   Diagnosis and management of dilated cardiomyopathy

Perry Elliott

Dilated cardiomyopathy is a heart muscle disorder defined by the presence of a dilated and poorly functioning left ventricle in the absence of abnormal loading conditions (hypertension, valve disease) or ischaemic heart disease sufficient to cause global systolic impairment. A large number of cardiac and systemic diseases can cause systolic impairment and left ventricular dilatation, but in the majority of patients no identifiable cause is found—hence the term "idiopathic" dilated cardiomyopathy (IDC). There are experimental and clinical data in animals and humans suggesting that genetic, viral, and immune factors contribute to the pathophysiology of IDC.

Diagnosis

Clinical presentation

The first presentation of IDC may be with systemic embolism or sudden death, but patients more typically present with signs and symptoms of pulmonary congestion and/or low cardiac output, often on a background of exertional symptoms and fatigue for many months or years before their diagnosis. Intercurrent illness or the development of arrhythmia, in particular atrial fibrillation, may precipitate acute decompensation in such individuals. Increasingly, IDC is diagnosed incidentally in asymptomatic individuals during routine medical screening or family evaluation of patients with established diagnosis.

A careful family history facilitates diagnosis of inherited causes of IDC by characterising the family phenotype, and also defines the scope of family screening.[1] At least 25% of patients have evidence for familial disease with predominantly autosomal dominant inheritance. Clinically, familial disease is defined by the presence of two or more affected individuals in a single family and should also be suspected in all patients with IDC and a family history of premature cardiac death or conduction system disease. A further 20% of relatives have isolated left ventricular enlargement that can progress to IDC in a minority of cases. Dilated cardiomyopathy can occur in a number of X linked diseases such as Becker's and Duchenne's muscular dystrophies and X linked IDC. It may also occur in patients with mitochondrial DNA mutations and inherited metabolic disorders. Thus when taking a family history, specific attention should be given to a history of muscular dystrophy, features of mitochondrial disease (for example, familial diabetes, deafness, epilepsy, maternal inheritance), and signs and symptoms of other inherited metabolic diseases. Inborn errors of metabolism usually present in infancy and childhood, but some may present in adulthood, in particular haemochromatosis. Nutritional deficiencies and endocrine abnormalities may produce heart failure, and a complete drug history is essential, both in relation to the administration of cardiotoxic drugs such as anthracyclines and with respect to the use of illegal substances. Cocaine abuse, in particular, can produce a chronic IDC picture as well as an acute cardiomyopathy. Exposure to HIV and other infectious agents such as hepatitis C may be relevant in some patients.

Causes of dilated cardiomyopathy

Young

- Myocarditis (infective/toxic/immune)
- Carnitine deficiency
- Selenium deficiency
- Anomalous coronary arteries
- Arteriovenous malformations
- Kawasaki disease
- Endocardial fibroelastosis
- Non-compacted myocardium
- Calcium deficiency
- Familial IDC
- Barth syndrome

Adolescent/adults

- Familial IDC
- X linked
- Alcohol
- Myocarditis (infective/toxic/immune)
- Tachycardiomyopathy
- Mitochondrial
- Arrhythmogenic right ventricular cardiomyopathy
- Eosinophilic (Churg Strauss syndrome)
- Drugs—anthracyclines
- Peripartum
- Endocrine
- Nutritional—thiamine, carnitine deficiency, hypophosphataemia, hypocalcaemia

Electrocardiography

The ECG in patients with IDC may be remarkably normal, but abnormalities ranging from isolated T wave changes to septal Q waves in patients with extensive left ventricular fibrosis, prolongation of atrioventricular (AV) conduction, and bundle branch block may be observed. Sinus tachycardia and supraventricular arrhythmias are common, in particular atrial fibrillation. Approximately 20–30% of patients have non-sustained ventricular tachycardia and a small number present with sustained ventricular tachycardia.

Echocardiography

An echocardiogram is essential for the diagnosis of IDC (fig 13.1). In patients with poor echo windows other imaging modalities such as radionuclide scans and magnetic resonance may be useful. Recently suggested echocardiographic criteria for IDC are shown in the adjacent box. When making the diagnosis of IDC it is important to take into account sex and body size. The most widely applied criteria in family studies are based on the Henry formulae, with a left ventricular cavity dimension of > 112% of predicted normal values used to define left ventricular enlargement and a shortening fraction of < 25% defining abnormal systolic function. These criteria have some limitations, in particular the use of only short axis dimensions and a relatively low specificity in young patients, but they are practical and reproducible. Recent European guidelines have suggested that when screening family members a more conservative cut off of > 117% of predicted values (2 SD plus 5%) should be used in order to increase specificity.[1]

Exercise testing

Symptom limited upright exercise testing is of considerable value when assessing functional limitation in patients with IDC, particularly when combined with respiratory gas analysis. Metabolic exercise testing provides an objective measure of exercise capacity, facilitates assessment of disease progression, helps assess prognosis, and is useful in selecting patients for cardiac transplantation. Metabolic exercise testing may also provide diagnostic information in patients with left ventricular impairment caused by primary metabolic abnormalities such as mitochondrial disease, by detecting severe acidaemia.

Viral serology

In children and adults with acute myocarditis, viral culture and serology may be useful in establishing a diagnosis of viral myocarditis by demonstrating rising titres of neutralising antibodies, or virus specific IgM class antibodies to enteroviruses indicative of recent infection. In adults with IDC the relation between viral infection and disease is more uncertain. Many studies purporting to demonstrate a positive association between viral infection and IDC are very small, and have failed to control for cross contamination with laboratory controls.[2] The source of disease and control populations is also important as the most commonly impli-

---

Diagnostic criteria for IDC

Ejection fraction < 0.45 and/or a fractional shortening of < 25%, and a left ventricular end diastolic dimension of > 112% predicted value corrected for age and body surface area.

Exclusion criteria:

- Absence of systemic hypertension (> 160/100 mm Hg)

- Coronary artery disease (> 50% in one or more major branches)

- Chronic excess alcohol (> 40 g/day female, > 80 g/day male for more than five years after six month abstinence

- Systemic disease known to cause IDC

- Pericardial diseases

- Congenital heart disease

- Cor pulmonale

Key

The criteria for left ventricular enlargement are based on data of Henry *et al* (*Circulation* 1980;**62**:1054–61). A value of > 112% of predicted represents 2 SDs from the mean corrected for body surface area and age given by the formula:

$(45.3 \times (\text{body surface area})^{1/3} - (0.03 \times \text{age}) - 7.2) \pm 12\%.$

Mestroni *et al* have suggested a more conservative cut off of > 117% (2 SDs + 5%) in order to increase specificity for family studies.[1] However, a value of 112% is probably just as predictive of disease if systolic function is also abnormal.

---

cated enterovirus, coxsackie B, is ubiquitous in most communities and causes small subclinical epidemics. At present, the detection of viral antibodies in patients with stable chronic IDC has little impact on management, but viral studies may become more important in the future if current trials suggest a role for immunosuppressive/modulatory treatments in IDC.

Endomyocardial biopsy

Although endomyocardial biopsy can be used to diagnose a wide range of myocardial diseases, most are rare causes of IDC and can often be diagnosed by other means. Even the detection of an inflammatory cardiomyopathy is of limited use, given the uncertainties and inconsistencies surrounding its diagnosis using conventional light microscope criteria. Endomyocardial biopsy may be of use in selected patients—for example, those with suspected cardiac haemochromatosis and other infiltrative or malignant diseases—but in general it should be confined to carefully conducted clinical trials. A number of immunohistological studies have already demonstrated increased numbers of T cells and increased expression of endothelial and interstitial MHC (major histo-

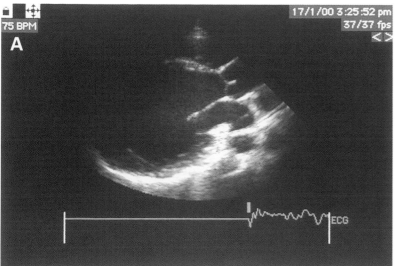

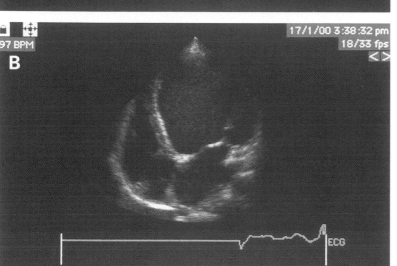

Figure 13.1. Parasternal long axis (A) and apical four chamber (B) cross sectional (two dimensional) echocardiograms in a 23 year old patient with IDC.

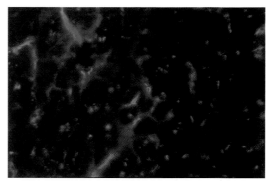

Figure 13.2. Myocardial section from a patient with IDC stained for the intercellular adhesion molecule 1 (ICAM-1) (green) and factor VIII (red). Dual staining in yellow indicates the presence of endothelial ICAM activity, indicative of chronic low grade inflammation. Reproduced with permission from Professor Michael Davies.

compatibility complex) antigens and cell adhesion molecules in IDC hearts, consistent with previous observations of immune activity in IDC (fig 13.2).[3] As our understanding of the clinical significance of immunohistochemical markers improves, it is likely that endomyocardial biopsy will become more important in guiding immunomodulatory treatment.

Treatment

Specific treatments are not available for most patients with IDC. Therefore, the primary aims of treatment are to control symptoms and to prevent disease progression and complications such as progressive heart failure, sudden death, and thromboembolism. Diuretics remain central to the management of congestive symptoms, but they should not be used as monotherapy as they exacerbate neurohumoral activation and may contribute to disease progression unless administered concomitantly with neurohumoral antagonists.

Recommended tests in adult patients with IDC

- Erythrocyte sedimentation rate (ESR)

- Creatine kinase (CK)

- Viral serology (if acute presentation)

- Renal function

- Liver function tests/calcium

- Serum ferritin/iron/transferrin

- Thyroid function tests

Only in specific indications:

- Coronary angiography

- Blood
    - autoantibodies
    - carnitine
    - lactate/pyruvate
    - selenium
    - pyruvate
    - acylcarnitine profile
    - drug screen
    - red cell transketolase (beri beri)
    - infective screen (HIV/hepatitis C, enteroviruses)

- Urine
    - organic acid/amino acids

- Skeletal muscle biopsy

- Endomyocardial biopsy

Angiotensin converting enzyme inhibitors

Activation of the renin–angiotensin–aldosterone system (RAAS) is central to the pathophysiology of heart failure of whatever underlying aetiology. For this reason, angiotensin converting enzyme (ACE) inhibitors are the mainstays of treatment in patients with IDC, irrespective of the severity of heart failure.[4] ACE inhibitors improve dyspnoea and exercise tolerance, reduce hospitalisation rates, and reduce cardiovascular mortality. They also prevent or slow disease progression in asymptomatic patients. A substantial proportion of patients who are given ACE inhibitors fail to reach the target doses reported in randomised studies. Recent evidence from the ATLAS study[5] suggests that maximum recommended doses of lisinopril (32.5–35 mg) are as well tolerated as low doses (2.5–5 mg), and are associated with a 12% greater reduction in the combined risk of death or hospitalisation. Although the comparative benefit of intermediate doses is still uncertain, it seems prudent to try to achieve recommended target doses in most patients.

Significant side effects are uncommon during ACE inhibitor treatment, the most frequent being hypotension, cough, and deterioration of renal function. Mild impairment of renal function (creatinine up to 265 µmol/l) in the absence of renal artery stenosis is not, however, an absolute contraindication for ACE inhibition. Similarly, a resting systolic pressure of 80–90 mm Hg during treatment is acceptable in the absence of postural symptoms. When side effects are problematic, the first step is to consider reducing the dose of other medications. In particular, diuretic doses can often be reduced in patients who no longer have congestive symptoms. When ACE inhibitors have to be discontinued, hydralazine–nitrate combination can be useful in treating congestive symptoms.

Angiotensin II receptor antagonists

Angiotensin II (AII) receptor antagonists have recently attracted much interest and controversy with regard to their place in the heart failure therapeutic armoury. AII receptor antagonists have haemodynamic effects broadly similar to those of ACE inhibitors, but may be slightly better tolerated and at least theoretically overcome the "escape" of angiotensin system blockade observed in some patients on ACE inhibitors. However, unlike ACE inhibitors, AII receptor antagonists do not inhibit bradykinin metabolism and thus lack a potentially beneficial vasodilatory effect. The ELITE-1 study[6] suggested that losartan may have a greater effect on mortality than captopril in elderly patients with mild to moderate heart failure. Preliminary data from the follow up to this study have failed to demonstrate a superior effect of losartan over captopril, but the study was not powered to detect equivalence between the two drugs. The recent RESOLVD study[7] has suggested that combination treatment with an ACE inhibitor and an AII antagonist may be more beneficial in reducing neurohumoral activation and in preventing ventricular remodelling than either drug alone. A number of trials (VALHEFT, CHARM) are currently addressing these and other issues regarding AII receptor treatment.

β Blockers

In spite of ACE inhibitor treatment, mortality continues to be high in patients with heart failure. This is perhaps not surprising given that ACE inhibitors act on only one aspect of the neurohumoral cascade (RAAS) that contributes to progressive left ventricular dysfunction. It has been recognised for some time that excess sympathetic activity contributes to the clinical syndrome of heart failure, but it was only recently that use of β blockers in heart failure patients gained widespread acceptance. Three recent multicentre placebo controlled studies, the US carvedilol studies,[8] CIBIS II (bisoprolol),[9] and MERIT-HF (metoprolol),[10] have demonstrated substantial reductions in sudden death and death from progressive heart failure in patients with predominantly New York Heart Association (NYHA) class II and III symptoms treated with β blockers. In CIBIS II and MERIT-HF, but not the US carvedilol study, subgroup analysis suggested a greater effect in patients with ischaemic heart failure compared to "non-ischaemic" heart failure. Nevertheless, when taken together with earlier studies, these data suggest that it is advisable to consider β blockers in IDC patients with mild to moderate symptoms in spite of maximal treatment with ACE inhibitors. Patients should not be started on β blockers if they have signs or symptoms of decompensated heart failure, and initial doses should be low (carvedilol 3.125 mg twice daily, bisoprolol 1.25 mg once daily, metoprolol SR 12.5 mg once daily). Doses should be increased gradually every 2–4 weeks, monitoring closely for hypotension, bradycardia or worsening heart failure until the target dose is achieved or side effects occur.

Spironolactone

High plasma concentrations of aldosterone are frequent in patients with moderate to severe heart failure and contribute to sodium retention, potassium loss, sympathetic activation, myocardial fibrosis, and baroreceptor dysfunction. ACE inhibition usually results in only a transient decrease in aldosterone concentrations, probably because a major source of aldosterone is reduced hepatic clearance rather than angiotensin dependent adrenal secretion. The recent RALES study[11] has shown that the addition of 25 mg of spironolactone to conventional treatment in patients with an ejection fraction < 35% and a history of NYHA class IV heart failure is associated with a 30% reduction in the overall risk of death. Hospitalisation rates for cardiac causes and functional status also improved, and serious hyperkalaemia was infrequent in patients with a serum creatinine < 221 µmol/l. The drug should be considered in all patients presenting with moderate to severe heart failure symptoms.

Novel potential pharmacological treatments

Natriuretic peptides

Atrial natriuretic peptide (ANP) is released from atrial myocytes in response to stretch, and induces diuresis, naturesis, vasodilatation, and suppression of the renin–angiotensin system. Circulating concentrations of ANP are increased in congestive cardiac failure and correlate with NYHA functional class and prognosis. Both ANP and brain natriuretic peptide are potent vasodilators and diuretics, but clinical trials have shown that tolerance frequently develops during intravenous ANP administration. This problem may be overcome by the development of drugs that inhibit neutral endopeptidase, the enzyme responsible for breakdown of natriuretic peptides.

Cytokine antagonists

Tumour necrosis factor α (TNFα) or cachectin is a proinflammatory cytokine released from activated macrophages, T cells, and failing myocardium. It circulates at high concentrations in patients with congestive cardiac failure and in experimental models causes pulmonary oedema, cardiomyopathy, cachexia, and reduced peripheral blood flow. Raised plasma concentrations of TNFα and other proinflammatory cytokines such as interleukin 6 have been interpreted as epiphenomena of heart failure, but it is increasingly thought that cytokines may promote heart failure progression. The experience with TNFα antagonists in heart failure is limited, but there are intriguing data on pentoxyfilline, a xanthine derivative that suppresses TNFα production,[12] and etanercept, a soluble P75 tumour necrosis factor receptor that binds irreversibly with TNFα.[13] Etanercept is currently being evaluated in two large multicentre studies (RENAISSANCE and RECOVER).

Endothelins are another family of locally acting peptides with profound vasoconstrictor effects found in high plasma concentrations in patients with heart failure. Experimental data using the endothelin antagonist bosentan have shown favourable haemodynamic effects in heart failure patients, although the drug is associated with dose related hepatic dysfunction, prompting the investigation of more selective endothelin antagonists.

Anticoagulants

Although the annual risk of thromboembolism in patients with IDC is relatively low, many patients are young and are exposed to an appreciable cumulative risk of systemic embolisation. At present there are no trial data to guide anticoagulant treatment in IDC, but warfarin is advised in patients with a history of thromboembolism or evidence of intracardiac thrombus. Patients with more than moderate ventricular dilatation and moderate to severe systolic dysfunction should also be advised to take warfarin.

Management of arrhythmia in IDC

There are substantial limitations to most currently available antiarrhythmic drugs in IDC, in particular their negative inotropic and proarrhythmic effects. Evidence from studies showing increased mortality in patients with advanced heart failure treated with class I agents suggest that these drugs should not be used to prevent arrhythmias of any origin in IDC except in an emergency. Two large scale trials have evaluated amiodarone in IDC, but only one, GESICA,[14] has demonstrated an improvement in overall prognosis. The second study, CHF-STAT,[15] did not demonstrate an improvement in overall survival, but there was a non-significant trend towards improved survival in patients with "non-ischaemic" cardiomyopathy. Dofetilide,[16] a more recently developed class III agent, has a neutral effect on overall survival but does reduce the incidence of atrial fibrillation. These data suggest that class III agents can be safely used to treat or prevent symptomatic supraventricular arrhythmias in IDC, but they cannot be recommended for sudden death prophylaxis. There are as yet no large scale randomised data of implantable cardioverter defribrillator (ICD) treatment in IDC, but it is reasonable to consider ICDs in patients with sustained haemodynamically unstable ventricular tachycardia/fibrillation. The role of ICDs in patients without symptomatic ventricular arrhythmia will hopefully be answered by ongoing trials (for example, SCD-HEFT).

Non-pharmacological treatment of advanced heart failure

Heterotopic heart transplantation is still the cornerstone of advanced heart failure management in patients with intractable heart failure symptoms and end stage disease. However, transplantation remains limited by the scarcity of suitable organs and the development of graft vasculopathy. In response to this dilemma several novel approaches are being evaluated.

Partial left ventriculectomy ("Batista" procedure)

Partial left ventriculectomy is based on the hypothesis that as wall tension is related to left ventricular diameter (Laplace's law), reducing the left ventricular size by excision of a portion of its circumference should reduce wall stress and improve ventricular haemodynamics. In the best centres results from this intervention were initially remarkably good given the nature of the procedure. It is clear, however, that even with careful patient selection many patients survive only with the benefit of left ventricular assist devices and subsequent transplantation.[17] Late sudden death is also described in a proportion of survivors. The difficulties associated with patient selection and subsequent postoperative care suggest that, at best, this form of treatment will be confined to a very small number of experienced centres.

Left ventricular assist devices

Left ventricular assist devices (LVADs) have recently received approval from the US Food and Drug Administration for use in patients with end stage heart failure as a bridge to cardiac transplantation. Experience in patients with IDC suggests that LVAD treatment can result in an apparent improvement in left ventricular function that may persist when the device is removed. However, there are as yet no reliable markers that distinguish the minority of patients that sustain useful recovery from the majority that deteriorate following explantation of the device. Technical advances in LVAD design now raise the possibility of using these devices as an alternative to transplantation in patients who are not transplant candidates. This mode of treatment is currently being evaluated in the REMATCH study,[18] which if positive will have substantial clinical and resource implications for centres managing advanced heart failure.

Multisite ventricular pacing

Many patients with advanced IDC have abnormal left ventricular activation that in turn results in prolonged and incoordinate ventricular relaxation. In some patients ventricular conduction delay is also associated with prolongation of atrioventricular conduction, resulting in a loss of atrioventricular synchrony and a predisposition to prolonged functional mitral regurgitation. Dual chamber pacing has been advocated as a method for restoring AV synchrony and improving left ventricular coordination in patients with severe congestive heart failure. Although initially favourable haemodynamic results using conventional right ventricular pacing were not confirmed by later studies, there has been a more consistent response in studies that have used biventricular pacing, the outcome depending critically on the native QRS duration and the paced AV delay.[19] Patients should be considered for biventricular pacing if they have QRS duration greater than 150 ms, PR interval prolongation, and symptoms refractory to conventional medical treatment.

Immunomodulation/immunosuppression

While there is considerable evidence to suggest that autoimmunity plays a significant role in the pathophysiology of IDC, there has been little evidence to suggest that immunosuppressive treatment is of any benefit. This lack of response is, perhaps, not that surprising given the limitations of criteria used to select patients for treatment in immunosuppresive studies and the heterogeneity of the underlying aetiology of the condition. Immunosuppression is also a rather indiscriminate weapon, as it may suppress potentially beneficial immune responses such as neutralising antibody production in patients with chronic viral myocarditis. New approaches to the diagnosis of chronic myocarditis and the treatment of inflammatory cardiomyopathy should improve this situation. There are already interesting preliminary data suggesting that high dose immunoglobulin[20] and immunoadsorption may result in short term improvement in left ventricular performance in patients with dilated and peripartum cardiomyopathy.

Trial acronyms

ATLAS: Assessment of Treatment with Lisinopril And Survival

CHARM: Candesartan in Heart Failure Assessment of Reduction in Mortality and Morbidity

CHF-STAT: Congestive Heart Failure: Survival Trial of Antiarrhythmic Therapy

CIBIS: Cardiac Insufficiency Bisoprolol Study

ELITE: Evaluation of Losartan in the Elderly study

GESICA: Grupo de Estudio de la Sobrevida en la Insuficiencia Cardiaca en Argentina

MERIT-HF: Metoprolol CR/XL Randomized Intervention Trial in Heart Failure

RALES: Randomized Aldactone Evaluation Study

RECOVER: Research into Etanercept: Cytokine Antagonism in Ventricular Dysfunction

REMATCH: Randomized Evaluation of Mechanical Assistance Therapy as an Alternative in Congestive Heart Failure

RENAISSANCE: Randomized Enbrel North American Strategy to study Antagonism of Cytokines

RESOLVD: Randomized Evaluation of Strategies for Left Ventricular Dysfunction

SCD-HEFT: Sudden Cardiac Death in Heart Failure Trial

VALHEFT: Valsartan Heart Failure Trial

The future

IDC is a disease of diverse causes and pathophysiology. Among the many challenges facing clinicians treating patients with the disorder are the detection of early disease, the identification of the predominant mechanism of left ventricular dysfunction, and the development of treatments that target the initiating mechanism of disease. Nevertheless, there have been major advances in our understanding of the genetic and immunological basis of IDC, and recent advances in the pharmacotherapy of heart failure have substantially improved the outlook for many patients. The rapid pace of current research and the development of new treatments for the management of both early and late disease augur well for the future.

1. **Mestroni L, Maisch B, McKenna WJ**, et al. Collaborative research group of the European human and capital mobility project on familial dilated cardiomyopathy. Guidelines for the study of familial dilated cardiomyopathies. Eur Heart J 1999;**20**:93–102.
• The inherited nature of IDC is often overlooked in the management of patients with IDC. This paper provides a set of practical guidelines for the clinical diagnosis of gene carriers.

2. **Baboonian C, Treasure T.** Meta-analysis of the association of enteroviruses with human heart disease. Heart 1997;**78**:539–43.
• This review discusses some of the potential reasons for the wide range of estimates for viral infection in patients with IDC. In many cases methodological considerations are just as important as genuine variation in the incidence of viral infection.

3. **Noutsias M, Seeberg B, Schultheiss H-P,** *et al.* Expression of cell adhesion molecules in dilated cardiomyopathy. Evidence for endothelial activation in inflammatory cardiomyopathy. *Circulation* 1999;**99**:2124–31.
- *The identification of immune activation in patients with IDC is likely to be of increasing importance in the diagnosis of disease in patients and their relatives. In particular it may help to identify patients who might benefit from immunomodulatory treatments.*

4. **European Society of Cardiology.** The treatment of heart failure. The task force of the working group on heart failure of the European Society of Cardiology. *Eur Heart J* 1997;**18**:736–53.
- *General review and guidelines for the management of congestive cardiac failure. These guidelines do not take into account recent data on β blockers, All receptor antagonists, and spironolactone.*

5. **Packer M, Poole-Wilson P, Armstrong P,** *et al.* The ATLAS study group 1. Comparative effects of low and high doses of the angiotensin-converting enzyme inhibitor, lisinopril, on morbidity and mortality in chronic heart failure. *Circulation* 1999;**100**:2312.
- *This paper shows that high dose ACE inhibitor treatment is superior to low dose with regard to hospitalisation rates for heart failure. The study did not evaluate moderate doses, but the paper provides clear evidence that it is desirable to aim as close as possible to maximum recommended doses of ACE inhibitors in heart failure patients.*

6. **Pitt B, Segal R, Martinez F, Meurers G,** *et al.* Randomised trial of losartan versus captopril in patients over 65 with heart failure (evaluation of losartan in the elderly study, ELITE). *Lancet* 1997;**349**:747–52.
- *First large study to demonstrate that angiotensin II antagonists are tolerated at least as well as ACE inhibitors. The trial also suggested that mortality was lower in the losartan group, but the trial was not powered to make this observation.*

7. **McKelvie RS, Yusuf S, Pericak D,** *et al.* Comparison of candesartan, enalapril and their combination in congestive cardiac failure. Randomized evaluation of strategies for left ventricular dysfunction (RESOLVD) pilot study. The RESOLVD pilot study investigators. *Circulation* 1999;**100**:1056–64.
- *This study suggests that the combination of an ACE inhibitor and an All receptor antagonist may be more effective than either agent alone in reducing neurohumoral activation and in preventing ventricular remodelling. Large scale trials are now underway to investigate this hypothesis.*

8. **Packer M, Bristow MR, Cohn JN,** *et al.* The effect of carvedilol on morbidity and mortality in patients with chronic heart failure. US carvedilol heart failure study group. *N Engl J Med* 1996;**334**:1349–55.
- *Although this study was in fact a composite of four smaller studies, the results of carvedilol treatment were impressive with a dramatic 65% reduction in mortality risk and a 38% reduction in the risk of death or hospitalisation. Similar reductions in mortality have now been observed with metoprolol and bisoprolol.*

9. **CIBIS-II Investigators.** The cardiac insufficiency bisoprolol study II (CIBIS-II): a randomised trial. *Lancet* 1999;**353**:9–13.
- *This study enrolled 2647 patients with stable class III/IV symptoms and ejection fraction less than 0.35. Bisoprolol treatment (target dose 10 mg) was associated with a mortality rate of 11.8% compared to 17.3% in the placebo arm.*

10. **MERIT-HF Investigators.** Effect of metoprolol CR/XL in chronic heart failure: metoprolol CR/XL randomised intervention trial in congestive heart failure (MERIT-HF). *Lancet* 1999;**353**:2001–7.
- *This study enrolled 3911 patients with stable class II–IV symptoms and ejection fraction less than 0.40. Mortality in the 1990 patients that received metoprolol CR/XL (target dose 200 mg) was 7.2% compared to 11% (p = 0.00009).*

11. **Pitt B, Zannad F, Remme WJ,** *et al.* The effect of spironolactone on morbidity and mortality in patients with severe heart failure. Randomized aldactone evaluation study investigators. *N Engl J Med* 1999;**341**:709–17.
- *First large scale study to show that aldosterone antagonism in patients with class III/IV symptoms already taking ACE inhibitors is associated with a substantial reduction in mortality. The benefit occurred with low dose treatment, without a high incidence of hyperkalaemia.*

12. **Sliwa K, Skudicky, Candy G,** *et al.* Randomised investigation of effects of pentoxifylline on left ventricular performance in idiopathic cardiomyopathy. *Lancet* 1998;**351**:1091 3.

- *Placebo controlled double blind study of 28 patients with idiopathic dilated cardiomyopathy. Treatment with pentoxifylline, an inhibitor of TNFα production, was associated with improvement in functional class, ejection fraction, and a reduction in TNFα concentrations.*

13. **Deswal A, Bozkurt B, Seta Y,** *et al.* Safety and efficacy of a soluble P75 tumor necrosis factor receptor (Enbrel, etanercept) in patients with advanced heart failure. *Circulation* 1999;**99**:3224–6.
- *Etanercept is a soluble P75 TNFα receptor fusion protein that binds to and inactivates circulating TNFα. In this study a single intravenous infusion resulted in improvement of six minute walk, ejection fraction, and quality of life score for two weeks. Etanercept is now being studied in large scale multicentre studies.*

14. **Dovai H, Nul D, Grancelli H,** *et al.* Gruppo de Estudio de la Sobrevida en la Insuficiencia en Argentina (GESICA). Randomised trial of low-dose amiodarone in severe congestive heart failure. *Lancet* 1994;**344**:493–8.
- *In this study, 516 patients with congestive cardiac failure were randomised to either placebo or amiodarone 300 mg daily. Amiodarone was associated with a 28% reduction in relative risk. Only 12 patients had to discontinue the drug because of side effects.*

15. **Massie BM, Fisher SG, Radford M,** *et al.* Effect of amiodarone on clinical status and left ventricular function in patients with congestive heart failure. CHF-STAT Investigators. *Circulation* 1996;**93**:2128–34.
- *In this study, 674 patients with class II–IV heart failure were randomised in a double blind fashion to either amiodarone or placebo. Amiodarone was associated with an improvement in ejection fraction, and a significant reduction in the composite end point of hospitalisation and cardiac death in patients with non-ischaemic heart failure. Compared to GESICA, many more patients in this study were withdrawn from treatment because of side effects. The difference in outcome may be explained by many factors including inclusion criteria, sex differences, prevalence of non-sustained ventricular tachycardia, and the aetiology and severity of heart failure.*

16. **Torp-Pedersen C, Moller M, Bloch-Thomsen P,** *et al.* The Danish investigations of arrhythmia and mortality on dofetilide study group. Dofetilide in patients with congestive heart failure and left ventricular dysfunction. *N Engl J Med* 1999;**341**:857–65.
- *This study demonstrates that dofetilide, a novel class III antiarrhythmic drug, is effective in reducing the incidence of atrial fibrillation in patients with congestive cardiac failure. The drug is limited by the requirement for in-hospital initiation of treatment in order to monitor for QT prolongation and torsades de pointes ventricular tachycardia.*

17. **McCarthy JF, McCarthy PM, Starling RC,** *et al.* Partial left ventriculectomy and mitral valve repair for end-stage congestive cardiac failure. *Eur J Cardiothorac Surg* 1998;**13**:337–43.
- *In this study 57 patients, 95% of whom had IDC and were listed for transplantation, underwent partial left ventriculectomy, together with mitral valve repair in 55 patients. Seventeen patients required left ventricular assist device rescue and only 50% were free from death or transplantation at one year. Seven patients died late after surgery.*

18. **Rose EA,** *et al.* The REMATCH trial: rationale, design, and end-points. *Ann Thorac Surg* 1999;**67**:723–30.
- *This paper outlines the rationale behind the REMATCH study. In particular it discusses the difficulties in adapting the now commonplace clinical trial model used in heart failure trials to the evaluation of surgical treatments.*

19. **Auricchio A, Stellbrink C, Block M,** *et al* for the Pacing Therapies for Congestive Heart Failure Study Group. The guidant heart failure research group. Effect of pacing chamber and atrioventricular delay on acute systolic function of paced patients with congestive heart failure. *Circulation* 1999;**99**:2993–3001.
- *Study demonstrating the beneficial effects of biventricular pacing in patients with heart failure. The major predictor of success is QRS duration.*

20. **McNamara D, Rosenblum W, Janosko K,** *et al.* Intravenous immune globulin in the therapy of myocarditis and acute cardiomyopathy. *Circulation* 1997;**95**:2476–8.
- *In this study, high dose immunoglobulin was given to 10 adults hospitalised with class III/IV heart failure. Of the nine patients that left hospital there was an improvement in functional class and ejection fraction. This was not a randomised trial and requires evaluation in a large scale randomised study.*

website extra

Additional references appear on the Heart website

14 Arrhythmogenic right ventricular cardiomyopathy: diagnosis, prognosis, and treatment

Domenico Corrado, Cristina Basso, Gaetano Thiene

Arrhythmogenic right ventricular cardiomyopathy (ARVC) is a myocardial disease, often familial, that is characterised pathologically by fibrofatty replacement of the right ventricular myocardium, and clinically by ventricular arrhythmias of right ventricular origin which may lead to sudden death, mostly in young people and athletes.[1-5] The term "dysplasia" was originally used to describe an entity that was considered to be the result of a developmental defect of the right ventricular myocardium.[1] A better understanding of clinical manifestations as well as morphologic findings does not support the theory of a congenital absence of the myocardium, but is in keeping with a non-ischaemic, ongoing atrophy of the right ventricular myocardium, most likely genetically determined, which becomes symptomatic in adolescents and young adults.[2-4] On the basis of its nature of progressive heart muscle disease of unknown aetiology, ARVC has been more appropriately included among the cardiomyopathies in the recent classification proposed by the task force of the World Health Organization/International Society and Federation of Cardiology. Although several theories have been advanced, the aetiopathogenesis of ARVC is still unknown.[5]

Pathologic features

The most striking pathologic feature of ARVC is the diffuse or segmental loss of the myocardium of the right ventricular free wall and its replacement by fibrofatty tissue (fig 1); it is frequently transmural and accounts for aneurysmal dilations of the diaphragmatic, apical, and infundibular regions (so called "triangle of dysplasia") in nearly 50% of the cases in the necropsy series.[2-4] A wave front progression of the pathological process occurs from the subepicardium to the endocardium, so that residual myocardium is confined to the inner subendocardial layer and to the trabeculae of the right ventricle, where islands of surviving myocardial cells are scattered throughout the fibrofatty tissue. Patchy acute myocarditis with myocyte death and round cell (mostly T lymphocytes) inflammatory infiltrates are present in nearly two thirds of the cases.

Two morphological variants of ARVC have been reported.[2] The *fatty* form is exclusively confined to the right ventricle and involves predominantly the apical and infundibular regions. It is characterised by partial or almost complete substitution of the myocardium by fatty tissue without wall thinning (4–5 mm). There is evidence of myocardial degeneration and death in about half of the cases, in the absence of significant fibrous tissue and inflammatory infiltrates. The left ventricle and the interventricular septum are typically spared. In the *fibrofatty* variant the adipose infiltration is associated with significant replacement type fibrosis, thinning of the right ventricular wall (< 3 mm) (fig 14.1A), aneurysmal dilatation, and inflammatory infiltrates. There is usually involvement of the diaphragmatic wall underneath the posterior leaflet of the tricuspid valve; the left ventricle and, more rarely, the ventricular septum may be involved to a lesser extent.

The replacement of the right ventricular myocardium by fibrofatty tissue has been related to three basic mechanisms[3]:
- Apoptosis or programmed cell death;
- Inflammatory heart disease with a spectrum of clinical presentations ranging from acute myocarditis to fibrous healing, which in severe forms may involve both right and left ventricles and may lead to congestive heart failure mimicking dilated cardiomyopathy;
- Myocardial dystrophy which might reflect a genetically determined atrophy.

In this setting, a genetic propensity to infectious and/or immune reaction may explain the occurrence of myocarditis.

Clinical diagnosis

The most common clinical manifestations of ARVC consists of ventricular arrhythmias with left bundle branch block (LBBB) morphology, ECG depolarisation/repolarisation changes mostly localised to right precordial leads, and global and/or regional dysfunction and structural alterations of the right ventricle.[1-6] However, patients with a clinical diagnosis of ARVC based on typical findings, such as right precordial ECG changes, right ventricular arrhythmias, and structural and functional right ventricular abnormalities, represent only one extreme of the disease spectrum. A number of cases are not recognised because they are asymptomatic until the first presentation with cardiac arrest or are difficult to diagnose through conventional non-invasive methods. In this regard, a prospective investigation on sudden death in the young in the Veneto region of Italy showed that nearly 20% of fatal events in young people and athletes were caused by concealed ARVC. At the other extreme of the spectrum are patients in whom the diagnosis of ARVC was not recognised at the onset of their symptoms, who present in later years with congestive heart failure with or without ventricular arrhythmias, and are often misdiagnosed as having dilated cardiomyopathy.[4]

Standardised diagnostic criteria have been proposed by the study group on ARVC of the working group on myocardial and pericardial disease of the European Society of Cardiology

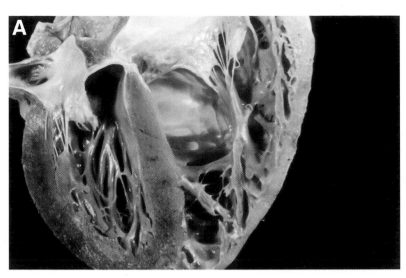

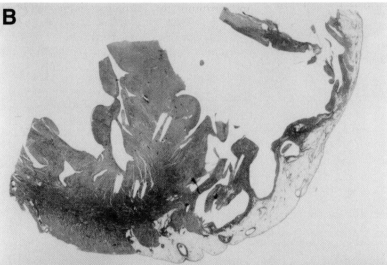

Figure 14.1. Morphologic features in a 25 year old man who died suddenly from arrhythmogenic right ventricular cardiomyopathy. (A) Four chamber view cut of the heart specimen showing the transmural fatty replacement of the right ventricular free wall and the translucent infundibulum. (B) Panoramic histologic view of the same heart confirming that the myocardial atrophy is confined to the right ventricle and substantially spares the interventricular septum as well as the left ventricular free wall (trichrome Heidenhain × 3). Reproduced from Basso C, Corrado D, Rossi L, et al. Morbid anatomy. In: Nava A, Rossi L, Thiene G, eds. Arrhythmogenic right ventricular cardiomyopathy—dysplasia. Elsevier, Amsterdam 1997, pp 71-86, with permission of the publisher.

and of the scientific council on cardiomyopathies of the International Society and Federation of Cardiology.[6] This task force was established because it was realised that the diagnosis of ARVC may be difficult because of several problems with the specificity of the ECG abnormalities, the different potential aetiologies of ventricular arrhythmias with an LBBB morphology, with the assessment of the right ventricular structure and function, and with the interpretation of endomyocardial biopsy findings. According to the task force guidelines, the diagnosis of ARVC is based on the presence of major and minor criteria encompassing genetic, electrocardiographic, arrhythmic, morphofunctional, and histopathologic factors (table 14.1). Based on this classification the diagnosis of ARVC would be fulfilled in the presence of two major criteria or one major plus two minor or four minor criteria from different groups. Although these guidelines represent a useful clinical approach to ARVC diagnosis, optimal assessment of diagnostic

criteria requires a prospective evaluation from a large patient population.

Genetics
A familial background have been demonstrated in nearly 50% of ARVC cases, with an autosomal dominant pattern of inheritance.[5 7] The involved genes and the molecular defects causing the disease are still unknown. However, seven ARVC loci have been identified so far, two of which are in close proximity of chromosome 14 (14q23-q24 and 14q12-q22),[8] and the others on chromosome 1 (1q42-q43), chromosome 2 (2q32.1-q32.2), chromosome 3 (3p23), and chromosome 10 (p12-p14). An autosomal recessive variant of ARVC that is associated with palmoplantar keratosis and woolly hair (so called "Naxos disease") has been mapped on chromosome 17. Genes encoding for actinin and keratin have been considered as potential candidates for the dominant and recessive variant of ARVC, respectively. It is noteworthy that in the Padua experience about 50% of the ARVC families undergoing clinical and genetic screening did not show linkage with any of the known chromosomal loci. Therefore, further genetic heterogeneity can be postulated. Although a preclinical diagnosis of ARVC by DNA characterisation is warranted, at the present time a genetic test for screening is not currently available.

Depolarisation/repolarisation abnormalities
ECG abnormalites are detected in up to 90% of ARVC patients.[5] The most common abnormality consists of T wave inversion in the precordial leads exploring the right ventricle (V1–V3) (fig 14.2). Inversion of T waves is often associated with a slight ST segment elevation (< 0.1 mV). These repolarisation changes are not specific and are considered only minor diagnostic criteria because they may be a normal variant in females and in children aged less than 12 years, or may be secondary to a right bundle branch block, either isolated or in the setting of a congenital heart disease accounting for a right ventricular overload.

The wide spectrum of ECG abnormalities reflecting a delayed right ventricular activation includes complete or incomplete right bundle branch block, prolongation of right precordial QRS duration, and postexcitation epsilon waves—that is, small amplitude potentials occurring after the QRS complex at the beginning of the ST segment. Correlation between surface ECG and epicardial mapping has shown that these ECG changes reflect an intraventricular myocardial ("parietal block") defect rather than a specialised conduction system ("septal block") conduction defect.[9] Both right precordial QRS prolongation and epsilon waves are deemed major diagnostic criteria. Localised prolongation of QRS complex in V1–V3 to more than 110 ms is a relatively sensitive and specific diagnostic marker; it mostly accounts for the QT dispersion across the 12 leads which has been reported to relate to the risk of sudden death. Epsilon waves are uncommon on standard 12 lead ECGs but can be detected in over 30% of ARVC patients in the form of late potentials by high resolution ECG and signal averaging techniques. Late potentials are fragmented low amplitude potentials in the terminal portion of the QRS complex. They reflect areas of slow intraventricular conduction which may predispose to re-entrant ventricular arrhythmias. The underlying substrate consists of islands of surviving myocardium interspersed with fatty and fibrous tissue, accounting for fragmentation of the electrical activation of the ventricular myocardium. In ARVC, late potentials are not specific for re-entrant ventricular arrhythmias and are better correlated with the extension of right ventricular involvement and with the disease progression over the time. Recently, a relation between late potentials, amount of replacement-type fibrous tissue, and degree of right ventricular dysfunction has been reported. Less common ECG abnormalities include P waves exceeding 2.5 mV in amplitude, low voltage QRS complex in peripheral leads, and T wave inversion in the inferior leads.

Ventricular arrhythmias

Although there are some asymptomatic ARVC patients who are recognised by chance or in the setting of a family screening, the most usual clinical presentation of the disease is as symptomatic ventricular arrhythmias of right ventricular origin, which characteristically occur during exercise. Related symptoms consist of palpitations, presyncope, and syncope. Ventricular arrhythmias range from isolated premature ventricular beats (fig 14.2) to sustained ventricular tachycardia (VT) with an LBBB morphology, or ventricular fibrillation (VF) leading to sudden cardiac arrest. The QRS morphology and the mean QRS axis during VT reflects its site of origin: an LBBB with inferior axis suggests the right ventricular outflow tract, while an LBBB with superior axis suggests the right ventricular inferior wall. It is not uncommon for patients with advanced ARVC to show several morphologies of VT, suggesting multiple right ventricular arrhythmogenic foci. VTs with LBBB pattern are not specific for ARVC.

In the presence of right ventricular tachycardias, the following structural heart disease characterised by right ventricular involvement should be ruled out before considering the diagnosis of ARVC: congenital heart disease, such as repaired tetralogy of Fallot, Ebstein anomaly, atrial septal defect, and partial anomalous venous return; acquired disease such as tricuspid valve disease, pulmonary hypertension, and right ventricular infarction; and bundle branch re-entry complicating a dilated cardiomyopathy. Once underlying structural right ventricular disease is excluded, the differential diagnosis should include a Mahaim pre-excited atrioventricular re-entry tachycardia or an idiopathic right ventricular outflow tract tachycardia. It is often difficult to differentiate ARVC from the latter condition, which is usually benign and non-familial. It is still debated whether right ventricular outflow

Table 14.1   Criteria for diagnosis of arrhythmogenic right ventricular cardiomyopathy (ARVC)[6]

I. Family history
   Major
      Familial disease confirmed at necropsy or surgery
   Minor
      Family history of premature sudden death (< 35 years) caused by suspected ARVC
      Family history (clinical diagnosis based on present criteria)

II. ECG depolarisation/conduction abnormalities
   Major
      Epsilon waves or localised prolongation (≥ 110 ms) of the QRS complex in the right precordial leads (V1–V3)
   Minor
      Late potentials seen on signal averaged ECG

III. ECG repolarisation abnormalities
   Minor
      Inverted T waves in right precordial leads (V2 and V3) in people >12 years and in the absence of right bundle branch block

IV. Arrhythmias
   Minor
      Sustained or non-sustained left bundle branch block type ventricular tachycardia documented on the ECG, Holter monitoring or during exercise testing
      Frequent ventricular extrasystoles (more than 1000/24 hours on Holter monitoring)

V. Global and/or regional dysfunction and structural alterations*
   Major
      Severe dilatation and reduction of right ventricular ejection fraction with no (or only mild) left ventricular involvement
      Localised right ventricular aneurysms (akinetic or dyskinetic areas with diastolic bulgings)
      Severe segmental dilatation of the right ventricle
   Minor
      Mild global right ventricular dilatation and/or ejection fraction reduction with normal left ventricle
      Mild segmental dilatation of the right ventricle
      Regional right ventricular hypokinesia

VI. Tissue characteristics of walls
   Major
      Fibrofatty replacement of myocardium on endomyocardial biopsy

*Detected by echocardiography, angiography, magnetic resonance imaging, or radionuclide scintigraphy.

tract tachycardia represents a minor form of ARVC, as suggested by the right ventricular structural abnormalities often detected by magnetic resonance imaging (MRI).

The true incidence of VF leading to sudden cardiac arrest in patients with ARVC remains unknown because many cases are discovered only at post mortem. VF is relatively rare in patients with known ARVC undergoing medical treatment of symptomatic ventricular tachycardia, although some cases of rapid, haemodynamically unstable or prolonged VT may degenerate into VF. On the other hand, abrupt VF is the most likely mechanism of instantaneous sudden death in previously asymptomatic young people and athletes with concealed ARVC.[10] Whether VF in this subset

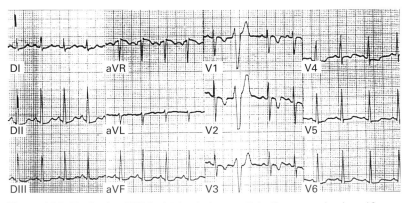

Figure 14.2. Twelve lead ECG obtained at preparticipation screening in a 19 year old football player who subsequently died from ARVC during a competitive game. Note the typical abnormalities consisting of inverted T waves from V1 to V4 and isolated premature ventricular beats with an LBBB morphology.

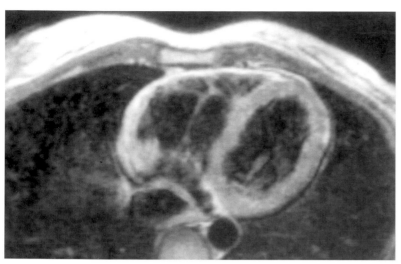

Figure 14.3. MRI findings in a 22 year old woman with a history of dizziness and sustained ventricular tachycardia with an LBBB pattern. Short axis view showing a dilated right ventricle with a brighter signal from a thin anterior free wall. Reproduced from Menghetti L, Basso C, Nava A, et al. Spin-echo nuclear magnetic resonance for tissue characterisation in arrhythmogenic right ventricular cardiomyopathy. Heart 1996;76:467–70, with permission of the publisher.

of patients is related to an acute phase of disease progression, either because of myocyte necrosis–apoptosis or inflammation, remains to be established.

Imaging of right ventricular morphofunctional abnormalities

Demonstration of right ventricular morphofunctional abnormalities by echocardiography, angiography, and MRI is a major criterion for diagnosing ARVC.[5] Functional and structural abnormalities consist of global right ventricular dilatation with or without ejection fraction reduction and left ventricular involvement; segmental right ventricular dilatation with or without dyskinesia (aneurysms and bulgings); and wall motion abnormalities such as ipoakinesia or dyskinesia.

All the imaging techniques are associated with significant limitations in the diagnostic accuracy for detecting right ventricular changes. Right ventricular angiography is usually regarded as the gold standard for the diagnosis of ARVC. Angiographic evidence of akinetic or dyskinetic bulgings localised in infundibular, apical, and subtricuspidal regions has a high diagnostic specificity (over 90%).[11] Large areas of dilatation akinesia with an irregular and "mamillated" aspect, most often involving the inferior right ventricular wall, are also significantly associated with the diagnosis of ARVC. However, considerable interobserver variability regarding the visual assessment of right ventricular wall motion abnormalities by contrast angiography have been reported.

Compared with right ventricular angiography, echocardiography is a non-invasive and widely used technique, and represents the first line imaging approach in evaluating patients with suspected ARVC or in screening family members. Echocardiography also allows serial examinations aimed to assess the disease progression during the follow up of affected patients. Furthermore, echocardiography is a reliable technique for differential diagnosis of ARVC by easily ruling out other right ventricular diseases such as Ebstein anomaly, atrial septal defect, etc. Other than a visual assessment of wall motion and structural abnormalities, a quantitative echocardiographic evaluation of the right ventricle, including measurements of end diastolic cavity dimensions (inlet, outlet, and mean ventricular body), wall thickness, volume, and function, is mandatory in order to enhance the diagnostic accuracy. In the presence of the typical echocardiographic features, contrast angiography or MRI may be avoided, whereas borderline or apparently normal findings in patients with suspected disease requires further examination.

MRI is an attractive imaging method because it is non-invasive and has the unique ability to characterise tissue, specifically by differentiating fat from muscle.[12] Recent studies have shown several limitations and a high degree of interobserver variability in the MRI assessment of free wall thinning and fatty deposition that are the most characteristic structural changes (fig 14.3). The right ventricular free wall is only 4–5 mm thick and the motion artifacts often result in insufficient quality/spectral resolution to quantify right ventricular wall thickness accurately. The normal presence of epicardial and pericardial fat also makes identification of true intramyocardial fat difficult. Some areas—such as the subtricuspidal region—are not easily distinguished from the atrioventricular sulcus which is rich in fat. There has been recent emphasis on functional methods such as right ventricular volume estimation with cine MRI. This approach also permits accurate assessment of right ventricular wall motion abnormalities and focal areas of dilatation with or without dyskinesia. In conclusion, although MRI is a promising technique for delineating right ventricular anatomy and function, as well as for characterising the composition of the right ventricular wall, its diagnostic sensitivity and specificity still need to be defined since the quality of images detected are, at the present time, largely subject to individual interpretation.

Radionuclide angiography is also an accurate non-invasive imaging technique for detection of global right ventricular dysfunction and regional wall motion abnormalities; its diagnostic concordance with right ventricular angiography is nearly 90%.

The diagnosis of ARVC at its early stages or in its concealed variants remains a clinical challenge by all imaging methods. Although these techniques appear to be accurate in detecting right ventricular structural and functional abnormalities in overt forms of ARVC, they are less sensitive in detecting subtle lesions.

Endomyocardial biopsy

A definitive diagnosis of ARVC relies on the histological demonstration of full thickness substitution of the right ventricular myocardium by fatty or fibrofatty tissue at postmortem examination. Transvenous endomyocardial biopsy has the potential for an "in vivo" demonstration of typical fibrofatty replacement of the right ventricular muscle and may increase the accuracy for the clinical diagnosis of ARVC, even though it has several diagnostic limitations. The sensitivity of endomyocardial biopsy is low owing to the segmental nature of the ARVC lesions and because the samples are usually taken from the septum for safety reasons, a region uncommonly involved by the disease. On the other hand, there is difficulty in differentiating ARVC from other causes of fatty infiltration of the right ventricular myocardium. In healthy subjects, particularly in the elderly, there is a normal amount of subepicardial adipose tissue which reflects the physiologic process of progressive involution of the right ventricle. Pathologic conditions which have been associated with fatty infiltration include chronic consummation of alcohol and inherited myopathies such as Duschenne/Backer muscular dystrophy. On the other hand, fibrosis can be observed in many cardiomyopathic and non-cardiomyopathic conditions. Histomorphometric criteria have been advanced in order to enhance the specificity of histopathologic diagnosis of ARVC at endomyocardial biopsy. A percentage of fat > 3% and of fibrous tissue > 40% with amounts of myocytes < 45% was considered a clear cut diagnostic border between ARVC and normal hearts or dilated cardiomyopathy.[13] Although biopsy cannot be routinely recommended, it represents a histologic validation of clinical findings and may improve the diagnostic accuracy by excluding other cardiomyopathy or myocarditis conditions, both idiopathic and specific.

Prognosis

Natural history

The natural history of ARVC is predominantly related to the ventricular electrical instability which can precipitate arrhythmic cardiac arrest at any time during the disease course. Moreover, there is clinical and pathological evidence that ARVC is a progressive heart muscle disease. Long term follow up data from clinical studies indicate that the right ventricle may become more diffusely involved with time.[14] Later in the natural history, the left ventricle may be progressively affected with subsequent biventricular failure. Recently a multicentred clinicopathologic investigation was carried out to define further the anatomoclinical profile of ARVC, with special reference to disease progression and left ventricular involvement.[4] By examining 42 affected whole hearts, including those removed at transplant, and correlating pathologic findings with the patient's clinical history, the study demonstrated that at least in this subgroup, representing an extreme of the disease spectrum, ARVC can no longer be regarded as an isolated disease of the right ventricle. Macroscopic or histologic involvement of the left ventricle was found in 76% of hearts with ARVC; it was age dependent, more common in patients with longstanding clinical history, and it was progressive as evaluated by serial echocardiographic examinations. Moreover, left ventricular

lesions were associated with clinical arrhythmic events, more severe cardiomegaly, inflammatory infiltrates, and heart failure.

At present, there is limited information about the clinical outcome of ARVC patients with overt disease and significant ventricular arrhythmias, and even less on asymptomatic affected family members. The following clinicopathologic phases can be considered[5]:

- "Concealed" phase characterised by subtle right ventricular structural changes, with or without minor ventricular arrhythmias, during which sudden death may occasionally be the first manifestation of the disease, mostly in young people during competitive sports or intense physical exercise.
- "Overt electrical disorder" in which symptomatic right ventricular arrhythmias possibly leading to sudden cardiac arrest are associated with overt right ventricular functional and structural abnormalities.
- "Right ventricular failure" caused by the progression and extension of right ventricular muscle disease that provokes global right ventricular dysfunction with a relatively preserved left ventricular function.
- Final stage of "biventricular pump failure" caused by pronounced left ventricular involvement. At this stage, ARVC mimics biventricular dilated cardiomyopathy of other causes leading to congestive heart failure and related complications such as atrial fibrillation and thromboembolic events.

Risk stratification

The main objective of management strategy is to prevent arrhythmic sudden death. However, there are no prospective and controlled studies assessing clinical markers which can predict the occurrence of life threatening ventricular arrhythmias. It has been established that sudden death may be the first manifestation of the disease, mostly in previously asymptomatic young subjects and athletes. Therefore all identified or suspected patients are at risk of sudden death even in the absence of symptoms or ventricular arrhythmias. The most challenging clinical dilemma is not whether to treat patients who already experienced malignant ventricular arrhythmias (secondary prevention), but to consider prophylactic treatment in patients with no or only minor symptoms in whom the disease has been diagnosed during family screening or by chance (primary prevention). Furthermore, ARVC is a progressive disease and the patient's risk of sudden death may increase with time.

The risk profile which emerges from retrospective analysis of clinical and pathologic series, including fatal cases, is characterised by young age, competitive sport activity, malignant familial background, extensive right ventricular disease with ejection fraction reduction and left ventricular involvement, syncope, and episodes of complex ventricular arrhythmias or VT.[2–4 10] The baseline clinical study for assessment of the risk of sudden death consists of non-invasive routine clinical study including detailed clinical history (mostly addressing familial background and previous syncope), 12 lead ECG, 24 hour

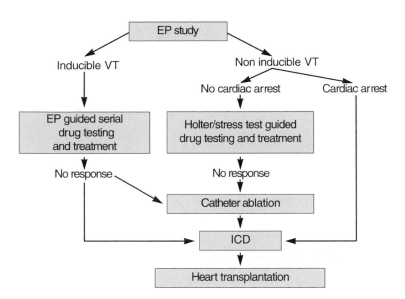

Figure 14.4. Treatment strategy in ARVC complicated by VT/VF.

ARVC is individualised and the strategies are based on the local experience of the different centres. Pharmacologic therapy is the first choice treatment of patients with well tolerated and non-life threatening ventricular arrhythmias. This subset of patients is usually treated empirically by β blockers and class I and III antiarrhythmic drugs. The evidence available suggests that either sotalol or amiodarone (alone or in combination with β blockers) are the most effective drugs with a relatively low proarrhythmic risk. The evaluation of efficacy of antiarrhythmic treatment may be based on symptom improvement, though a more reliable approach involves guiding treatment by serial 24 hour Holter monitoring and/or stress testing by demonstrating reduction in arrhythmic events.

In patients with sustained VT or VF, antiarrhythmic drug treatment guided by programmed ventricular stimulation with serial drug testing is the most effective therapeutic strategy, although its ability to prevent sudden death has not been proven. Non-pharmacological treatment is reserved for those patients with life threatening ventricular arrhythmias in whom drug treatment either is ineffective, is not applicable because of the inability to induce the clinical ventricular arrhythmias during electrophysiologic study, or is associated with serious side effects. Figure 14.4 is a flow chart outlining the management of ARVC patients with VT or VF. Patients with inducible VT during programmed ventricular stimulation undergo drug testing (mostly class I and III antiarrhythmic drugs) guided by serial electrophysiologic study. If a drug regimen can be found that prevents the induction of VT, the patient is discharged on the effective drug. Patients who remain inducible on different antiarrhythmic drugs are treated non-pharmacologically by an ICD (fig 14.5), except for rare cases with localised disease in whom catheter ablation of the VT may be an alternative option. Among patients with non-inducible VT, those who experienced spontaneous, haemodynamically well tolerated VT may be treated empirically by antiarrhythmic drug treatment, which is subsequently tested by serial 24 hour Holter monitoring and exercise stress testing. In case of no drug response, pace mapping directed catheter ablation may be attempted before implanting a prophylactic defibrillator. In patients with previous syncope or cardiac arrest and no inducible VT, the automatic cardioverter defibrillator represents the first option.

Sotalol has been reported to be the most effective antiarrhythmic drug in the treatment of both inducible and non-inducible VT in ARVC, with overall efficacy rates of more than 68% and 82%, respectively.[15] However, its efficacy in preventing sudden death remains to be established.

Catheter ablation

Although acute success rates of 60–90% have been reported with catheter ablation, VT recurrences are common (up to 60% of the cases) and may lead to sudden arrhythmic

Holter monitoring, exercise stress testing, and signal averaged ECG. All affected patients, either symptomatic or asymptomatic, should undergo this first line evaluation, even if its positive predictive value for subsequent malignant ventricular arrhythmias remains to be established. Invasive, intracardiac electrophysiologic study with programmed ventricular stimulation should be reserved for patients symptomatic for sustained VT or VF, patients with syncopal episodes in whom non-invasive evaluation was negative, and asymptomatic patients with strongly positive findings such as history of premature sudden death, non-sustained ventricular tachycardia, and depressed right ventricular function. The major aims of electrophysiologic study are: (1) to assess the disease's arrhythmogenic potential by induction of VT or VF during the basic pacing protocol or after isoproterenol; (2) to evaluate haemodynamic consequences of sustained VT and its propensity to degenerate into VF; and (3) to establish the susceptibility of VT to be interrupted by antitachycardia stimulation, and its reinducibility in view of serial electropharmacologic studies or implantation of an automatic defibrillator. The value of electrophysiologic study in arrhythmic risk stratification of patients with ARVC remains to be validated by prospective investigations.

Treatment

Since the assessment of sudden death risk in patients with ARVC is still not well established, there are no precise guidelines to determine which are the patients who need to be treated and which is the best management approach.[5] The therapeutic options include β blockers, antiarrhythmic drugs, catheter ablation, and implantable cardioverter defibrillator (ICD). At the present time, it is unclear how to best predict the efficacy of both pharmacological and non-pharmacological treatment in patients with ARVC; management of patients with

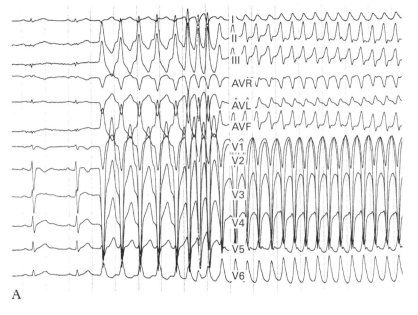
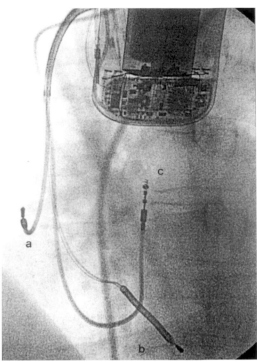

A

B

Figure 14.5. A 24 year old man affected by ARVC complicated by severe ventricular arrhythmias, with a recent family history of sudden death. (A) Twelve lead ECG during programmed ventricular stimulation: the first two beats at sinus rhythm show a low voltage QRS complex in the peripheral leads and T wave inversion in right precordial leads. After a drive of five paced ventricular beats, three extrastimuli induce a sustained ventricular tachycardia with an LBBB pattern and a cycle length of 250 ms, which was promptly interrupted by DC shock caused by the rapid haemodynamic deterioration. Serial antiarrhythmic drug testing, including sotalol, failed to identify any effective drug. (B) Chest radiography (60° left anterior oblique) of the same patient after implantation of a transvenous prophylactic automatic cardioverter defibrillator. Besides the atrial lead (a) and the double coil ventricular lead (b) for cardioversion, a third lead (c) was screwed onto the mid septum to assure a reliable sensing and pacing function.

death. The progressive nature of the underlying disease which predisposes to the occurrence of new arrhythmogenic foci over time may explain this discrepancy between acute and long term follow up success rates. In this regard, recurring VTs usually show a QRS morphology other than that previously ablated. Therefore, catheter ablation should be reserved for particular clinical conditions such as drug refractory incessant VT or frequent recurrences of VT after defibrillator implantation. Haemodynamically stable and well tolerated VT, which is not inducible or is not suppressed by electrophysiologic study directed pharmacologic treatment, may represent a further indication, in the presence of very localised cardiomyopathic changes and a still preserved right ventricular function.

Implantable cardioverter defibrillator

The ICD is the most effective safeguard against arrhythmic sudden death. However, its precise role in changing the natural history of ARVC by preventing sudden and non-sudden death needs to be evaluated by a prospective study of a large series of patients. The implantable defibrillator is the treatment of choice in patients resuscitated from a cardiac arrest caused by rapid VT or VF. Other indications include: patients with symptomatic VT non-inducible at electrophysiologic study; patients in whom electrophysiologic study guided drug treatment is ineffective or is associated with severe side effects; patients with severe right ventricular involvement and poor tolerance of VT; and sudden death of a close family member. Although ICD may confer a survival benefit of

up to 50% in patients with ARVC, there are potential complications associated with the device implantation which are related to the distinctive pathologic changes of the right ventricular wall. The very thin free wall predisposes to right ventricular perforation by the transvenous lead. The loss of the right ventricular myocardium with fibrofatty replacement underlies the difficulty in obtaining adequate R waves and pacing thresholds at the time of implantation (fig 14.5B). Moreover, undersensing or pacing exit block may occur during the follow up as a consequence of the progression of the myopathic process, leading to right ventricular myocardial disappearance. Finally, inappropriate treatment owing to sinus tachycardia and lead dislodgement has been described in more active young patients undergoing implantation of the device.

Heart failure

In patients in whom ARVC has progressed to severe right ventricular or biventricular systolic dysfunction with risk of thromboembolic complications, treatment consists of current therapy for heart failure, including diuretics, angiotensin converting enzyme inhibitors, and digitalis, as well as anticoagulants. In case of refractory congestive heart failure, the patients may become candidates for heart transplantation.

1. **Marcus FI, Fontaine G, Guiraudon G,** *et al.* Right ventricular dysplasia. A report of 24 adult cases. *Circulation* 1982;**65**:384–98.
• *This paper is the first clinical report in the English literature of arrhythmogenic right ventricular cardiomyopathy in adults.*

2. **Thiene G, Nava A, Corrado D,** *et al.* Right ventricular cardiomyopathy and sudden death in young people. *N Engl J Med* 1988;**318**:129–33.
- *This paper describes the clinicopathologic features of arrhythmogenic right ventricular cardiomyopathy in young sudden death victims.*

3. **Basso C, Thiene G, Corrado D,** *et al.* Arrhythmogenic right ventricular cardiomyopathy. Dysplasia, dystrophy, or myocarditis? *Circulation* 1996;**94**:983–91.
- *A detailed description is provided of the morphologic findings of arrhythmogenic right ventricular cardiomyopathy together with critical analysis of several pathogenetic theories.*

4. **Corrado D, Basso C, Thiene G,** *et al.* Spectrum of clinicopathologic manifestations of arrhythmogenic right ventricular cardiomyopathy/dysplasia: a multicenter study. *J Am Coll Cardiol* 1997;**30**:1512–20.
- *The left ventricular involvement and natural history of arrhythmogenic right ventricular cardiomyopathy are addressed.*

5. **Nava A, Rossi L, Thiene G.** *Arrhythmogenic right ventricular cardiomyopathy—dysplasia.* Amsterdam: Elsevier, 1997.
- *The first book devoted to arrhythmogenic right ventricular cardiomyopathy with comprehensive chapters on pathobiology, aetiopathogenesis, clinical diagnosis, and management strategies.*

6. **McKenna WJ, Thiene G, Nava A,** *et al.* Diagnosis of arrhythmogenic right ventricular dysplasia/cardiomyopathy. *Br Heart J* 1994;**71**:215–18.

7. **Nava A, Thiene G, Canciani B,** *et al.* Familial occurrence of right ventricular dysplasia: a study involving nine families. *J Am Coll Cardiol* 1988;**12**:1222–8.

8. **Rampazzo A, Nava A, Danieli GA,** *et al.* The gene for arrhythmogenic right ventricular cardiomyopathy maps to chromosome 14q23-q24. *Human Molecular Genetics* 1994;**3**:959–62.

9. **Fontaine G, Frank R, Tonet JL,** *et al.* Arrhythmogenic right ventricular dysplasia: a clinical model for the study of chronic ventricular tachycardia. *Jpn Circ* 1984;**48**:515–38.

10. **Corrado D, Thiene G, Nava A,** *et al.* Sudden death in young competitive athletes: clinicopathologic correlation in 22 cases. *Am J Med* 1990;**89**:588–96.

11. **Daliento L, Rizzoli G, Thiene G,** *et al.* Diagnostic accuracy of right ventriculography in arrhythmogenic right ventricular cardiomyopathy. *Am J Cardiol* 1990;**66**:741–5.

12. **Auffermann W, Wichter T, Breithardt G,** *et al.* Arrhythmogenic right ventricular disease: MR imaging vs angiography. *Am J Roentgenol* 1993;**161**:549–55.

13. **Angelini A, Basso C, Nava A,** *et al.* Endomyocardial biopsy in arrhythmogenic right ventricular cardiomyopathy. *Am Heart J* 1996;**132**:203–6.

14. **Blomström-Lundqvist C, Sabel CG, Olsson SB.** A long term follow up of 15 patients with arrhythmogenic right ventricular dysplasia. *Br Heart J* 1987;**58**:477–88.

15. **Wichter T, Borggrefe M, Hoverkamp W,** *et al.* Efficacy of antiarrhythmic drugs in patients with arrhythmogenic right ventricular disaese. Results in patients with inducible and noninducible ventricular tachycardia. *Circulation* 1992;**86**:29–37.

SECTION IV: VALVE DISEASE

15 Worldwide perspective of valve disease

Jordi Soler-Soler, Enrique Galve

Valvar heart disease is a paradigm of the changing aetiology of human disease. In particular, we have witnessed dramatic changes in the incidence of rheumatic heart disease (fig 15.1); such changes have been limited mostly to industrialised countries, highlighting the role of factors other than microorganisms in this disease. Interestingly, the frequency of valvar heart disease is still high in industrialised countries, as new types of valve disease become increasingly prevalent (fig 15.2). The most important of them is degenerative valve disease, which relates directly to the increased lifespan of people living in industrialised countries compared to those in developing countries. On the other hand, aetiologies related to the relative wealth of industrialised countries have also appeared, the most dramatic example being valve disease related to appetite suppressant drugs.

Rheumatic valve disease

Although rheumatic fever was thought to be nearly eradicated from developed countries, it continues to be a challenge because of its high prevalence in the developing world. In addition, new aspects have emerged and are a cause of concern, as indicated by the recent outbreaks in industrial countries.

A variety of epidemiologic studies have shown that the incidence of rheumatic fever and the prevalence of rheumatic heart disease have declined dramatically over the last decades in the developed countries. A number of reasons (table 15.1) have been postulated to explain such a decrease: improvement in living standards, better access to medical care, wider use of antibiotics, as well as natural changes in the streptococcal strains.

In the USA, in the mid 1980s the medical community was surprised by the resurgence of a disease that had been considered to have virtually disappeared. Although the first outbreak was documented in the Intermountain area,[1] a nationwide survey of paediatric cardiologists indicated that a definite increase in rheumatic valve disease had occurred in 24 states. The resurgence was very intense in certain areas, where the incidence was similar to that occurring in the early 1960s. After the outbreak, a general decline in new cases was observed, but the disease did not totally disappear. Some disturbing features of the outbreak were that in the majority of cases there was not the antecedent of a sore throat, and that in some patients who had the typical symptomatology,

they had taken the recommended treatment for streptococcal pharyngitis (oral penicillin for 10 days). In contrast with what might be expected, the resurgence was not restricted to socioeconomically deprived groups. The unresolved questions are whether the disease returned because of an emergence of modified strains, a breakdown of immunity, or simply a slackening of public health vigilance. The most likely explanation for the outbreak is that highly rheumatogenic strains of group A streptococci accounted for local increases in acute rheumatic fever.[2] Viewed now in retrospect, through the enormous publicity that accompanied the outbreak, a nationwide survey of all children's hospitals and general hospitals of more than 600 beds in the USA revealed that rheumatic fever was no more common than Kawasaki disease, with approximately 5000 cases of each occurring over four years (from 1984 to 1987), and with no increasing trend.

In the developing countries, the situation is similar to that of industrialised nations in the early 20th century, when rheumatic fever was still one of the leading causes of death and disability in young people. An accurate evaluation of trends of rheumatic fever in these countries is not possible because of a lack of reliable health statistics, but there is overwhelming evidence that the disease continues unabated. The existing information indicates that the magnitude of the problem may not have changed during the last years or may have actually increased in the last 50–60 years. Worldwide estimates of chronic rheumatic heart disease in school age children and young adults range from 4.9 to 30 million.[3] Hospital statistics from most developing nations reveal that about 10–35% of all cardiac admissions are for patients with rheumatic fever or chronic rheumatic heart disease (table 15.2). Accordingly, valve replacement accounts for the majority of cardiac surgery in these countries.

Unfortunately, the notion that rheumatic fever is a disease of the poor and the underprivileged is still true at the beginning of the new millennium. The absence of factors that account for the sharp decline of the disease in the industrialised countries explains its persistence in the developing world. The difficulties in accessing health care rapidly may explain why streptococcal sore throat (the most important primary cause of this disease) is not treated adequately. A report from Costa Rica shows that a single dose of penicillin benzathine administered to all patients with sore throat could reduce significantly the incidence of rheumatic fever.[4] Another additional problem is that secondary prophylaxis is rarely done, and recurrences are frequent. Changes in the standard of living in these countries, with crowding in urban areas with poor living status (slum areas), has accelerated the propagation of the disease, since streptococcal infection spreads in these type of conditions. At the present time, prevalence of rheumatic heart disease is higher among the urban poor than the rural poor population.

Fortunately, group A streptococcus remains sensitive to penicillin, but it may be only a matter of time before it becomes resistant (resistance to erythromycin, the second drug of choice, is common and seems to be increasing). Recently, important progress towards the development of an effective vaccine to protect against streptococcal nasopharyngeal infection opens up the possibility of better control of rheumatic fever.[5]

Degenerative valve disease

Although there has been a dramatic reduction in rheumatic valve disease in the industrialised countries over the past 30 years, there has not been a similar reduction in valve surgery. This is because the types of patients being referred for surgery have changed. The significant increase in life expectancy in developed countries partly accounts for this change in aetiology, especially in aortic valve disease. In one surgical series over a five year period (from 1981 to 1985), it was found that while the proportion of patients with congenitally bicuspid aortic stenosis remained stable (from 37% to 33%), postinflammatory valve disease decreased from 30% to 18% while degenerative valve disease increased from 30% to 46%.[6]

Although the incidence of degenerative valve disease increases with age, aging does not seem to be the only factor, as valve disease is not present universally in the elderly (25–45% of octogenarians do not have aortic calcification). Moreover, and most intriguing, the initial lesion of calcific aortic valve disease appears to involve an active process with some similarities to atherosclerosis, including lipid deposition (apo B, apo(a), and apo E), macrophage infiltration, and production of osteopontin and other proteins.[7-9] In the Cardiovascular Health Study[7] the relation between aortic sclerosis or aortic stenosis and clinical risk factors for atherosclerosis was evaluated in 5201 subjects aged 65 years or more; aortic valve sclerosis was found in 26% and aortic stenosis in 2% of the entire cohort. Independent clinical factors associated with both types of degenerative valve disease included age (twofold increased risk for each 10 year increase in age), male sex (two fold excess risk), and a history of hypertension (20% increase in risk); other significant factors included high lipoprotein Lp (a) and low density lipoprotein (LDL) cholesterol concentrations.

Another study found an association between atherosclerotic risk factors and mitral annulus calcification, and stenotic and non-stenotic aortic valve calcification.[8] The analysis was done from a prospective database of 8160 consecutive patients and showed that age (odds ratio (OR) varying from 5.78 to 10.4, depending on age class), hypertension (OR 2.38), diabetes mellitus (OR 2.85), and hypercholesterolaemia (OR 2.95) were strongly and significantly associated with aortic valve calcification, as were age (OR varying from 8.82 to 67, depending on age class), hypertension (OR 2.72), diabetes mellitus (OR 2.49), and hypercholesterolaemia (OR 2.86) with mitral annu-

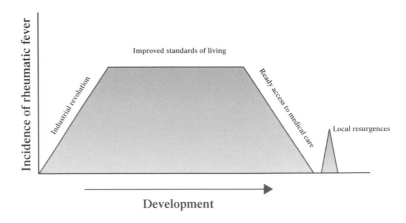

Figure 15.1. Changes in the incidence of rheumatic fever. Rheumatic fever increased during the period of the industrial revolution, possibly because of overcrowding in urban areas. Later on, it reached a steady state as living standards began to improve. Finally, in the postindustrial period, the decline in incidence was associated with an easier access to medical care, widespread use of antibiotics, and reduced overcrowding. At the present time, when the disease is considered to be nearly eradicated, isolated outbreaks continue to occur.

lar calcification. The most important consequence of this process is aortic calcification and/or aortic stenosis, but the same calcific deposits may be located in the undersurface of the posterior mitral leaflet and, if extensive enough, can cause mitral incompetence and, more rarely, mitral stenosis.

The results of these studies suggest that degenerative valve disease does not have to be regarded as an inevitable consequence of aging, and that these findings might be translated to preventive measures. Taking into consideration that atherosclerotic heart disease, at least coronary heart disease, is to a certain extent a preventable condition, in which efforts have to be made to modify the natural (or unnatural course), the same principles would apply to degenerative valve disease. Accordingly, early forms of aortic stenosis and, probably, of aortic sclerosis and mitral annulus calcification should be considered as indicators to implement measures generally used to treat atherosclerotic vascular disease, including diet modification, tobacco consumption cessation, plasma lipid determinations, and blood pressure control.

The prevalence of degenerative valve disease is not known in underdeveloped countries. Presumably, it is low as life expectancy is much shorter and atherosclerotic heart disease is much less prevalent than in industrialised countries.

Emerging valve disease

During the last 20 years, the medical community has witnessed the appearance of new forms of cardiac valve disease. There are three main sources of these "modern" types of valve involvement: (a) new infectious diseases such as AIDS; (b) drug related diseases resulting from the overuse of drugs that, in many cases, are specifically linked to problems only found in developed countries (for example, appetite suppressant drugs); and (c) new types of

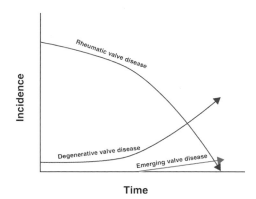

Figure 15.2. Evolution of different types of valve disease in the developed world. Rheumatic valve disease has witnessed an abrupt decline, which has been matched in part by an increase in degenerative valve disease, related to aging. Meanwhile, new types of valve disease have emerged, although they account for a minority of all cases in comparison with the old incidence of rheumatic valve disease or the current incidence of degenerative valve disease.

idiopathic diseases (for example, the antiphospholipid syndrome).

Infectious diseases: AIDS

Cardiac disease is not a common complication of AIDS, but the incidence of AIDS related heart involvement will increase as this infection becomes more prevalent and patients live longer.[10] [11] Valve involvement is less common than myocardial or pericardial disease in AIDS patients, unless a predisposing factor such as intravenous drug abuse exists.[12] In these cases, endocarditis is caused by *Staphylococcus aureus* or *Streptococcus pneumoniae*, but can also be caused by fungi or HACEK (*Haemophilus* species, *Actinobacillus actinomycetencomitans*, *Cardiobacterium hominis*, *Eikenella corrodens*, and *Kingella* species). It has been reported that the degree of immunosupression caused by the HIV infection increases the severity of valve disease and the resulting mortality.[13]

The other type of valve involvement is non-bacterial thrombotic or marantic endocarditis, in a manner similar to other wasting diseases such as cancer. The incidence ranges from 4–7% in necropsy series. Vegetations are composed of sterile verrucae attached to coaptation points of the valves and comprise fibrin–platelet masses. When vegetations reach a size

greater than 2 mm they can be detected and the condition diagnosed by means of echocardiography. Any valve can be involved and, from a clinical viewpoint, the most common phenomena are embolic. There is no specific treatment.

Drug related diseases
Ergot alkaloid heart disease
Methysergide and ergotamine are two classical drugs that are used in the prophylaxis and treatment of migraine headaches. Ergotamine is believed to relieve migraine by inducing vasoconstriction of the cerebrovascular bed, while methysergide achieves a similar effect by its antiserotoninergic properties. They are ergot alkaloid derivatives, and both share a common chemical structure to the neurohormone serotonin. Serotonin is the agent responsible for valve disease in the carcinoid syndrome, involving endocardial fibrosis.

It has been reported that chronic ingestion of methysergide or ergotamine can induce endocardial thickening that results in valve dysfunction.[14] The endocardial involvement comprises a fibrotic reaction that coats valves, chordae, papillary muscles, and all the endomyocardial surface. Fibrosis causes valve and chordae retraction that results in either stenosis or regurgitation. The process is similar to that described in the carcinoid syndrome, but while carcinoid associated valve disease is restricted to the right sided valves (except in the case of bronchial carcinoid), in ergot alkaloid associated valve disease, although all four valves can be involved, the aortic and mitral valves are most often damaged.

The pathophysiologic underlying mechanism that explains why these lesions develop after the chronic ingestion of these drugs is unknown. Ergot alkaloid valve heart lesions only occur after very prolonged exposure: all patients diagnosed had received this treatment for a minimum of six years (usually 20 years). The incidence and importance of cardiac lesions are directly correlated to doses and time of exposure.

The incidence of this type of valve disease is unknown because no studies have evaluated large numbers of ergot alkaloid consumers, just sporadic cases. Thus, there are no reports on the natural history of the condition. A small series from the Mayo Clinic included five patients symptomatic enough to require valve surgery.[14] All the patients developed symptoms after long periods of drug consumption but, once the symptomatology was established, its progression was rapid, to the point of requiring valve replacement within six months to four years. One patient that continued using ergot alkaloid suppositories after mitral and aortic surgery developed severe tricuspid involvement shortly after, which was not present preoperatively.

The treatment of ergot alkaloid valve disease is very simple. The most important measure is, of course, to stop the drug treatment. Occasionally, the interruption of therapy may be followed by diminution of the murmurs associated with the valve disease, but this has not

Table 15.1 Suggested reasons for the decline of rheumatic fever in industrialised nations[2]

Reasons	Possible mechanism of benefit	Evidence
Improved standards of living	• Less overcrowding • Improved nutrition	• Declining incidence of RF before the antibiotic era
Greater access to health care and widespread use of antibiotics	• Prompt treatment of symptomatic streptococcal infections • Reduced occurrence of epidemics of streptococcal sore throat • Prevention of recurrence of RF through secondary prophylaxis	• Studies examining the effect of improved health care availability in poor urban areas • Fourfold decline in reported national mortality from RF after introduction of penicillin
Diminished streptococcal virulence and fewer "rheumatogenic" subtypes	• Less rapid spread of streptococcal infections • Reduced prevalence of specific "rheumatogenic" strains	• No direct evidence, diminishing incidence of RF in the face of unchanged prevalence of streptococcal infection

RF, rheumatic fever.

been confirmed by echocardiography. These patients have to be managed conventionally, with appropriate medical and surgical interventions as used to treat rheumatic or degenerative valve disease.

Appetite suppressants drugs and cardiac valve disease

Reports on the efficacy of the combination of fenfluramine and phentermine in the treatment of obesity appeared in 1992. Dexfenfluramine, the d-isomer of fenfluramine, was approved by the US Food and Drug Administration (FDA) in 1996. These drugs were very successful, and by 1997 approximately 14 million prescriptions had been written (although a concern was raised on their association with pulmonary hypertension). However, in July 1997, Connolly and colleagues reported a series of 24 patients who had taken the fenfluramine-phentermine combination for an average of 11 months, and found a high incidence of cardiac valve regurgitation; five patients in the study need valve surgery, with findings similar to those occurring in serotonin related carcinoid syndrome (although in these patients they were left sided).[15] Immediately afterwards, a series of retrospective echocardiographic studies found that the prevalence of aortic or mitral regurgitations in patients treated with these drugs ranged from 20–30%, and as a result the drugs were withdrawn from the market.

Three reports published simultaneously in the *New England Journal of Medicine* confirmed the association between the cardiac valve disease and the drugs, although the reports differed in the estimate of risk magnitude.[16–18] The prevalence of echocardiographic valvar regurgitation (FDA criteria) varied from 6.9–25%, depending on the study, the type of appetite suppressant drug, and the duration of treatment. The incidence of clinically detected cardiac valve disease was much lower (reflecting the insensitivity of clinical evaluation in diagnosing mild to moderate valve regurgitation). Other conclusions were that the probability of developing valve disease was related to longer times of exposure and higher doses.

The lesson in this case is similar to that learned with ergot alkaloid cardiac valve disease. Drugs that act via the serotonin pathways are potentially dangerous. Phentermine,

which acts via the catecholamine pathway, has escaped incrimination as a cause of valve damage when given alone. The main difference between what happened with the appetite suppressant drugs and the ergot alkaloid drugs was that in the former the valve damage occurred after only a few months of treatment, while in the latter the valvar involvement was described only after years of treatment.

Cardiac valve disease associated with the antiphospholipid syndrome

The antiphospholipid (aPL) syndrome is an entity characterised by vascular thrombosis with frequent heart involvement, particularly valvar lesions.[19] The syndrome is caused by the appearance of circulating aPL antibodies, which are spontaneously acquired circulating immunoglobulins directed against negatively charged phospholipids. aPL antibodies were initially found in sera of patients with systemic lupus erythematosus. They have since been found occasionally in other connective tissue diseases, as well as in drug induced, malignant, and infectious disorders. In addition, they have been found in subjects without any underlying disorder.

aPL antibodies are associated with an intriguing effect on blood coagulation. In vitro they act as an anticoagulant that prolongs the whole blood clotting time, although no specific deficiency of the clotting factors is detectable. Despite its anticoagulant behaviour in vitro, the paradox comes from the clinical manifestations associated with the aPL phenomenon, as these patients present with a high incidence of arterial and venous thrombosis. The combination of a laboratory finding— that is, the presence of aPL antibodies—and of a clinical finding—that is, the presence of either arterial or venous occlusive events—has been termed the antiphospholipid syndrome.

aPL antibodies are associated with a wide variety of clinical manifestations, but the vast majority of them share in common the characteristic of being part of the hypercoagulopathic state. The most frequent features are thrombosis either in the venous or in the arterial bed as deep vein thrombosis, commonly multiple and bilateral, pulmonary embolism, secondary pulmonary chronic hypertension, stroke, transient ischemic attacks, multiple visceral arterial occlusions, and other large vessel occlusions— for example, of the subclavian artery. No portion of the vasculature is spared from thrombotic events.

Cardiac involvement is frequently seen under the broad umbrella of the aPL syndrome, and it can be present in many diverse ways.[20] Initially, aPL antibodies were significantly associated with the finding of valve lesions in lupus patients. Nevertheless, systemic lupus is a complex disease in which multiple inflammatory, thrombotic, and degenerative phenomena are involved. Thus, the best model to determine whether aPL antibodies and valve lesions are related is the primary antiphospholipid syndrome, namely, those patients with antibodies to phospholipids, thrombotic manifestations, but no other disease that

Table 15.2   Hospital admissions for rheumatic heart disease.[2]

Country	Admissions as percentage of all cardiac admissions
Asia	
Bangladesh	34.0
Burma	30.0
India	16.5–50.6
Mongolia	30.0
Pakistan	23.0
Thailand	34.0
Africa	
Ethiopia	34.8
Ghana	20.6
Malawi	23.0
Nigeria	18.1–23.0
South Africa	25.0
Tanzania	9.7
Uganda	24.7
Zambia	18.2

may account for the antibodies. Subsequently, valvar involvement has been demonstrated in patients with the primary aPL syndrome.[20] Lesions are found by means of Doppler echocardiography in 38% of patients, involving the mitral and the aortic valve; they are regurgitant, and in some cases the valvar regurgitation is so severe as to require surgery. The lesions appear as irregular, localised valve thickenings, not vegetative. The pathogenesis of these endocardial lesions is as yet unknown. Some investigators have found thrombi over the involved valves. In order to link the thrombotic occlusions of the vessel and the valve involvement in these patients, it could be hypothesised that the initial valve lesions are thrombi deposits that subsequently promote an unspecific anti-inflammatory response and ultimately become organised.

The isolated finding of aPL antibodies in the absence of clinical manifestations does not require treatment, but patients with thrombotic manifestations have to be fully anticoagulated. It is unknown whether the finding of valve heart disease should be treated, but the tendency is not to give specific therapy to asymptomatic subjects. Nevertheless, these patients should probably receive infective endocarditis prophylaxis.

1. **Veasy LG, Wiedmeier SE, Orsmond GS**, et al. Resurgence of acute rheumatic fever in the Intermountain area of the United States. N Engl J Med 1987;**316**:421–7.
* The paper reports an outbreak of acute rheumatic fever that occurred in 74 children during a 18 month period (from January 1985 to June 1986) at one centre in Salt Lake City. The children were predominantly white and from middle class families with above average incomes and ready access to medical care. There was no apparent increase in the incidence of streptococcal disease or other explanation for the major increase in rheumatic fever. In the previous 10 year period the average incidence had been six cases per year.

2. **Narula J, Virmani R, Reddy KS, Tandon R, eds.** Rheumatic fever. Armed Forces Institute of Pathology, Washington: American Registry of Pathology, 1999.
* This book is a comprehensive multidisciplinary review of the state of the art of rheumatic fever at the present time. The monograph comprises aspects such as history, epidemiology, microbiology of group A streptococci, clinical manifestations, the problem of the resurgence of rheumatic fever, treatment, and prevention (including the progress on the vaccine development).

3. **World Health Organization.** Rheumatic fever and rheumatic heart disease. WHO Technical Report Series no. 764. Geneva: WHO, 1988.

4. **Arguedas A, Mohs E.** Prevention of rheumatic fever in Costa Rica. J Pediatr 1992;**121**:569–72.

5. **Dale JB.** Group A streptococcal vaccines. Infect Dis Clin North Am 1999;**13**:227–43.

6. **Passik CS, Ackermann DM, Pluth JR**, et al. Temporal changes in the causes of aortic stenosis: a surgical pathologic study of 646 cases. Mayo Clin Proc 1987;**62**:119–23.

7. **Stewart BF, Siscovick D, Lind BK**, et al. Clinical factors associated with calcific aortic valve disease. Cardiovascular Health Study. J Am Coll Cardiol 1997;**29**:630–4.
* Clinical factors associated with aortic sclerosis and stenosis were evaluated in older subjects (> 65 years of age) enrolled in the Cardiovascular Health Study. Independent clinical factors found to be associated with these types of degenerative valve disease were age, male sex, present smoking, and hypertension, while high Lp(a) and LDL cholesterol concentrations were other significant factors.

8. **Boon A, Cheriex E, Lodder J**, et al. Cardiac valve calcification: characteristics of patients with calcification of the mitral annulus or aortic valve. Heart 1997;**78**:472–4.

9. **Wilmshurst PT, Stevenson RN, Griffiths**, et al. A case-control investigation of the relation between hyperlipidemia and calcific aortic valve stenosis. Heart 1997;**78**:475–9.
* A case control study designed to evaluate the relation of hyperlipidaemia to calcific aortic valve stenosis. The presence of a stenosed tricuspid aortic valve was associated with a significant increase in total plasma cholesterol, while for bicuspid valves the degree of elevation was less and not significant.

10. **Michaels AD, Lederman RJ, MacGregor JS**, et al. Cardiovascular involvement in AIDS. Curr Probl Cardiol 1997;**22**:109–48.

11. **Ribera E, Miro JM, Cortes E**, et al. Influence of human immunodeficiency virus 1 infection and degree of immunosuppression in the clinical characteristics and outcome of infective endocarditis in intravenous drug users. Arch Intern Med 1998;**158**:2043–50.

12. **Acierno LJ.** Cardiac complications in acquired immunodeficiency syndrome (AIDS): a review. J Am Coll Cardiol 1989;**13**:1144–54.
* This review emphasises that the most common endocardial lesion seen in AIDS is non-bacterial thrombotic bacterial endocarditis (so-called marantic endocarditis). This type of involvement is probably due to the long-term wasting characteristics of AIDS.

13. **Milei J, Grana D, Fernandez Alonso G**, et al. Cardiac involvement in acquired immunodeficiency syndrome—a review to push action. The committee for the study of cardiac involvement in AIDS. Clin Cardiol 1998;**21**:465–72.

14. **Redfield MM, Nicholson WJ, Edwards WD**, et al. Valve disease associated with ergot alkaloid use. Echocardiographic and pathologic correlations. Ann Intern Med 1992;**117**:50–2.
* This is a report of the clinical, echocardiographic, and pathologic findings of five patients with valvar disease associated with long term ingestion of ergot alkaloids. Valvar disease was sufficiently symptomatic to necessitate valve replacement in all cases. Patients were identified because gross pathologic findings were unusually severe for rheumatic disease.

15. **Connolly HM, Crary JL, McGoon MD**, et al. Valvular heart disease associated with fenfluramine-phentermine. N Engl J Med 1997;**337**:581–8.
* Investigators at the Mayo Clinic describe 24 women in whom valvar heart disease developed after an average of 12 months of treatment with fenfluramine and phentermine. Eight women also had newly documented pulmonary hypertension. At the time of the report valve surgery was needed in five cases of the series. This paper was the first to arouse concern about this relation and prompted other studies that finally confirmed the association.

16. **Khan MA, Herzog CA, St Peter JV**, et al. The prevalence of cardiac valvular insufficiency assessed by transthoracic echocardiography in obese patients treated with appetite-suppressant drugs. N Engl J Med 1998;**339**:713–8.
* Echocardiograms from 257 obese patients that had taken or were taking fenfluramine, dexfenfluramine or phentermine were reviewed, and compared against 239 matched controls. A total of 1.3% of the controls and 22.7% of the patients met the case definition of valvar regurgitation (FDA criteria).

17. **Jick H, Vasilakis C, Weinrauch LA**, et al. A population-based study of appetite-suppressant drugs and the risk of cardiac valve regurgitation. N Engl J Med 1998;**339**:719–24.

18. **Weissman NJ, Tighe JF, Gottdiener JS**, et al, **for the Sustained-Release Dexfenfluramine Study Group.** An assessment of heart-valve abnormalities in obese patients taking dexfenfluramine, sustained-release dexfenfluramine, or placebo. N Engl J Med 1998;**339**:725–32.
* An echocardiogram was performed in 1072 patients who had participated in a randomised double blind trial comparing dexfenfluramine and placebo. Although the period of treatment was very short (only 72 days) and the recording was performed a median of one month after the discontinuation of treatment, the prevalence of either aortic or mitral regurgitation was significantly higher in those patients that had taken dexfenfluramine, although in most cases the valve insufficiency was considered as trace or mild.

19. **Asherson RA, Cervera R.** Antiphospholipid antibodies and the heart. Lessons and pitfalls for the cardiologist. Circulation 1991;**84**:920–3.
* Although an editorial, this article is also a good review which summarises the relations between antiphospholipid antibodies and cardiac disease with a very appropriate clinical sense. With respect to valvar involvement, clues to differentiating antiphospholipid lesions from infective endocarditis are provided.

20. **Galve E, Ordi J, Barquinero J**, et al. Valvular heart disease in the primary antiphospholipid syndrome. Ann Intern Med 1992;**116**:293–8.
* A series of 28 consecutive patients with primary antiphospholipid syndrome, and 28 age and sex matched healthy controls, studied by Doppler echocardiography. Valvar involvement was found in 38% of patients, lesions being of the regurgitant type (no stenoses were found), and appearing as irregular, localised valve thickening, not vegetative.

16 Timing of aortic valve surgery

Catherine M Otto

The timing of aortic valve surgery is described for patients presenting with two conditions: aortic stenosis and chronic aortic regurgitation.

Aortic stenosis

Aortic stenosis may be caused by rheumatic disease, a congenital bicuspid valve or calcification of a trileaflet valve. In Europe and North America, the aetiology of aortic stenosis most often is increased leaflet stiffness, without commissural fusion, caused by lipo-calcific deposits on the aortic side of the valve leaflets. This active disease process affects both congenitally bicuspid and normal trileaflet aortic valves and represents the extreme of a spectrum of disease that includes both aortic sclerosis without outflow obstruction and severe valvar aortic stenosis. Aortic valve sclerosis and stenosis are the most common valve diseases in Europe and North America, with sclerosis present in about 25% of all people over age 65 years and stenosis present in 2–7% of this population.[1] Significant outflow obstruction tends to occur at a younger age in patients with a bicuspid valve, possibly related to increased mechanical stress on the valve leaflets.

At the tissue level, aortic valve stenosis is characterised by focal areas of displacement of the subendothelial elastic lamina on the aortic side of the leaflet; there is protein and lipoprotein deposition and an inflammatory cell infiltrate with macrophages, T lymphocytes, and production of proteins, such as osteopontin, that are associated with tissue calcification. Ongoing studies of this active disease process will further clarify mechanisms of disease.

Aortic sclerosis

The initial phase of the disease process leading to aortic stenosis is mild leaflet thickening without obstruction to ventricular outflow, defined as aortic sclerosis. Although these patients do not have cardiac symptoms, they still are at increased risk for adverse cardiovascular outcomes. In the population based Cardiovascular Health Study, subjects with aortic sclerosis on echocardiography and no known cardiovascular disease had an approximately 50% increased risk of myocardial infarction and cardiovascular death over an average follow up of 5.5 years.[2] Clearly, valve surgery is not indicated in these subjects as there is no outflow obstruction. Although there have been no studies of medical treatment to decrease cardiovascular risk in these subjects,

the prudent physician will evaluate and treat conventional coronary risk factors.

Haemodynamic progression

Once mild aortic stenosis is present (defined as an aortic jet velocity > 2.5 m/s), a gradual increase in the severity of outflow obstruction is seen in most patients (fig 16.1). Overall, the average annual rate of increase in aortic jet velocity is 0.3 m/s per year, with an increase in mean transaortic pressure gradient of 7 mm Hg per year and a decrease in valve area of 0.1 cm^2 per year.[3] However, there is wide individual variability in the rate of haemodynamic progression. Some patients have little change in the degree of outflow obstruction over several years, while others have a relatively rapid rate of disease progression. Factors that predict the rate of haemodynamic progression in an individual patient have not yet been identified.

Symptom onset

At some point, the degree of outflow obstruction prevents an adequate increase in cardiac output with exertion, and the patient becomes symptomatic. Interestingly, some patients develop clear symptoms with obstruction that traditionally has not been considered "critical", while others remain asymptomatic with apparently severe obstruction. We now recognise that there is substantial overlap in haemodynamic severity between symptomatic and asymptomatic patients, even though clinical outcome is most dependent on the presence or absence of symptoms. Thus, a difficult clinical problem is the patient who has symptoms compatible with aortic stenosis but has outflow obstruction that traditionally would be considered only moderate. In this situation it can be difficult to separate symptoms caused by outflow obstruction from symptoms caused by other comorbidity. Exercise testing can be helpful in providing an objective measure of exercise tolerance and in documenting the haemodynamic response to exercise in these patients. However, it is incumbent on the physician to assume that symptoms are caused by aortic stenosis unless other explanations are evident or the degree of stenosis is so mild that

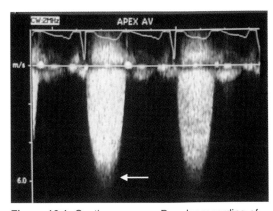

Figure 16.1. Continuous wave Doppler recording of aortic jet velocity in an elderly patient with severe aortic stenosis. Non-invasive Doppler evaluation of jet velocity, mean pressure gradient, and valve area are key to the evaluation and management of adults with aortic stenosis.

> **Indications for surgery in valvar aortic stenosis**
>
> - Definite indications:
>   - symptoms caused by aortic stenosis (even if mild)
>   - asymptomatic severe aortic stenosis with left ventricular systolic dysfunction
>   - severe aortic stenosis at the time of other cardiac surgery
>
> - Selected patients:
>   - asymptomatic patients with severe stenosis and anticipated high levels of exertion, plans for pregnancy, poor access to medical care, etc
>   - patients with moderate aortic stenosis undergoing coronary bypass surgery
>
> - Not accepted:
>   - prevention of sudden death in asymptomatic patients

valve replacement would not improve haemodynamics.

There is widespread agreement that valve replacement is indicated for symptomatic severe aortic stenosis. Both historical series before the availability of valve surgery and more recent series of patients who refused intervention for severe symptomatic aortic stenosis show that outcome is extremely poor, with survival rates as low as 50% at two years and 20% at five years after symptom onset.

The three classical symptoms of aortic stenosis are angina, heart failure, and syncope. However, in patients followed prospectively, symptom onset is insidious and may not be recognised by the patient or physician unless a careful, directed history is performed. Specifically, the physician needs to ask what activities the patient is doing now compared to 1–3 years ago. If there has been any decrease in physical activity, the possibility of symptom onset should be considered. Patients often ascribe their decrease in activity to "the flu" or "getting old", rather than recognising the subtle symptoms that led to their change in lifestyle.

The most common initial symptom in adults followed prospectively is a decrease in exercise tolerance or dyspnoea on exertion. Angina also is common but may not be recognised as such unless the physician has educated the patient about the significance of chest "discomfort" or "heaviness". When severe aortic stenosis is present on echocardiography, surgical intervention should be performed promptly once even these minor symptoms occur. Symptoms of pulmonary oedema and syncope are late manifestations of the disease process, most often occurring in patients without appropriate access to medical care or who have ignored earlier symptoms. If the symptom status of the patient is unclear, exercise testing is helpful to determine exercise duration and the haemodynamic response to exercise. A fall or only minimal rise in blood pressure indicates symptomatic disease.

Valve replacement for symptomatic aortic stenosis

Aortic valve replacement remains the definitive treatment for symptomatic aortic stenosis. In recent surgical series, operative mortality averages 2–9 % with long term survival rate of 80% at three years (table 16.1). Aortic stenosis in adults is rarely amenable to repair although commissurotomy may be an option in carefully selected young adults with non-calcified valves. Alternative procedures, such as balloon aortic valvuloplasty and surgical or ultrasonic valve debridement have not been successful. The choice of valve substitute in an individual patient is based on the balance between the durability of a mechanical valve compared to a tissue valve versus the need for long term anticoagulation. Newer, stentless tissue valves offer improved haemodynamics and the promise of increased longevity without the need for anticoagulation, although long term outcome data are not yet available. Other options include an aortic homograft in young women desiring pregnancy and the pulmonic autograft procedure in carefully selected younger patients at some experienced centres.

Table 16.1 Aortic valve replacement for aortic stenosis in the elderly and in those with impaired left ventricular function (selected series)

Series			n	30 day operative mortality	Event free survival
Culliford 1991	Age ≥ 80 years	AVR	35	5.7%	93.3% at 1 year
		AVR+CABG	36	19.4%	80.4% at 3 years
Azariades 1991	Age ≥ 80 years	AVR±CABG	88	16%	5 years 64 (7)%
Olsson1992	Age ≥ 80 years	AVR±CABG	44	14%	2 years 73%
	Age 65–75years	AVR±CABG	83	4%	2 years 90%
Elayda1993	Age ≥ 80 years	AVR	77	5.2%	1 year 90.8%
		AVR+CABG	75	24%	5 years 76%
Logeais1994	Age ≥ 75 years	AVR±CABG	675	12.4%	
Connolly 1997	EF ≤ 35%	AVR±CABG	154	9%	EF improved in 76%

AVR, aortic valve replacement; CABG, coronary artery bypass graft; MI, myocardial infarction; EF, ejection fraction.
Sources: Culliford AT, *et al. Am J Cardiol* 1991;**67**:1256–60; Azariades M, *et al. Eur J Cardiothorac Surg* 1991;**5**:373–7; Olsson M, *et al. J Am Coll Cardiol* 1992;**20**:1512-16; Elayda MA, *et al. Circulation* 1993;**88**:II-1–6; Logeais Y, *et al. Circulation* 1994;**90**:2891–8; Connolly HM. *Circulation* 1997;**95**:2395–400.

Aortic stenosis in the elderly

Aortic valve replacement is indicated for symptomatic severe aortic stenosis, regardless of age. In comparison with outcome on medical treatments, operative mortality rates are acceptable even in octogenarians (5–15%). Comorbid conditions are common in the elderly and some patients have strong preferences regarding surgical intervention—both are factors that need to be taken into account in decision making in this patient group. On the other hand, the rate of calcification of tissue valves decreases with age so that long term anticoagulation usually can be avoided by using a tissue valve with an expected longevity greater than the patient's expected survival.

Despite the compelling evidence that aortic valve replacement is both appropriate and feasible in the elderly, recent studies have highlighted its underuse. Elderly adults with severe symptomatic aortic stenosis often are not referred for surgical consideration because of misconceptions about the risks and benefits of valve replacement. Many primary care physicians are unaware that elderly patients with aortic stenosis and heart failure are the most likely to benefit from relief of outflow obstruction. It also is important to review tables of expected longevity for the patient's current age, as many patients (and physicians) are not aware of the expected further life span. For example, an 80 year old woman can expect to live an additional 10 years. Quality of life also is improved, even when operative mortality and morbidity are considered.

Aortic stenosis with left ventricular systolic dysfunction

Another difficult clinical situation is the patient with aortic stenosis and left ventricular systolic dysfunction. When stenosis is severe and there is a high pressure gradient across the aortic valve (maximum gradient > 50 mm Hg), surgery is indicated regardless of the degree of left ventricular systolic dysfunction. In the series from the Mayo clinic of 154 patients with an ejection fraction ≤ 35%, operative mortality was only 9% and overall survival was 69% at five years in those with coexisting coronary artery disease, compared to 77% in those with isolated aortic stenosis (fig 16.2).[4] Since left ventricular afterload is increased when aortic stenosis is present, with relief of obstruction, ventricular function improved in 76% of patients, with an increase in mean (SD) ejection fraction from 27 (6)% to 39 (14)%.

Aortic stenosis with a low pressure gradient and left ventricular dysfunction is even more problematic. If the low pressure gradient is associated with severe stenosis resulting in left ventricular dysfunction and a low transaortic volume flow rate, the patient will improve after aortic valve replacement. However, if the pressure gradient is low because of moderate aortic stenosis with concurrent primary myocardial dysfunction, valve replacement is less likely to be beneficial. Distinguishing these two groups of patients is not easy as both have a small calculated valve area since, in both cases, valve opening is impaired. Dobutamine stress echo-

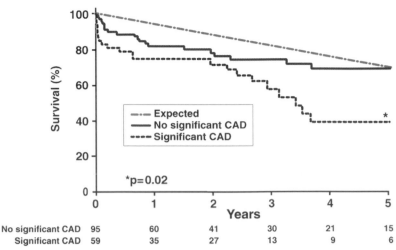

Figure 16.2. Kaplan–Meier survival curves for patients with aortic stenosis and reduced left ventricular function with and without significant coronary artery disease (two vessel disease or greater or left main coronary disease) in comparison with expected survival. Number of patients alive at each point is shown on the x axis. CAD, coronary artery disease. Reproduced with permission from Connolly HM, et al. Circulation 1997;95:2395–400.

> **Evaluation of the patient with aortic stenosis and left ventricular dysfunction**
>
> - Calculate standard measures of stenosis severity and left ventricular ejection fraction
>
> - Look at the severity of aortic valve calcification
>
> - Consider the risk:benefit ratio of valve replacement in this patient
>
> - Undertake dobutamine stress echocardiography to assess leaflet flexibility in selected cases

---

cardiography, with measurement of pressure gradient and valve area at baseline and at an increased flow rate (typically with 10 μg/min/kg of dobutamine), has been advocated for evaluation of these patients. If there is an increase in valve area with an increase in stroke volume, the valve leaflets are flexible and stenosis is not severe. Conversely, if valve area remains fixed despite an increase in flow rate, severe stenosis is present. However, this approach has not yet been validated on the basis of clinical outcome. In addition, if stroke volume fails to increase, it remains unclear whether the primary problem is increased valve stiffness or myocardial dysfunction.

A pragmatic approach in this patient group is to look at the degree of valve calcification, either by transthoracic or transoesophageal echocardiography or by fluoroscopy. Severe valve calcification is consistent with severe stenosis. Focal areas of thickening or only mild calcification suggest that valve surgery is not indicated. Unfortunately, patients with low gradient aortic stenosis have a poor outcome with both medical and surgical treatment. Given this prognosis, my bias is to err on the side of surgical intervention, in the hope that ventricular function will improve at least to the extent that afterload is reduced.

Mild to moderate aortic stenosis in patients undergoing coronary artery bypass surgery

Recent prospective studies have demonstrated that about 75% of patients with initially asymptomatic aortic stenosis develop symptoms requiring valve replacement within the next five years. This observation has led to the suggestion that valve replacement be performed at the time of coronary artery bypass surgery when mild to moderate stenosis is present to preclude the need for repeat surgery in the next few years. Surgical mortality rates for repeat surgery for aortic valve replacement are high (14–30%), further supporting the suggestion that "prophylactic" valve replacement be considered. However, we need to be cautious in applying this approach without consideration of the clinical factors in each patient. The likelihood of progression to symptoms is strongly correlated with the baseline aortic jet velocity. Those with a velocity < 3.0 m/s have a five year event free survival of 84 (16)% suggesting that valve replacement is not necessary, while those with a jet velocity > 4.0 m/s have a five year freedom from valve replacement of only 21 (18)%, suggesting that valve replacement is appropriate (fig 16.3). The decision about valve replacement in those patients with intermediate jet velocities (3–4 m/s) should be individualised, based on the risk of valve surgery, expected prosthetic valve haemodynamics and longevity, the extent of valve calcification, and patient preferences. In the future, it is possible that aggressive medical treatment to slow disease progression will provide an alternative to valve replacement in this patient group.

Rationale for surgery before symptom onset

There clearly are a few situations in which aortic valve replacement is appropriate in asymptomatic patients. Examples include patients with evidence of left ventricular systolic dysfunction caused by aortic stenosis, young women with severe stenosis who desire pregnancy, patients with asymptomatic severe disease who plan activities that involve severe exertion or who live in areas remote from medical care, and adults with very severe stenosis, in whom symptom onset is inevitable in the short term and in whom an elective procedure is preferred.

However, some investigators have suggested that valve replacement be performed in patients with severe aortic stenosis before symptom onset in order to prevent irreversible left ventricular hypertrophy and left ventricular systolic and diastolic dysfunction, and to decrease the risk of sudden death. There are little convincing data to support this approach. The most important predictor of postoperative left ventricular systolic function is preoperative systolic function, and most patients with aortic stenosis show an increase in ejection fraction after valve replacement. It is clear that diastolic dysfunction persists for years after aortic valve surgery, with histologic studies showing persistence of increased myocardial fibrosis.[5] However, it is unclear how early the intervention would need to be performed in order to prevent these changes, and there have been no trials demonstrating clinical benefit of early intervention. The risk of sudden death in the absence of antecedent symptoms is extremely low in adults with aortic stenosis and certainly is lower than the operative mortality of valve replacement surgery.

At this time, it is difficult to advocate routine early surgery in asymptomatic adults with severe aortic stenosis. This issue is further confused by our changing understanding of the definition of severe stenosis. Some patients develop symptoms at a pressure gradient and valve area that traditionally have been considered moderate, while other patients with apparent severe stenosis remain asymptomatic. Thus, it is problematic to define a specific numerical measure of stenosis severity that could be used to justify earlier surgical intervention. Of course, the other side of the risk-benefit equation in the timing of aortic valve replacement includes operative mortality and morbidity and the suboptimal haemodynamics and longevity of prosthetic valves. As surgical techniques improve and better valve substitutes are developed the argument for early surgery may become more persuasive.

Chronic aortic regurgitation

Chronic aortic regurgitation may be caused by abnormalities of the valve leaflets, most often a congenitally bicuspid valve, or by enlargement of the aortic root (fig 16.4). When aortic root disease is the cause of aortic regurgitation, timing of surgical intervention is more dependent on aortic root pathology than on the severity of aortic regurgitation. For example, in a patient with Marfan syndrome, the extent and rate of aortic root dilation are the primary determinants of the timing of aortic root and valve replacement. Acute aortic regurgitation differs from chronic disease both in clinical presentation and management. Acute aortic regurgitation may be caused by leaflet destruction (for example, endocarditis) or by lack of commissural support (for example, aortic dissection). Acute aortic regurgitation caused by aortic dis-

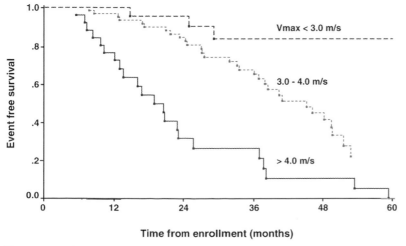

Figure 16.3. Cox regression analysis showing event free survival in 123 initially asymptomatic adults with valvar aortic stenosis, defined by aortic jet velocity at entry (p < 0.001 by log rank test). Reproduced with permission from Otto CM, et al. Circulation 1997;95:2262–70.

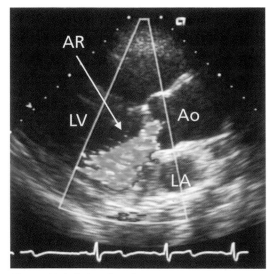

Figure 16.4. Colour flow Doppler image showing severe aortic regurgitation with a broad regurgitant jet and dilated left ventricle in a patient with a bicuspid aortic valve. Doppler measures of regurgitant severity are most helpful in identifying patients in whom periodic evaluation of left ventricular size and systolic function is warranted.

section is a surgical emergency. Severe aortic regurgitation caused by endocarditis also should be treated promptly with surgical intervention as outcome with medical treatment alone is poor.

Symptom onset

Patients with chronic aortic regurgitation may remain asymptomatic for many years despite haemodynamically significant backflow across the valve. The increased volume load on the left ventricle leads to a gradual increase in left ventricular dimension so that a normal forward stroke volume is maintained. Most patients eventually develop symptoms as a result of aortic regurgitation, with an average rate of symptom onset of 5–6% per year in prospective studies.[6 7] The most common initial symptom is dyspnoea on exertion or a decrease in exercise tolerance. In previously asymptomatic patients with severe aortic regurgitation, there is a small risk of sudden death occurring in 2–4% of patients over 7–8 years of follow up, typically in patients with severe left ventricular dilation.

Echocardiography provides a useful non-invasive approach to risk stratification in adults with chronic aortic regurgitation since the rate of symptom onset is directly related to the extent of left ventricular dilation. In one study, patients with an initial end systolic dimension < 40 mm had an annual rate of symptom onset of 0%, compared to 6% in those with an end systolic dimension of 40–49 mm and 19% in those with an end systolic dimension > 50 mm.[6] In another study, the strongest predictor of clinical outcome in chronic aortic regurgitation was the change in left ventricular ejection fraction from rest to exercise, normalised for the exercise change in end systolic wall stress.[7] However, measurement of this parameter is difficult and cumbersome in the clinical setting, as it requires both echocardiographic and radionuclide data acquisition

during exercise testing. The simpler measure of the exercise left ventricular ejection fraction is also strongly predictive of clinical outcome, with an exercise ejection fraction > 56% indicating a low rate of symptom onset (0% per year) compared to those with an exercise ejection fraction < 50% in whom symptoms occurred at a rate of 8.8% per year.

There have been no prospective studies showing that quantitative evaluation of the severity of regurgitation is predictive of clinical outcome. Of course, these studies only included patients with "severe" regurgitation as defined by clinical and echocardiographic criteria. As with aortic stenosis, the availability of non-invasive quantitative measures of valve disease is changing our understanding of the relation between regurgitant severity and clinical outcome. Many patients with "severe" aortic regurgitation remain asymptomatic with little change in ventricular size or function for many years. Thus, severe chronic aortic regurgitation should be defined as the degree of backflow across the aortic valve that results in progressive left ventricular dilation in association with adverse clinical outcomes. Doppler criteria alone should not be used to define severity until prospective studies are available that show the value of these quantitative measures in predicting clinical outcome.

On the other hand, Doppler measures of aortic regurgitant severity are extremely helpful when the degree of left ventricular dilation seems out of proportion to the severity of regurgitation. Quantitative measurements may then allow distinction between severe aortic regurgitation resulting in left ventricular dilation and mild to moderate aortic regurgitation with concurrent primary myocardial dysfunction caused, for example, by myocarditis or ischaemic disease. When clinical and Doppler data are discordant, evaluation of aortic regurgitation in the catheterisation laboratory also can be helpful.

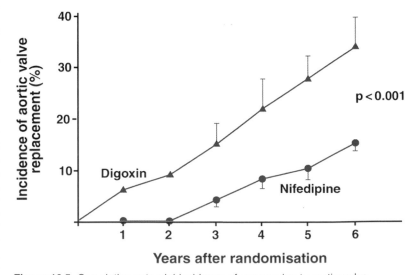

Figure 16.5. Cumulative actuarial incidence of progression to aortic valve replacement in 143 initially asymptomatic patients with severe aortic regurgitation randomised to treatment with digoxin 0.25 mg daily or nifedipine 20 mg twice a day. Reproduced with permission from Scognamiglio et al.[8]

Table 16.2 Timing of valve replacement in chronic aortic regurgitation

Study	n	Symptoms at entry	Mean (range) age (years)	Conclusions
Henry 1980	49	Yes	46 (19–68)	Pre-op ESD > 55 mm and FS < 25% were associated with poor outcome post AVR
Henry 1980	37	No	35 (17–64)	ESD and FS predicted which patients became symptomatic and required AVR
Bonow 1983	77	No	37 (16–67)	AVR is not needed until symptoms or LV dysfunction occurs
Bonow 1984	37	Yes	41 (20–46)	Duration of pre-op LV dysfunction is an important predictor of reversibility of LV function
Taniguchi 1987	62	Yes	43 (18–64)	Pre-op LV-ES volume index was most important predictor of subsequent cardiac death
Bonow 1988	61	Yes	43 (19–72)	Long term improvement in LV function is related to early reduction in EDD post-op
Siemienczuk 1989	50	No	48 (16)*	Patients can be risk stratified for "early progression to AVR" based on measurement of LV size and function
Taniguchi 1990	35	Yes	43 (15–60)	The post-op increase in EF correlated with the decrease in ESS. Contractile dysfunction persisted
Bonow 1991	104	No	36 (17–67)	Multivariate predictors of outcome (death, ventricular dysfunction or symptoms) were age, initial ESD, and rate of change in ESD and rest EF
Pirwitz 1994	27	Yes	(18–72)	The peak systolic pressure to ESV ratio was the strongest predictor of postoperative (post-op) functional class
Klodas 1996	31	Yes	50 (15)*	Pre-op EF (not EDD) predicted late survival and post-op EF. Severe LV dilation is not a contraindication to surgery
Borer 1997	104	No	46 (15)*	Change in EF from rest to exercise (normalise to the change in wall stress) was the strongest predictor of outcome
Dujardin 1999	264	No	56 (19)*	Predictors of outcome were age, functional class, comorbidity, AF, and ESD

AF, atrial fibrillation; AVR, aortic valve replacement; EF, ejection fraction; EDD, end diastolic dimension; ESD, end systolic dimension; ESS, end systolic stress; ESV, end systolic volume; FS, functional shortening; LV, left ventricular; *SD.
Sources: Henry WL, et al. Circulation 1980;**61**:71–483; Henry WL, et al. Circulation 1980;**61**:484–92; Bonow RO. Circulation 1983;**68**:509–17; Taniguchi K, et al. J Am Coll Cardiol 1987;**10**:510–18; Bonow RO. Circulation 1988;**78**(II):108–20; Siemienczuk D, et al. Ann Intern Med 1989;**110**:587–92; Taniguchi K, et al. Circulation 1990;**82**:798–807; Bonow RO. Circulation 1991;**84**:1625–35; Pirwitz MJ, et al. J Am Coll Cardiol 1994;**24**:1672–7; Klodas E, et al. J Am Coll Cardiol 1996;**27**:670–7; Borer JS, et al. Circulation 1997; **97**: 525–34; Dujardin KS, et al. Circulation 1999; **99**:1851–7.

Medical treatment

Medical treatment has been shown to be effective in slowing the rate of left ventricular dilation and delaying the timing of surgical intervention in adults with chronic aortic regurgitation. Aortic regurgitation represents both a volume and pressure overload state of the left ventricle as the increased stroke volume is ejected into the high resistance aorta. Thus, it makes physiologic sense that afterload reduction might decrease the severity of regurgitation and prevent progressive ventricular dilation. Several small studies have shown that angiotensin converting enzyme (ACE) inhibitors can slow the rate of left ventricular dilation. Further, in a randomised study of adults with severe aortic regurgitation and left ventricular dilation, treatment with nifedipine was associated with a six year event free survival rate of 85% compared to 65% in those treated with digoxin (fig 16.5).[8] Afterload reduction treatment now is standard in patients with severe aortic regurgitation and evidence of left ventricular dilation.

Asymptomatic ventricular systolic dysfunction

In patients with chronic aortic regurgitation, valve replacement is indicated at symptom onset. However, a small number of patients develop irreversible left ventricular systolic dysfunction in the absence of symptoms. The ideal measure of left ventricular systolic function would reflect contractility and be relatively independent of loading conditions, such as the end systolic pressure-volume relation or elastance. However, measurement of contractility is an elusive goal and measures that approximate this goal are impractical in the clinical setting. Thus, clinical decision making is based on parameters that have been shown to be predictive of postoperative outcome in series of patients undergoing valve replacement.

In studies of symptomatic patients who underwent valve replacement for severe aortic regurgitation, baseline predictors of postoperative left ventricular dysfunction include: (1) increased left ventricular size at end systole, defined either as end systolic dimension or end systolic volume index; (2) the duration of left ventricular dysfunction; (3) end systolic wall stress; and (4) ejection fraction. In a smaller number of studies that prospectively followed asymptomatic patients with chronic aortic regurgitation, the same factors (ventricular size and contractile function) were found to predict

17 Cardiac valve surgery in the octogenarian

René Prêtre, Marko I Turina

As the human lifespan increases and healthcare quality improves, more people are reaching an advanced age only to present with cardiac disorders that are usually treated uneventfully in young patients. The balance between enhanced initial risks and reduced eventual benefits in the elderly has often led to difficult medical decisions, and at times painful ethical and economical considerations.

Although there may be, on an individual basis, a substantial discrepancy between chronological and physiological age, the ability of elderly patients to withstand a major physiological insult such as cardiac surgery is reduced because of associated comorbidities, limited functional reserve of vital organs, and diminished defence and adaptation capacities. In the 1970s, an increase in mortality after cardiac surgery was apparent in patients older than 70 years. With the development of less traumatic heart–lung machines, more effective myocardial protection strategies, and improved perioperative care, mortality in the more robust patients—that is, the septuagenarians—dropped to levels of younger age groups.[1] Nowadays, the range of benefit of cardiac surgery remains narrow in patients 80 years of age or older, the age group discussed here.

Epidemiology

In the early 1990s, 7.4 million people (3% of the population) in the USA were older than 80 years. With a current life expectancy of 6.9 years for octogenarian men and 8.7 years for women, the number of octogenarians is expected to exceed 10 million (4.3 % of the population) by the year 2000. In England, the number will be 2 million. It is estimated that 40% of octogenarians have serious symptomatic heart disease. The number of elderly patients undergoing open heart surgery is increasing in all institutions. Because women outlive men by 6.9 years the ratio of women to men undergoing surgery increases and comes close to 1:1 in the older groups.

General considerations

Frailty of the elderly

Elderly patients with valve disease present with associated comorbidities (table 17.1) as well as reduced defence and adaptation capabilities. The aging process and atherosclerosis have undermined the reserve of many organs that are bound for postoperative dysfunction, or have already induced altered function. Furthermore, atherosclerosis frequently involves the aorta. Any manipulation of the aorta (cannulation for arterial inflow during cardiopulmonary bypass, cross clamping, and placement of a de-airing vent) may fragment a plaque and induce embolisation. Intraoperative transoesophageal and/or epiaortic echocardiography, which should routinely complement palpation of the aorta in the elderly, has shown that 20% of patients older than 75 years have protruding, sometimes mobile, atheromatous plaques in the ascending aorta and aortic arch.[2] The risk of embolisation can be reduced by avoiding cross clamping of the aorta and performing the operation (sometimes with endarterectomy or resection of the ascending aorta and aortic arch) during a period of deep hypothermic circulatory arrest. This formidable undertaking is, however, inappropriate in an old patient, and gentle manipulation of the aorta remains the sole practical preventive measure.

Table 17.1 Prevalence of comorbidities in octogenarians with cardiac valve disease

Coronary artery disease	40–60%
Obstructive lung disease	15–25%
Renal insufficiency	5–10%
Peripheral vascular disease	2–10%
Cerebrovascular disease	5–25%
Hypertension	20–50%
Diabetes	10–20%

Malperfusion of the brain is another complication of diffuse atherosclerosis that may occur during cardiopulmonary bypass. The lack of pulsatility of the bypass flow, uneven distribution of blood because of atherosclerosis, and impaired cerebral autoregulation may result in global or local underperfusion of the brain. Delayed awakening, agitation, and incomplete return of cognitive function are possible consequences of poor global brain perfusion. Together, diffuse and focal neurological deficits may affect 15–20% of elderly patients after heart surgery and are particularly devastating; they initiate a protracted postoperative course which often turns out to be fatal or leads to permanent institutionalisation.

Surgical risk:benefit ratio in the elderly

The true influence of age on early mortality after cardiac surgery is difficult to estimate, because of the high prevalence of other confounding factors. Although age appears in all scoring systems as an incremental risk factor

---

Principles of cardiac surgery in octogenarians

- Consider only symptomatic patients

- Liberal indications for independent and motivated patients

- Select the simplest operation and accept incomplete repair

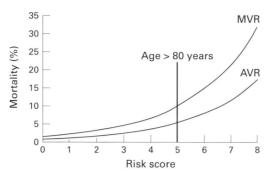

Risk factor	Weighting index
Age >80	5
LV ejection fraction 30–50%	2
Reoperation	2
Valve + CABG	2
Emergent operation	2
LV ejection fraction < 30%	5
Chronic renal failure	
Creatinine > 200 µmol/l	5
Dialysis	6
Critical situations	4–13

Figure 17.1. Mortality rates of aortic and mitral valve surgery according to the cumulated risk score. Critical situations include urgent operations (acute aortic dissection, postinfarction ventricular septal defect or papillary muscle avulsion) and necessity to operate within 48 hours after myocardial infarction. AVR, aortic valve replacement; MVR, mitral valve replacement; CABG, coronary artery bypass graft; LV, left ventricular.

for postoperative mortality, some studies found that it had no or only a marginal influence in relatively simple operations like isolated aortic valve replacement.[3] Most scoring systems in open heart surgery have shown that mortality increases logarithmically with the progression of the risk score. Figure 17.1, which is derived from the French score,[1] represents the mortality of mitral and aortic valve surgery in relation to the risk score. Age over 80 years shifts the patient to the right, where the steep rise in mortality starts. Without the addition of another risk factor, the operative risk of an octogenarian seems acceptable for almost any cardiac operation. The addition of one single moderate risk factor (with a score of 2 in fig 17.1) doubles the mortality rate of the cardiac operation. The addition of two moderate or one serious risk factor (with a score of 5) more than triples the rate and should warn against surgery.

The expected benefit of an intervention should not be viewed in terms of prolonging life, but of improving the quality of life; octogenarians seek surgery only to preserve their fading activity, threatened independence, or both. Therefore, only symptomatic and motivated patients should be considered for surgery, and the increase in wellbeing must be substantial to justify the operative risk. Obviously, conditions such as dementia or protracted depression that prevent an improvement in quality of life, and disorders such as advanced cancer or organ failure that reduce length of survival, make even low risk cardiac surgery inappropriate. Likewise, prophylactic operations or operations that yield a benefit only after a long survival, such as the "Maze" operation for chronic atrial fibrillation or the Ross procedure for aortic valve disease, should never be considered in the elderly. Not only does the addition of any comorbidity lead to a steep increase in the operative risk, it also reduces survival prospects in the elderly. In such a situation, the surgeon is well advised to opt for a technically and physiologically less demanding operation, even at the cost of an incomplete repair, with reduced mid-term benefit. Acceptance of a residual aortic stenosis in case of a small aortic annulus, mild mitral regurgitation (with or without repair) or revascularisation limited to the major coronary arteries are examples of incomplete yet appropriate management in the sick elderly.

A fair and objective discussion regarding operative risk and subsequent improvement in quality of life will allow most elderly patients, their family and doctor to reach a decision regarding further treatment. The decision will, however, be difficult to reach in the case of acute cardiac failure, because the patient may no longer be able to assess critically his or her needs and wishes.

Preoperative investigations

A decision regarding the necessity for valve repair or replacement can be based on clinical and echocardiographic findings alone. Atherosclerosis is, however, so conspicuous in the elderly that coronary angiography is appropriate in almost every patient. The risk of this examination, although increased, is not overwhelming (procedural mortality and morbidity are around 0.5% and 5%, respectively) and the benefit of appropriate coronary revascularisation is undisputable. Likewise, to reduce the high rate of postoperative stroke, a Doppler ultrasound of the carotid artery bifurcation should be obtained in every patient. Carotid endarterectomy before or at the time of heart surgery should be considered for symptomatic or bilateral high grade stenosis. The presence of an asymptomatic carotid stenosis or occlusion should lead the surgeon to work with

---

Comorbidities advising against valve surgery

- Coronary artery disease and left ventricular ejection fraction < 30%

- Creatinine concentration > 200 µmol/l

- Chronic obstructive pulmonary disease with FEV_1 < 800 ml

- Neurological deficit restricting patient's independence, outside activity, or both

- Debilitating psychiatric disorders (dementia, protracted depression)

- Cancer reducing quality of life, survival, or both

FEV_1, forced expiratory volume in 1 second

higher perfusion pressures, some will add some degree of systemic hypothermia, during the period of cardiopulmonary bypass.

Aortic valve disease

Aortic valve stenosis
Indication for surgery
Calcific aortic stenosis is the most common valve disorder encountered in octogenarians, and accounts for 60–70% of the valve surgery caseload.[4 5] In a population based study, significant aortic stenosis was found in 2.9% of randomly selected people aged 75–86 years, half of whom had symptoms. This figure predicts a yearly potential need for 3500 aortic valve replacements in octogenarians in a country like England.

Replacement of a stenotic aortic valve (and myocardial revascularisation limited to major coronary trunks) in elderly patients should be considered when symptoms occur. Most surgeons, however, will also consider valve replacement for only moderate stenosis (with a transvalvar gradient between 20–30 mm Hg and a valve orifice surface between 1–1.2 cm^2) in patients undergoing coronary revascularisation. This prophylactic replacement seems warranted on the grounds that the replacement only marginally increases the operative risk and progression of an aortic stenosis in an elderly person can be rapid, quickly negating the benefit of isolated bypass surgery.

Choice of prosthesis
Because the life expectancy of an octogenarian is shorter than the expected functional time of a biological prosthesis, most surgeons select a tissue valve for aortic valve replacement. Even if the thromboembolic risk of a mechanical valve in the aortic position can be controlled with a low anticoagulation dosage, the risk of bleeding remains a concern in the elderly patient. A few surgeons argue that the risk is extremely low and warrants implantation of mechanical prostheses in small aortic annuli. These prostheses have a smaller transvalvar gradient than bioprostheses and provide better haemodynamics and unloading of the left ventricle in annuli smaller than 21 mm in diameter.[6] In this situation, however, most surgeons accept the higher residual gradient of a bioprosthesis, or choose to enlarge the aortic annulus with a patch to accommodate a larger biological valve, or implant a stentless biological valve. The stentless valves are devoid of a sewing ring and, therefore, offer the largest opening surface and smallest transvalvar gradient. They are, however, more difficult to implant (they require two separate suture lines) and require longer cross clamp and cardiopulmonary bypass times. Furthermore, the suturing of the commissures of the prosthetic valve may be dangerous on a calcified aortic root, as is often encountered in old patients.

Results of surgery
The majority of patients with aortic stenosis have a preserved left ventricular function and half have normal coronary arteries. Postoperative mortality rates of 5–10% (only slightly higher than the rates of 2–3% for younger populations) are regularly reported for isolated valve replacement in this age group.[3-5 7] Associated coronary artery disease requiring coronary grafting raises the mortality rate to 15–20%. Although these good operative results were achieved on a selected population of fit elderly patients, it must also be acknowledged that the great majority were operated on at an advanced stage of valve disease, and a significant proportion had congestive heart failure, a condition known to increase operative mortality.[4 5] After successful surgery, survival is similar to a control population with rates of 95%, 80%, and 70% at one, three, and five years, respectively (fig 17.2).[7] The great majority of patients (up to 90%) return to their homes and lead an independent life, and those not limited by other comorbidities are able to perform moderate to vigorous activity.[8] These excellent results contrast with the grim natural history of symptomatic aortic stenosis. The survival rate of a matched population of patients who refused surgery (not of patients to whom surgery was not offered) was 57%, 37%, and 25% at one, two, and three years, respectively, and their quality of life was severely reduced.[9]

Percutaneous balloon angioplasty
Percutaneous balloon angioplasty has been proposed to relieve aortic stenosis in the elderly patient. Yet stenotic aortic valves in octogenarians exhibit rock hard calcification of the leaflets with no discernible commissures, and are the least suitable valves for dilatation. The results of balloon dilatation in this age group are disappointing with a significant rate of serious complications, including death, stroke, aortic rupture, and aortic insufficiency, and a high prevalence of residual or early recurrent severe stenosis.[10] Persistence of stenosis accounts for the lack of improvement in survival

---

Appropriateness of valve operations in octogenarians

- Aortic valve replacement for severe stenosis — +++
- Mitral valve repair or replacement for severe insufficiency — ++
- Aortic valve replacement for moderate stenosis during CABG — ++
- Mitral valve repair for moderate insufficiency during CABG — +
- Percutaneous balloon valvoplasty of the mitral valve — +
- Mitral valve replacement for moderate insufficiency during CABG — 0
- Combined aortic and mitral valve replacement — 0
- Percutaneous balloon valvoplasty of the aortic valve — 0
- Composite graft or homograft replacement of the aortic root — −
- Ross procedure (pulmonary autograft) — − −

+++ highly recommended; ++ recommended; + acceptable; 0 not recommended; − should be avoided; − − has no indication.

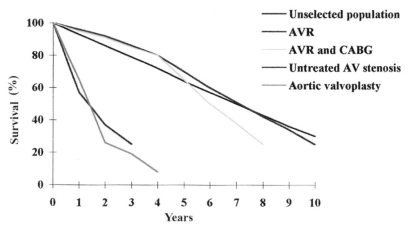

Figure 17.2. Survival rates of octogenarians with aortic valve stenosis. AV, aortic valve; R, replacement; CABG: coronary artery bypass graft.

Aortic valve stenosis in octogenarians

- Aortic valve replacement is well tolerated

- Only severe associated comorbidities should contraindicate surgery

- Calcification of the ascending aorta produces cerebral embolisation in 10% of patients

- Tissue valves are best

- Postoperative survival is similar to a control population

- Survival without operation in symptomatic patients is extremely short

- Indications for percutaneous balloon dilatation are limited

rates. That the results of valve replacement after failed percutaneous valvoplasty are also good (according to the US registry, the operative and two year survival rates after failed valvoplasty were 88% and 71%, respectively[11]) suggest that the reluctance to operate on aortic stenosis in the elderly is often exaggerated and the counselling for treatment options too often slanted towards valvoplasty. Valvoplasty might be considered as an initial step to alleviate stenosis in patients presenting with acute decompensation and progressive renal, hepatic, and respiratory failure. Although it is unclear whether this bridging valvoplasty is more effective than urgent surgery, it has the advantage of postponing major surgery until the patient can give a considered decision about his or her destiny.

Aortic valve regurgitation

Aortic valve insufficiency is rare in this age group and represents only 3–5% of the valve surgery caseload.[5] Chronic forms are found in patients with longstanding hypertension, in patients with progressive dilatation of the ascending aorta, and in patients who previously received an aortic bioprosthesis that has degenerated. Medical treatment, centred on the administration of vasodilators, often succeeds in stabilising or slowing progression of regurgitation. While surgery is advised prophylactically in young patients for echocardiographic signs of early ventricular deterioration or for when the diameter of the ascending aorta exceeds 6 cm, it should be deferred in octogenarians to when symptoms occur. In case of dilatation of the ascending aorta, a reduction plasty of the aorta reinforced with a synthetic mesh combined with the aortic valve replacement is a valuable alternative to the more radical but also more dangerous composite graft replacement. Acute forms of aortic valve insufficiency occur with endocarditis and aortic dissection. Emergency replacement of the aortic root with a valve homograft (with reimplantation of the coronary arteries) is the procedure of choice in endocarditis not responding to medical treatment in young persons. The magnitude of the operation, however, is excessive for the ill prepared and septic elderly. Debridement of the annulus and replacement of the valve with a prosthesis can be a better alternative, even if the risk of persistent or recurrent endocarditis is higher. Aortic insufficiency in aortic dissection is caused by the loss of commissural support of the valve and can usually be corrected by appropriate resuspension of the commissures. Resection of the dissected aorta should be limited to the ascending aorta in octogenarians; deep hypothermic circulatory arrest for simultaneous aortic arch replacement should be avoided if the aortic arch does not threaten to rupture.

Mitral valve disease

Mitral valve regurgitation
Indication for surgery

Chronic mitral valve insufficiency is the second most common operated valve disorder in the elderly, and represents 30–35% of the valvular surgery caseload.[4 5] Although chronic regurgitation causes damage to the left ventricle before symptoms occur, surgery in octogenarians should not be considered in asymptomatic patients. Chronic regurgitation is usually caused by myxomatous degeneration of the valve or by ischaemic dysfunction of the left ventricle.[12] With time, the mitral annulus dilates and regurgitation worsens. Degenerative regurgitation is typically caused by prolapse of the leaflets and ischaemic regurgitation by restricted motion of the leaflets. The distinction is, however, at times difficult; mild degrees of myxomatous degeneration and coronary artery disease frequently coexist in this age group. The distinction is not relevant when the valve needs be repaired or replaced on because the same surgical techniques are used. It is, however, important in patients operated on primarily for coronary artery disease and presenting mild to moderate degrees of regurgitation. Regurgitation may regress with improved myocardial perfusion and contractility. In these patients, intraoperative transoesophageal echocardiography provides a convenient way to assess the valve. If regurgitation is mild after induction of anaesthesia, it should be left untouched and later handled with vasodilators if systemic afterload is increased. If it is moderate, some surgeons will opt for the same conservative management while others will choose to implant an annuloplastic ring. If it is severe, correction is required.

Repair or replacement of the mitral valve
Repair of mitral insufficiency caused by myxomatous degeneration can often be achieved by application of simple and reliable techniques. Resection of the part of the leaflets that prolapses (with readaptation of the leaflet) and remodelling the annulus with a ring are often successful. The ring reduces the increased anteroposterior diameter of the mitral valve and brings the two leaflets closer together and improves their coaptation. Replacement of the mitral valve can be performed with preservation of the subvalvar apparatus in cases of myxomatous degeneration, but frequently requires its sacrifice in ischaemic regurgitation (and in mitral stenosis). Preservation of the subvalvar apparatus prevents the unfavourable globular remodelling of the left ventricle. This remodelling and fixation of the posterobasal part of the ventricle to the valve acutely diminishes ventricular systolic function.

The choice of prosthesis in the mitral position is debatable. Many surgeons select a biological prosthesis, which allows avoidance of anticoagulation or maintenance of anticoagulation at a low level when atrial fibrillation and massive dilatation of the atria coexist. Implantation of these prostheses is, however, more difficult than implantation of mechanical ones. For this reason (and especially in case of atrial fibrillation) some surgeons opt for a mechanical prosthesis. Finally, the stented commissures of a bioprosthesis protrude into the left ventricular outflow tract after implantation, and may create a subaortic obstruction when the left ventricle is not dilated. In the case of a small left ventricle, as occurs in acute forms of mitral regurgitation and in pure mitral stenosis, implantation of a low profile mechanical valve is a safer alternative.

Repair or replacement of the mitral valve can be technically challenging when the annulus is heavily calcified. The calcifications often extend to the epicardium of the atrioventricular groove. Overzealous decalcification can result in a non-repairable atrioventricular disconnection or in a delayed rupture of the left ventricle, which typically occurs a few hours after vigorous ventricular contraction. Partial decalcification of the annulus may lead to paraprosthetic leaks caused by the poor adaptation of the prosthesis ring to the rugged annulus.

Results of surgery
Mitral valve repair for regurgitation usually yields excellent results and should be attempted in the majority of elderly patients, even if only a less than perfect repair can be achieved. In a series of 100 patients older than 65 years, operative mortality was 4% and survival rate at one year was 90% after mitral valve repair.[12] The impact of valve repair on

---

Mitral valve regurgitation in octogenarians

- Surgery only in symptomatic patients

- Functional regurgitation in ischaemic cardiomyopathy often regresses with myocardial revascularisation

- Repair is often obtained with simple manoeuvres and provides more superior results than replacement

- Mild residual regurgitation after repair should be accepted

- Severe annular calcification is an additional risk for valve replacement

- Bioprostheses are more difficult to implant and their superiority over mechanical prostheses is marginal

---

survival and quality of life in octogenarians is currently unknown because of the small number of patients reported. Replacement of the mitral valve is not so well tolerated. The mortality rate in octogenarians fluctuates between 10–20%, and subsequent survival rates are 80%, 64%, and 41% at one, three, and five years, respectively.[13 14]

Mitral valve stenosis

Mitral valve stenosis is rare in octogenarians (1% of the valve surgery caseload), but still prevalent in septuagenarians. Valvar morphology is often not favourable for repair because of extensive calcification, rigidity, and retraction of all the valve components. Again, surgery is best recommended to patients with disabling symptoms only. Percutaneous balloon commissurotomy has been proposed as an alternative to surgery in high risk patients. In experienced hands, the procedural mortality in patients older than 70 years was 5% and improved transvalvar haemodynamics (mitral valve opening area > 1.5 cm^2 with mitral regurgitation $\leqslant 2+$) was achieved immediately in 50% of patients and persisted for three years in 30%.[15] Surgery, however, with an increased mortality to 20%, was necessary in 50% of patients within three years. Although better than on the aortic valve, the haemodynamic improvement after mitral valvoplasty vanishes rapidly and can be considered only as a palliative, often temporary measure.

1. **Roques F, Gabrielle F, Michel P,** *et al.* Quality of care in adult heart surgery: proposal for a self-assessment approach based on a French multicenter study. *Eur J Cardiothorac Surg* 1995;**9**:433–9.
- *This prospective multicentred study validated the French scoring system for assessment of the operative risk in open heart surgery. The French score showed a better predictive accuracy in operative mortality than the much used Parsonnet score. Area under the relative operative characteristic curve (so called ROC curve) was 0.75 for the French and 0.65 for the Parsonnet score.*

2. **Katz ES, Tunick PA, Rusinek H,** *et al.* Protruding aortic atheromas predict stroke in elderly patients undergoing cardiopulmonary bypass: experience with intraoperative transesophageal echocardiography. *J Am Coll Cardiol* 1992;**20**:70–7.
- *This study showed that direct palpation of the aorta is unreliable in detecting patients at risk for plaque material embolisation during manipulation of the aorta. Transesophageal echocardiography more reliably detects dangerous, friable atheromatous plaques.*

3. **Culliford AT, Galloway AC, Colvin SB,** *et al.* Aortic valve replacement for aortic stenosis in persons aged 80 years and over. *Am J Cardiol* 1991;**67**:1256–60.
- *This retrospective study reports excellent early and late results in 71 octogenarian patients after aortic valve*

replacement alone or with associated coronary artery bypass surgery.

4. Freeman WK, Schaff HV, O'Brien PC, et al. Cardiac surgery in the octogenarian: perioperative outcome and clinical follow-up. *J Am Coll Cardiol* 1991;**18**:29–35.
- *General overview of the results of open heart surgery in 191 octogenarian patients. Follow up extended to five years (mean 22 months). The authors state that cardiac surgery improved longevity in all subsets of patients surviving operation.*

5. Akins CW, Daggett WM, Vlahakes GJ, et al. Cardiac operations in patients 80 years old and older. *Ann Thorac Surg* 1997;**64**:606–14.
- *Excellent retrospective study on 600 consecutive octogenarian patients undergoing valve or coronary artery surgery, or both. Overall mortality was 8% and overall postoperative stroke rate 7%.*

6. Elayda MA, Hall RJ, Reul RM, et al. Aortic valve replacement in patients 80 years and older. Operative risks and long-term results. *Circulation* 1993;**88**(part 2):11–16.
- *One of the largest series of aortic valve replacement in octogenarian patients (171 patients). Mortality for isolated AVR was 5.2%, for AVR and CABG 24%, and for AVR and MVR 35%. The authors recommend a mechanical prosthesis for annuli ≤ 23 mm because of superior haemodynamic characteristics compared to bioprosthesis. Many authors have achieved better results with combined procedures.*

7. Gehlot A, Mullany CJ, Ilstrup D, et al. Aortic valve replacement in patients aged eighty years and older: early and long-term results. *J Thorac Cardiovasc Surg* 1996;**111**:1026–36.
- *Largest series (322 patients), spanning 20 years of aortic valve replacement in octogenarians. Risk factors for early death included female sex, creatinine concentration > 150 mg/l, concomitant CABG, reduced left ventricular ejection fraction < 35%, and chronic obstructive pulmonary disease. Extensive analysis of long term survival. Overall, survival (including early mortality) was 83% and 60% at one and five years, respectively.*

8. Shapira OM, Kelleher RM, Zelingher J, et al. Prognosis and quality of life after valve surgery in patients older than 75 years. *Chest* 1997;**112**:885–94.
- *One of the few studies that analyses quality of life after surgery. Most patients reported that their health status had improved and rated it to be between good and excellent. Postoperative stroke (4.8% of patients) had a devastating effect on the quality of life.*

9. O'Keefe JH Jr, Vlietstra RE, Bailey KR, et al. Natural history of candidates for balloon aortic valvuloplasty. *Mayo Clin Proc* 1987;**62**:986–91.

10. Bernard Y, Etievent J, Mourand JL, et al. Long-term results of percutaneous aortic valvuloplasty compared with aortic valve replacement in patients more than 75 years old. *J Am Coll Cardiol* 1992;**20**:796–801.
- *The long term results of aortic balloon valvuloplasty turned out to be disappointing, with a significant early mortality (6.5%), an additional 52% mortality rate at three years, and a need to operate on 35% of surviving patients within 35 months. This report sharply contrasts with that of another group in France, which claimed a 0% postprocedural mortality and a 73% survival rate at one year (Eltchaninoff et al. Eur Heart J 1995;16:1079–84). Other reports are in keeping with Bernard's experience.*

11. Otto CM, Mickel MC, Kennedy JW, et al. Three-year outcome after balloon aortic valvuloplasty. Insights into prognosis of valvular aortic stenosis. *Circulation* 1994;**89**:642–50.

12. Bolling SF, Deeb GM, Bach DS. Mitral valve reconstruction in elderly, ischemic patients. *Chest* 1996;**109**:35–40.
- *This group showed that mitral valve repair was an excellent treatment in elderly patients with ischaemic mitral regurgitation. Unfortunately, very few operative data have been included (methods of repair, time of myocardial ischemia have not been reported). The consequences of the ventricular–annular distortion following mitral valve replacement are well explained.*

13. Asimakopoulos G, Edwards MB, Brannan J, et al. Survival and cause of death after mitral valve replacement in patients aged 80 years and over: collective results from the UK heart valve registry. *Eur J Cardiothorac Surg* 1997;**11**:922–8.
- *The UK heart valve registry reported an early mortality after mitral valve replacement in 86 octogenarians of 10% and subsequent survival rates at one, three, and five years of 80%, 64%, and 41 %, respectively. The registry has the advantage of presenting the average results for the country, while the literature favours publication of reports with good results. It does not, however, inform on the prevalence of other risk factors such as associated coronary artery disease, which could explain the disappointing midterm result.*

14. Davis EA, Gardner TJ, Gillinov AM, et al. Valvular disease in the elderly: influence on surgical results. *Ann Thorac Surg* 1993;**55**:333–7.
- *Concomitant CABG increased early mortality from 3.3% (AVR alone) to 7.2% (AVR and CABG) and raises the question of how aggressively revascularisation should be pursued. A more advanced myocardial dysfunction in patients requiring concomitant CABG was probably responsible for the increased mortality. Limiting revascularisation to the major coronary trunks could be the answer to this puzzling question.*

15. Iung B, Cormier B, Farah B, et al. Percutaneous mitral commissurotomy in the elderly. *Eur Heart J* 1995;**16**:1092–9.
- *Improvement of valve function was only moderate, and subsequent functional deterioration frequent after percutaneous mitral commissurotomy. This palliative approach should not be enthusiastically presented, even to elderly patients, when the surgical risk lies within acceptable limits.*

18 Anticoagulation in valvar heart disease: new aspects and management during non-cardiac surgery

Christa Gohlke-Bärwolf

The indications for oral anticoagulant treatment have been extended over the last 10 years. The detection of new congenital thrombophilic risk factors, the studies on non-valvar atrial fibrillation, and the increase in valvar heart surgery have all led to a rise in the number of patients being treated. In 1997, 64 000 valve operations were performed across Europe; in two thirds of these operations mechanical prostheses were used, subsequently requiring lifelong oral anticoagulant treatment.[w1]

New developments in anticoagulation

Several recent developments in the management of anticoagulation with vitamin K antagonists can potentially improve the efficacy and safety of this treatment.

- The introduction of the international normalised ratio (INR) as a measure of the intensity of anticoagulation has provided a reliable parameter for monitoring oral anticoagulant treatment, independent of the responsiveness of the thromboplastin used.[1 w2 w3] All the expert committees have recommended the use of the INR instead of prothrombin time, although its acceptance has varied from country to country.
- The development of the concept of risk factor adjusted, prosthesis specific intensity of anticoagulation[2 w4] has influenced the management of patients with mechanical valve prosthesis and valvar heart disease in general, allowing risk stratification and lower anticoagulation intensities in certain lower risk groups of patients.
- The results of prospective, randomised studies evaluating the effect of different intensities of anticoagulation on thromboembolic and haemorrhagic events allow a more targeted approach.[3 4 w5 w6]
- The development of simple anticoagulation monitors has dramatically improved the quality of anticoagulation control.[5 6]
- The guidelines developed by the working group on valvar heart disease of the European Society of Cardiology on the management of antithrombotic treatment in heart valve disease,[2] together with the guidelines of the British Society of Haematology[1] and the American Heart Association/American College of Cardiology (AHA/ACC),[7] have provided the basis for the following discussion.

Indication for oral anticoagulant treatment

The indications for lifelong anticoagulation are listed in table 18.1. Anticoagulation is indicated for the first three months after valve replacement with bioprostheses, even when sinus rhythm is present. This also applies to mitral valve repair. Oral anticoagulation is indicated 3–4 weeks before and after cardioversion.

Concept of risk factor adjusted, prosthesis specific intensity of anticoagulation

The concept of risk factor adjusted, prosthesis specific intensity of anticoagulation was first proposed by Butchart[w4] in regard to mechanical valve prosthesis, and was included in the recommendations by the working group on valvar heart disease.[2] Within certain limits the degree of reduction in thromboembolic events is higher with increasing intensity of anticoagulation, yet at the expense of an exponential rise in bleeding risk with increasing intensity.

There is only a narrow range of intensity of anticoagulation in which the reduction in thromboembolic events is as pronounced as possible and the bleeding risk is as low as possible. This optimal range of INR or target INR varies from patient to patient, and can be illustrated by comparing two patients at the extreme ends of thromboembolic risk:

- A young man with a valve prosthesis of low thrombogenicity such as the St Jude Medical valve or the Medtronic Hall valve in aortic position, in sinus rhythm, with normal left ventricular function and size, without heart failure and other risk factors, has a thromboembolic risk of about 1% per year with moderate anticoagulation intensity.[1 3 8]
- A 70 year old patient with a first generation Starr-Edwards prosthesis in the mitral position, with atrial fibrillation, large left atrium, and congestive heart failure, has a thromboembolic risk of about 5% per year.[8 w4] Thus the intensity of anticoagulation used in this latter patient should be higher than in the former.

Three major groups of risk factors for thromboembolic events and strokes should be taken into account when defining the intensity of oral anticoagulant treatment in valvar heart disease. These risk factors are related to the

Table 18.1 Absolute indication for lifelong oral anticoagulation

All patients with:
- Mechanical prostheses
- Chronic or intermittent atrial fibrillation in the presence of
  - native valve disease
  - bioprostheses
  - valve repair
  - valvuloplasty
- Native valve disease and previous emboli
- Mitral valve stenosis, independent of rhythm, with
  - high valve gradients
  - thrombus in left atrium
  - spontaneous echo contrast in left atrium
  - large left atrium > 50 mm
  - low cardiac output
  - congestive heart failure

general and cardiac status of the patient, to the prosthesis being used, and to the time interval from the operation.

Patient related risk factors

The incidence of stroke and systemic embolism rises with increasing age, smoking, hypertension, diabetes, hyperlipidaemia, increasing fibrinogen, and acquired or congenital abnormalities of the coagulation system.

The type and severity of the underlying valve disease are important risk factors. Patients with the highest risk for thromboembolism are patients with mitral stenosis, particularly those who develop atrial fibrillation. In these patients the risk of thromboembolism increases to 20% per year. Atrial fibrillation is a very potent risk factor for thromboembolic events, particularly in patients with heart valve disease and after valve replacement. Whereas atrial fibrillation without associated heart disease is associated with a minimal increase in thromboembolic risk to 0.5% per year, the association with other cardiovascular diseases such as hypertension increases the risk of stroke to about 4–6% per year. Atrial fibrillation associated with mitral valve disease leads to an 18 fold increase in embolic risk.

Decreased ventricular function, low cardiac output, and congestive heart failure, as well as left atrial enlargement, are risk factors for thromboembolic events; even loss of atrial contraction in the presence of electrophysiologically normal sinus rhythm carries an increased risk. The degree of mitral stenosis is an important determinant of embolic risk. Patients with severe mitral stenosis are prone to thromboembolism even in sinus rhythm. A history of previous peripheral emboli is associated with a 20% recurrence rate within the first year.

Prothesis related risk factors

Prosthesis related risk factors are defined by the type and localisation of the prosthesis. While bioprostheses in general have a lower thromboembolic risk than mechanical prostheses, a further differentiation can be made on the basis of localisation and design. Prostheses in the aortic position have a lower thromboembolic risk than in the mitral position.

Furthermore, first generation prostheses like the Starr-Edwards, the older Björk-Shiley standard, and the Omniscience prostheses have a higher thromboembolic risk than the second generation protheses such as the St Jude Medical or the Medtronic Hall valves.

With anticoagulation, generally most second generation prostheses have a thromboembolic risk of 0.5–2.2% per year in the aortic position and 2–3% per year in the mitral position.[7-9]

Of further importance is the time interval from the operation. The thromboembolic rate is highest in the first three months following surgery. Twenty per cent of all thromboembolic complications occur during the first month,[9] when a pronounced hypercoagulable state is present which decreases with time. The endothelialisation process of a newly implanted valve takes several weeks. The valve ring with the sutures are prone to platelet deposition and thrombus formation. This is the basis for the recommendation to anticoagulate patients with bioprostheses during the first three months after surgery.

Intensity of anticoagulation, therapeutic range of INR, target INR

Among the most recent recommendations for anticoagulation in patients with mechanical valves, opinions differ in regard to the desired intensity of anticoagulation.

On the basis of the concept of risk factor and prostheses adjusted oral anticoagulation, the European Society of Cardiology[2] recommends intense anticoagulation with an INR of 3.0–4.5 in patients with the older first generation prostheses such as the Starr-Edwards (table 18.2). However, the British Society of Haematology[1] considers a target INR of 3.5 to be sufficient for all mechanical valves, as does the AHA/ACC although the addition of aspirin 80–100 mg is suggested.[7] Only for high risk patients who cannot tolerate additional aspirin does the AHA/ACC recommend an INR of 3.5–4.5.[7]

Whether an INR > 3.5 is indeed required in high risk patients with first generation mitral valves or other high risk patients has not been investigated prospectively. Such a decision

Table 18.2 Intensity of anticoagulation

	European Society of Cardiology 1995[2] INR range	British Society of Haematology[1] target INR	AHA/ACC 1998[7] INR range
Mechanical valve: first generation (eg. Starr-Edwards, Björk-Shiley standard); second generation (St Jude Medical, Medtronic Hall, BS Monostrut)		3.5 in all patients with mechanical prostheses	2.5–3.5
Aortic position	2.5–3.0		2.0–3.0*
Mitral position	3.0–3.5		2.5–3.5
Bioprostheses sinus rhythm			
Aortic position	2.5–3.0		Aspirin 80–100 mg
Mitral position	3.0 3.5	2.5	Aspirin 80–100 mg
	No AC after 3 months	No AC after 3 months	No AC after 3 months
Bioprostheses and atrial fibrillation	3.0–4.5	2.5	AVR + RF 2.0–3.0 MVR + RF 2.5–3.5
Rheumatic valvar heart disease and atrial fibrillation	3.0–4.5	2.5	
Patients with recurrent emboli under adequate anticoagulation	3.0–4.5 + 100 mg aspirin		
Non-valvar atrial fibrillation with risk factors	2.0–3.0	2.5	

*With RF 2.5–3.5; AC, anticoagulation; AVR, aortic valve replacement; MVR, mitral valve replacement; RF, risk factors

should be taken on an individual basis, particularly in view of the increased bleeding risk.

Patients with the St Jude Medical valve, the Medtronic Hall valve, and the Monostrut valve need less intense anticoagulation. The European guidelines[2] recommend a target INR of 3.0–3.5 in the mitral position and 2.5–3.0 in the aortic position. This may need to be adjusted if other underlying risk factors for thromboembolism and stroke are present.

The AREVA study[3] compared two different intensities of oral anticoagulation (INR 2.0–3.0 v 3.0–4.5) in low risk patients with aortic valve replacement, mostly with the St Jude Medical valve. A mean INR of 2.7 was achieved in the first group and 3.2 in the second group. The moderate anticoagulation group with an INR of 2–3 had a significantly lower haemorrhagic event rate (11.2 per 100 patient years) than the group with an INR of 3–4.5 (20.5 per 100 patient years). This was not associated with an increased rate of thromboembolic events (3.1% v 2.4%). Since the median INR for each patient was between 2.5 and 3.5 in 72% of all patients, this study may not support an INR target level of < 2.5 in patients with low risk aortic valve prostheses.

A retrospective analysis revealed that if the INR falls below 2.5 in patients with mechanical heart valves a rather pronounced rise in the thromboembolic rate occurs.[10]

The importance of risk factors for determining the intensity of anticoagulation is also addressed in patients with bioprostheses. As long as patients remain in sinus rhythm, they only need anticoagulation for three months and none thereafter. The AHA/ACC guidelines recommend lifelong low dose aspirin.[7] Whether this is necessary in patients without associated coronary artery disease and only aortic valve bioprosthesis is still undecided.

Yet when atrial fibrillation occurs, patients with bioprostheses also require anticoagulation. In the mitral position an INR of 3.0–4.5 is recommended by the European guidelines[2]; in the aortic position an INR of 2.5–3.5 is recommended. Generally, in those patients with atrial fibrillation as a risk factor for thromboembolic events, the intensity of anticoagulation should be adjusted according to the underlying pathological condition and the risk associated with it.

If atrial fibrillation occurs in patients with rheumatic mitral valve disease, particularly in severe mitral stenosis, the risk for stroke and other thromboembolic complications is high—at least 5% per year—thus an INR of 3.0–4.5 is recommended. In aortic valve disease the risk is less, thus an INR of 2.5–3.5 can be considered sufficient. In patients with non-valvar atrial fibrillation and risk factors, an even less intense anticoagulation with an INR of 2–3 is sufficient.

In patients with previous emboli despite adequate anticoagulation the risk of recurrent thromboembolism is higher. Therefore for these patients an INR of 3.0–4.5, in addition to aspirin 100 mg daily, is recommended if no other cause for the recurrent emboli can be identified. Most of these patients with recurrent emboli have, however, inadequate anticoagulation. Furthermore, other risk factors for thromboembolic events—such as hyperlipidaemia, smoking, hypertension, diabetes—are frequently present which also need to be better controlled. Many studies have shown that lipid lowering in patients with coronary artery disease leads to a reduction in stroke rate by 30%.[11] Cardiologists have universally accepted that risk factor modification is an established part of the treatment of coronary patients. However, there are no studies in patients with valvar heart disease or mechanical protheses. This concept can at least be applied to patients with valve disease and associated coronary artery disease. Because of the profound effects of atherosclerotic risk factors on the coagulation system, leading to a hypercoagulable state,[w7] it seems logical to implement a strict risk factor modification programme for all patients with valvar heart disease or mechanical prostheses in order to reduce the likelihood of stroke and general thromboembolic events in these patients.

Modification of anticoagulant treatment for specific procedures

Patients receiving anticoagulant treatment require adjustments in their anticoagulation when undergoing different types of non-cardiac surgery or diagnostic procedures. This most commonly arises when patients undergo dental procedures, but anticoagulant adjustment is also required for ophthalmic and minor or major surgical procedures, either on an elective or emergency basis. Patients may need to undergo interventional cardiac procedures such cardiac catheterisation, coronary angioplasty, and the implantation of pacemakers or defibrillators, which also necessitate alteration in anticoagulation. Adjustment is also needed in the event of conditions such as cerebral haemorrhage and certain gastrointestinal disorders such as bleeding ulcer. Randomised studies are not available for most of these situations,[w8] and there are only a few prospective observational studies[w9] to guide management. Much of the available information comes from retrospective analyses, and opinions differ over what is felt to be the safest level of anticoagulation for various procedures[9] [w10–12] and on the estimation of the thromboembolic risk that exists.[w13]

In studies concerning non-cardiac surgery in patients with mechanical valves the incidence of thromboembolic events varied between 0–2% in patients with aortic valve replacement and 11–20% in patients with mitral valve replacement.[7] [8] [12] [w9] [w14]

Thus the risk to be anticipated in case of interruption of anticoagulation during non-cardiac surgery may be appreciably higher than calculated, depending upon the individual risk factors for thromboembolic events, which are related to patients, protheses, procedures, and pathology (table 18.3).

Table 18.3   Risk assessment for non-cardiac surgical procedures

According to risk factors related to:	Low risk	High risk
Patients		
Atrial fibrillation		+
Previous thromboembolism		+
Hypercoagulable congenital or acquired conditions		+
Left ventricular dysfunction		+
Heart failure		+
Prostheses design		
Ball valve		+
Tilting disk	+	
Bileaflet	+	
Prostheses position		
Aortic	+	
Mitral		+
Procedures		
Dental, ophthalmic	+	
Skin	+	
Gastrointestinal		+
Pathology		
Tumour		+
Infection		+

Different management strategies have been suggested, including:

- discontinuation of oral anticoagulation until normalisation of the INR without heparin replacement;
- discontinuation of oral anticoagulation until normalisation of the INR with heparin replacement as soon as the INR is < 2.0;
- lowering the intensity of anticoagulation while oral anticoagulation is maintained;
- continuing a therapeutic level of anticoagulation.

The choice of which regimen should be followed should be based on the individual risk for thromboembolic events, the time interval required to be off or at low anticoagulation levels, and the risk of haemorrhage determined by the procedure.

Thus the concept of risk factor adjusted intensity of anticoagulation can also be used to determine the most appropriate and safest strategy.

Patient related risk factors (table 18.3) increase thromboembolic risk by a factor of 5–20. Also prosthesis design and position have to be taken into account. Discontinuation of anticoagulation for one week leads to a significant thromboembolic risk in patients with mitral valve replacement varying between 10–20%, whereas the incidence of thromboembolism in patients with aortic valve replacement is 0–2%.[12 w9 w14]

The prothrombotic state of the surgical procedure itself may increase the risk for thromboembolic events.

All stages of haemostasis can be altered during and after surgery—with increased platelet aggregation and activation, conversion of fibrinogen to fibrin, and depressed fibrinolysis by decreased activators and increased inactivators—thus potentially increasing the thromboembolic risk of the prosthetic valve patient. The level of hypercoagulable changes correlates with the magnitude and duration of surgery, and postoperative changes and complications such as infection. The underlying disease which first led to the surgical procedure—such as a tumour—is a further risk factor. In a large general surgical population 68% (11/16) of thromboembolic events occurred among patients who were operated on because of a tumour.[12]

The time interval necessary to discontinue anticoagulation before non-cardiac surgical procedures depends on: the half life of the oral anticoagulant used; the actual INR; the desired INR for the specific procedure; and the individual vitamin K pool.[13]

If warfarin is used, the guidelines of the AHA/ACC[7] and the British Society of Haematology[1] suggest discontinuation for 72 hours before routine non-cardiac surgical procedures. The INR should be closely monitored, because the decrease in INR may vary greatly among different patients.

Dental surgery

Dental surgery is one of the procedures with the lowest risk for thromboembolic complications. A recent literature review[14] covering 2014 dental surgical procedures and 1964 extractions showed that thromboembolic complications occurred in five (0.9%) of 493 patients in whom anticoagulation was discontinued. However, four of the five thromboembolic complications were lethal. In contrast, continuation of anticoagulation in 774 patients was not associated with any thromboembolic events. Bleeding complications occurred in 1.6% patients, and none were fatal. All bleedings occurred with an INR > 4.5.[14]

Thus dental surgical procedures do not require major changes in the intensity of anticoagulation. Continuation of anticoagulation at an INR of 2.0–2.5 is the safest approach for dental surgery; even full mouth extractions have a low risk for bleeding, which can easily be treated with local measures (table 18.4).[2 w15 w16] Heparin, as suggested by Peuten[w17] is not necessary.

Interventional cardiac procedures

For left heart catheterisation by the brachial route, the INR should be < 2.5, and by the femoral route it should be < 1.8.[2 w15]

Surgical procedures

Minor surgical procedures can be performed while the INR is just < 2 and oral anticoagulation can be resumed on the day of surgery. Robinson[w10] and Bartley[w11] suggested it was not necessary to discontinue oral anticoagulation before cataract extractions and other oculoplastic surgical procedures, provided the INR was not above the therapeutic range.

Table 18.4   Anticoagulation before diagnostic and surgical procedures (European Society of Cardiology)[2]

	INR
Left heart catheterisation (Sones)	< 2.5
Left heart catheterisation (Judkins)	< 1.8
Tooth extraction	< 2.5
Minor surgical procedure	< 2.0
Major surgical procedure	< 1.5
Replace with heparin when INR:	< 2.5 in high risk patients
Replace with heparin when INR:	< 2.0 in average risk patients

Major surgical procedures require lowering of the INR to < 1.5. In these cases anticoagulation needs to be maintained with heparin. Heparin should be started when the INR is < 2.5 in high risk patients (for example, in patients with mitral mechanical valves) and < 2.0 in patients with aortic mechanical valves. The activated partial thromboplastin time (aPTT) should be prolonged to 1.5–2.0 of the control value. Heparin should be continued until six hours before surgery and resumed 6–12 hours after surgery, when surgically feasible. It should be continued until INR is > 2. Oral anticoagulation can be resumed 1–2 days after surgery.[1][2][7]

Management before emergency surgery

In the event of emergency surgery, oral anticoagulation needs to be neutralised by infusion of prothrombin complex concentrate or fresh frozen plasma, the dose of which needs to be individualised. Additional repeat small doses of vitamin K may be given intravenously or orally.[15][16] Complete reversal of oral anticoagulants with vitamin K in large doses may lead to prolonged resistance to oral anticoagulants and the possibility of valve thrombosis and thromboemboli.

Low molecular weight heparin

Recently it has been suggested that low molecular weight heparin (LMWH) can be used for the interim maintenance of anticoagulation. Although it is not approved for application in patients with mechanical prosthesis, and no studies are available for non-cardiac procedures, it is already used for this purpose in some countries. Montalescot[17] reported the use of LMWH in the immediate postoperative period after valve surgery. In 102 patients there were two major bleedings and one thromboembolic event, which did not differ from the incidence of bleeding and thromboembolic events in a group of patients previously treated with unfractionated heparin. The study was not randomised and was conducted for only 14 days without further follow up or echocardiographic studies.

If follow up is short after discontinuation of anticoagulation, and echocardiographic studies are not performed routinely, significant thromboembolic events may be missed. Valve thrombosis may develop slowly and insidiously and may not be evident for 1–2 months.

No definite information on the safety and efficacy of LMWH is available at this time to guide its use. Because of the longer half life, requiring only 1–2 doses per day in randomised studies on unstable angina pectoris, LMWH appears to have a promising role in the perioperative management of non-cardiac surgery. Randomised studies, aimed at defining doses in different patient groups, are necessary.

The optimal management of anticoagulation during non-cardiac surgery requires careful risk assessment of patients and procedures. Self testing and self management of anticoagulation

---

Management of oral anticoagulant treatment can be improved by:

- Following the concept of risk factor adjusted indication for and intensity of oral anticoagulant treatment

- Use of the INR for monitoring the intensity of anticoagulation

- Intensive education of the patient about anticoagulation

- Implementing self testing by suitable patients

- Increasing the frequency of testing

The risks associated with interruption of oral anticoagulant treatment during non-cardiac surgery can be reduced by:

- Performing dental procedures at an INR between 2–2.5

- Using local measures to treat bleeding in the dental surgery

- Replacing oral anticoagulant treatment with heparin before major surgery, when INR is < 2.5 in high risk patients with mechanical mitral valves, and < 2.0 in patients with aortic valves, up to six hours before surgery

- Discontinuing warfarin 72 hours before surgery, but observing factors influencing the time interval required for reduction in INR

- Resuming heparin 6–12 hours postsurgery and maintaining until INR > 2.5

---

by the patient can facilitate management and reduce risks.

Outlook for better anticoagulation control

Physicians and patients should become more informed about anticoagulation control. Patients need verbal and written information about the purpose of their anticoagulation treatment and its effects, the desired INR range and target INR, side effects, drug interference, diet, and signs and symptoms of overdose (bleeding) and underdosing (valve thrombosis and thromboembolism), as well as other complications.

Self monitoring of anticoagulation by patients has improved their anticoagulation control[5] and thus their quality of life. Modification of atherosclerotic risk factors is important for all patients with diseased native and prosthetic heart valves to reduce thromboembolic and stroke risk.

Future research should be directed towards evaluation of alternatives to conventional anticoagulation in non-cardiac surgery, such as LMWH.

Methods for improved risk assessment and risk stratification in different patient groups should be developed, including family history and laboratory studies for congenital or acquired risk factors for thromboembolic events.

1. **British Society of Haematology.** British committee for standards in haematology guidelines on oral anticoagulation, 3rd ed. *Br J Haematol* 1998;**101**:374–87.
• *This is a thorough review of clinically important topics in anticoagulation and recommendations for management.*

2. **Gohlke-Bärwolf C, Acar J, Oakley C,** *et al.* Guidelines for prevention of thromboembolic events in valvular heart disease. Study group of the working group on valvular heart disease of the European Society of Cardiology. *Eur Heart J* 1995;**16**:1320–30.
• *These guidelines provide a delineation of the concept of risk factor adjusted anticoagulation in patients with various native valvar heart diseases and following all types of valve operations, and present recommendations for management in various clinical situations.*

3. **Acar J, Iung B, Boissel JP,** *et al.* AREVA: multicenter randomized comparison of low-dose versus standard-dose anticoagulation in patients with mechanical prosthetic heart valves. *Circulation* 1996;**94**:2107–12.
• *This was the first multicentre randomised study to compare two different target ranges of anticoagulation (INR 2–3 v 3–4) in low risk patients after aortic valve replacement with St Jude Medical valves.*

4. **Turpie AG, Gent M, Laupacis A,** *et al.* A comparison of ASS with placebo in patients treated with warfarin after heart valve replacement. *N Engl J Med* 1993;**8**:524–9.

5. **Bernardo A.** Experience with patient self-management of oral anticoagulation. *J Thromb Thrombolysis* 1996;**2**:321–5.

6. **Sawicki PT for the Working Group for the Study of Patient Self-Management of Oral Anticoagulation.** A structured teaching and self-management program for patients receiving oral anticoagulation: a randomised controlled trial. *JAMA* 1999;**281**:145–50.

7. **Bonow RO, Carabello B, DeLeon AC,** *et al.* ACC/AHA guidelines for the management of patients with valvular heart disease. *J Am Coll Cardiol* 1998;**32**:1486–8.

• *This is a comprehensive review of the management of valvar heart disease, setting the current standard of care.*

8. **Cannegieter SC, Rosendaal FR, Briët E.** Thromboembolic and bleeding complications in patients with mechanical heart valve prostheses. *Circulation* 1994;**89**:635–41.

9. **Butchart EG, Bodnar E, eds.** *Thrombosis, embolism and bleeding.* London: ICR Publishers, 1992: 293–317.

10. **Cannegieter SC, Rosendaal F, Wintzen A,** *et al.* Optimal oral anticoagulant therapy in patients with mechanical heart valves. *N Engl J Med* 1995;**333**:11–17.

11. **Pedersen TR.** Randomised trial of cholesterol lowering in 4444 patients with coronary heart disease: the Scandinavian simvastatin survival study (4S). *Lancet* 1994;**344**:1383–9.

12. **Carrel TP, Klingenmann W, Mohacsi PJ,** *et al.* Perioperative bleeding and thromboembolic risk during non-cardiac surgery in patients with mechanical prosthetic heart valves: an institutional review. *J Heart Valve Dis* 1999;**8**:392–8.

13. **White R, McKittrik T, Hutchinson R,** *et al.* Temporary discontinuation of warfarin therapy: changes in the international normalized ratio. *Ann Intern Med* 1995;**122**:40–4.
• *This is a clinically important study on the time sequence of INR decrease after discontinuation of warfarin and factors that influence it.*

14. **Wahl MJ.** Dental surgery in anticoagulated patients. *Arch Intern Med* 1998;**158**:1610–16.
• *This article presents a review of studies published during the last 40 years on thromboembolic and bleeding complications associated with different anticoagulation regimens before dental surgery, showing that continuation of anticoagulation is associated with lower thromboembolic risk without increasing bleeding significantly.*

15. **Shetty HGM, Backhouse G, Bentley DB,** *et al.* Effective reversal of warfarin-induced excessive anticoagulation with low dose vitamin K1. *Thromb Haemost* 1992;**67**:13–15.

16. **Weibert RT, The Le D, Kaiser SR,** *et al.* Correction of excessive anticoagulation with low-dose oral vitamin K1. *Ann Intern Med* 1997;**125**:959–62.

17. **Montalescot G, Polle V, Collet J,** *et al.* Low molecular weight heparin after mechanical heart valve replacement. *Circulation* 2000;**101**:1083–6.

19 Interface between valve disease and ischaemic heart disease

Bernard Iung

The association of coronary artery disease with heart valve disease is frequently encountered and it can be expected that this association will become more common because of the evolution in the epidemiology of valvar diseases. Degenerative lesions are now the most frequent cause of valve disease in western countries and they frequently occur in old patients, who are also at higher risk for atherosclerotic disease. The association of calcified aortic stenosis and coronary heart disease is the main problem, because it is the most frequently encountered association and because it raises specific questions, particularly in regard to the detection and management of both pathologies. Despite many reports in the literature, recently published guidelines point out the fact that concern remains regarding the optimal strategies for diagnosis and treatment of coronary artery disease in patients with valve disease.[1]

Calcific aortic stenosis associated with coronary artery disease

Frequency of coronary artery disease in patients with calcified aortic stenosis

The frequency of coronary artery disease in patients with calcified aortic stenosis can be correctly assessed only in studies comprising systematic coronary angiography, regardless of the symptoms. The frequency of associated coronary disease varies according to the characteristics of the population involved, in particular age and, to a lesser degree, the geographic origin. Series of patients with calcific aortic stenosis whose mean age is between 60 and 70 years reported 30–50% of associated significant coronary artery disease (at least one stenosis > 50% or 70% of vessel diameter). Coronary artery disease has been reported in more than 50% of patients aged $\geq$ 70 years[2] and, of patients aged $\geq$ 80 years, in 65% in series from the USA[3] and 41% in a British series.[4]

Series published in the 1960s and '70s led certain authors to suggest that aortic stenosis could have a protective role against coronary atherosclerosis. This was in fact probably only the consequence of a selection bias in series in which the indication of coronary angiography depended on the symptoms. Patients with aortic stenosis and coronary disease became symptomatic earlier in the course of their disease, which could explain the lower incidence and severity of coronary disease than in patients without valve lesions. More recent studies including systematic coronary angiography report frequent association of coronary disease, with a majority of multivessel disease, and therefore do not support this hypothesis of a protective effect.

Calcific aortic stenosis and coronary atherosclerosis were initially considered as two independent diseases, their association being interpreted only as a consequence of their increasing frequency with age. Immunohistochemical analysis of stenotic aortic valves with different levels of severity have shown that early lesions of aortic stenosis have several common features with atherosclerosis, in particular inflammatory cell infiltrates, lipoproteins, and calcium deposits. This is further confirmed by a prospective population based study, in which predictive factors of aortic sclerosis or stenosis were also predictors of atherosclerosis, such as older age, male sex, history of hypertension, smoking, and low density lipoprotein cholesterol.[5] The possibility that calcific aortic stenosis and atherosclerosis could share predisposing factors underlines the importance of assessing coronary status in patients with aortic stenosis.

There are few data regarding the consequence of coronary disease on the adaptation of the left ventricle to aortic stenosis. It seems that patients with coronary disease have a higher systolic wall stress because of a less pronounced hypertrophy, than patients with aortic stenosis and normal coronary arteries.[6] The negative effect of hypertrophy on left ventricular function would therefore appear earlier in the course of aortic stenosis if coronary disease is associated.

Diagnosis of associated coronary stenosis in patients with aortic valve stenosis
Clinical assessment
Angina pectoris has a low positive predictive value of coronary disease in patients with aortic stenosis. Less than 50% of patients with aortic stenosis and typical angina have significant coronary lesions. In the others, myocardial ischaemia can be explained by chronic increased afterload, including increased wall stress, wall thickening, and the modifications in coronary microcirculation encountered in left ventricular hypertrophy. There is no controversy as regards the indications for coronary angiography in patients with aortic stenosis and angina.

On the other hand, the negative predictive value of angina was thought to be high, and some authors in the 1980s recommended not performing coronary angiography in patients with aortic stenosis without angina. However, patients with aortic stenosis can have significant coronary artery stenosis without any chest pain. Left main stenosis or three vessel disease was reported in 14% of the patients with aortic stenosis and no angina.[7]

Non-invasive assessment
Stress tests have been used to detect coronary lesions in patients with aortic valve disease, in particular in conjunction with radionuclide

myocardial perfusion imaging using thallium. Such examinations generally have a rather low specificity, because of the possibility of a false positive result related to myocardial hypertrophy. Moreover, sensitivity is < 100%, meaning significant coronary artery disease can be missed. However, the main concern about the use of stress tests on patients with aortic valve stenosis is safety. Stress tests may be performed with specific protocols in patients with asymptomatic aortic stenosis, in order to evaluate their functional capacity accurately. Nevertheless, the presence of symptomatic aortic stenosis remains a contraindication for a stress test in current guidelines. Tests using dipyridamole have the same limitations regarding specificity, sensitivity, and also safety. Stress echocardiography has also been shown to be non-specific of coronary disease in patients with aortic stenosis. The detection of thoracic aortic plaque by transoesophageal echocardiography is a strong predictor of coronary artery disease in patients with aortic stenosis, but 10% of the patients without aortic plaque have significant coronary artery disease. Combined assessment of carotid atherosclerosis using echography could enhance sensitivity, although this remains < 100%. Transoesophageal echocardiography can therefore not be considered as a reliable examination to eliminate associated coronary artery disease. Electron beam computed tomography enables high grade coronary artery stenosis to be detected non-invasively. High sensitivity and specificity have been reported but this examination suffers limitations in availability and feasibility.

Coronary angiography
Given the limitations of non-invasive techniques, the only method for the definite diagnosis of coronary artery disease is coronary angiography. The risk of coronary angiography is very low in patients with aortic stenosis when there is no associated cardiac catheterisation. Echocardiography-Doppler generally allows an accurate evaluation of aortic valve disease and a haemodynamic evaluation is seldom required. North American guidelines recommend performing coronary angiography in patients with heart valve disease where there is chest pain, objective evidence of ischaemia, decreased left ventricular systolic function, history of coronary artery disease or coronary risk factors (including age).[1] The age above which coronary angiography should be systematically performed in the preoperative evaluation of valvar heart disease is difficult to set definitely. North American guidelines recommend coronary angiography in men over 35 years old, in premenopausal women aged over 35 and with coronary risk factors, and in postmenopausal women. A threshold commonly used in Europe is 40 years for men and 50 years for women. With the current predominance of degenerative valve disease, coronary angiography should therefore be considered in nearly all patients with calcific aortic stenosis.

> ## Detection of coronary artery disease associated with heart valve disease
>
> - The sensitivity of stress tests is below 100% and they can therefore miss significant coronary artery disease.
>
> - The main concern of stress tests is their safety in current practice.
>
> - Methods using imaging (transoesophageal echocardiography, electron beam computed tomography) give promising results, but still have limits in feasibility and reliability.
>
> - Coronary angiography is the only current means to ensure a reliable detection of coronary artery disease associated with heart valve disease.
>
> - Coronary angiography should be systematic in preoperative evaluation of heart valve diseases in men aged > 40 years old and women > 50 years old.

Treatment of aortic stenosis associated with coronary arteriosclerosis
It is widely accepted that the treatment for symptomatic aortic stenosis is aortic valve replacement (AVR). Balloon dilatation provides only a limited and transient improvement and does not influence the natural history of the disease. However, concern remains as regards the optimal treatment of aortic stenosis and associated coronary artery disease according to the respective severity of both pathologies.

Symptomatic aortic stenosis associated with significant coronary artery disease
Although the benefits are not irrevocably proven, it is generally accepted that patients with significant aortic stenosis associated with significant coronary artery disease (stenosis > 50% or 70% of vessel diameter) should be treated by combined AVR and coronary artery bypass grafting (CABG).[1] Many series have reported immediate and late results of combined valvar and coronary surgery in patients with aortic and coronary disease and compared these results with those obtained after isolated AVR in patients with aortic stenosis without coronary lesions. It is difficult to summarise the results of all these series, because they are heterogenous in regard to the type of aortic valve disease (aortic stenosis or mixed aortic stenosis and regurgitation), the severity of coronary disease, and the period of operation (table 19.1).[7–12] Patients treated in the 1980s and '90s were older and had more frequent coronary diseases.[2] This evolution may explain the persistence of a relatively high operative mortality of combined AVR and CABG, between 5–10% in most series. The improvement of perioperative management is probably partly counterbalanced by the increasing proportion of elderly patients with comorbidities.

Comparative studies most often reported higher perioperative mortality rates after combined surgery than after AVR alone. The relevance of such comparisons is, however, limited by the fact that patients with or without coronary artery disease differ by many characteristics. In particular, patients with coronary artery disease are generally older, more symptomatic, and more frequently have left ventricular dysfunction. We attempted to diminish the effect of these confounding factors in a study comparing patients undergoing combined aortic and coronary surgery with patients having normal coronary arteries and undergoing isolated AVR, who were matched for age, sex, functional class, left ventricular ejection fraction, and the date of operation.[11] Despite matching in some important predictive factors, there remained a trend towards a higher operative mortality (10.4% v 4.9%, p = 0.08) in patients undergoing combined aortic and coronary surgery. In multivariate analysis taking into account other patient characteristics, combined CABG is associated with a lower increase in operative mortality than in univariate analysis.[2] These findings do not indicate that CABG in itself increases the risk of AVR, but should be interpreted as the adverse influence of an associated atherosclerotic disease on the result of cardiac surgery.

Long term results after AVR associated with CABG are generally good, with survival rates > 60% at nine and 10 years in recent studies, despite the high risk profile of the patients (table 19.1).[10 11] The comparison of late results after isolated AVR in patients with normal coronary arteries reveals the same limitations as the comparison of early mortality, because of the differences in the patients involved. In matched populations, mortality was not significantly higher in patients undergoing combined surgery up to nine years after the postoperative period.[11] Relative survival, compared with a standard population, was not influenced by CABG until 10 years after surgery in another series.[2] Apart from survival, late functional results are excellent in most series, most patients being in New York Heart Association (NYHA) class I–II, without a low incidence of angina and acute coronary events.[9–11]

Despite a trend towards an increase in perioperative mortality compared with patients with normal coronary arteries, the immediate results of AVR associated with CABG are satisfying according to the characteristics of the patients involved. These results support the current practice which is to bypass significant coronary artery stenosis (50% for left main and 50–70% for other arteries) when possible in

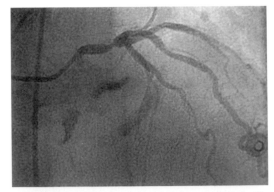

Figure 19.1. Calcified aortic stenosis associated with a 50% distal left main stem stenosis.

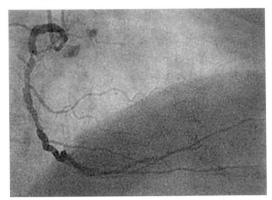

Figure 19.2. Calcified aortic stenosis with a tight stenosis on the second segment of a diffusely atherosclerotic right coronary artery.

patients who should have AVR for aortic valve stenosis (figs 19.1 and 19.2).[1] The extrapolation of large series on CABG suggests that the use of the left internal mammary artery should be recommended for the grafting of the left anterior descending artery in those patients more frequently operated on at an advanced age, and for whom late reoperation should be avoided.

Isolated AVR in patients with coronary artery stenosis

Published series comprise only a few patients who had coronary stenosis associated with aortic stenosis and who underwent isolated AVR without CABG. Moreover, these patients constitute a particularly heterogeneous group, because the absence of CABG can be related to very different situations, whether it is deliberate in moderate stenosis (approximately 50%) or impossible in significant stenosis because of anatomical conditions. The absence of CABG was deliberate in all cases only in the Bonow series,[13] which reported a favourable outcome

Table 19.1 Results of aortic valve replacement combined with coronary artery bypass grafting in patients with aortic valve disease associated with coronary artery disease

Series	Years of operation	AVR+ CABG (n)	AS (n)	Mean age (years)	3 vessel or LM (%)	Operative deaths (%)	Late survival (%)
Mullany[7]	1967–76	112	–	–	34	6.3	49 at 10 years
	1982–83	99	–	–	48	4.01	
Lytle[8]	1967–91	500	–	62	23	5.8	52 at 10 years*
Czer[9]	1969–84	233	–	67	52	8.2	41 at 10 years
Lund[10]	1975–86	–	55	64	47	3.6	62 at 10 years
Iung[11]	1979–92	–	144	69	31	10.4	67 at 9 years
Flameng[12]	1980–92	449	–	65	30	7.6	–

*Among postoperative survivors.
AVR, aortic valve replacement; AS, aortic stenosis; CABG, coronary artery bypass grafting, LM, left main stenosis.

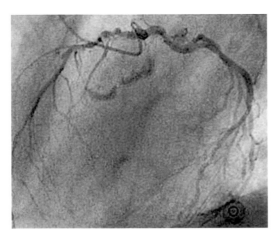

Figure 19.3. Calcified aortic stenosis with atherosclerosis of left anterior descending and circumflex arteries, no stenosis being more than 50%.

but whose interpretation should take into account the majority of mono-vessel diseases and the short follow up. In our experience, mid term outcome after isolated AVR in patients who had aortic stenosis associated with moderate coronary artery stenosis (40–60%) is excellent and identical to patients with normal coronary arteries (fig 19.3).[11] As regards patients who had aortic stenosis and significant coronary disease which could not be bypassed for technical reasons, there was a trend towards a higher postoperative mortality and a more rapid decrease of the survival curve after a four year follow up.[7 10 11] However, mid term survival was satisfying (60% at five years) and functional results were good, with more than 90% of the patients being free from angina in the absence of CABG.[11] It is necessary to be cautious given the small number of patients, but these results strongly suggest that AVR should be performed in patients with symptomatic aortic stenosis, even if they have significant coronary lesions which cannot be bypassed for technical reasons. Immediate and late results seem less satisfying than those in patients who underwent combined aortic and coronary surgery but are far better than the natural history of aortic stenosis. Future studies are needed to evaluate the association of transmyocardial laser revascularisation with AVR in such patients.

Moderate aortic stenosis associated with significant coronary artery disease

In patients who have moderate aortic stenosis and significant coronary artery disease for which there is an indication for revascularisation, percutaneous coronary angioplasty should be considered if possible. In patients who have coronary artery disease requiring CABG, the therapeutic choice is between :

- associating AVR and CABG, which is a radical treatment but exposes the patient to a higher operative risk and, later, to prosthetic related complications;
- performing only CABG, which will expose the patient to a subsequent AVR in case of progression of the aortic stenosis.

The mean rate of progression of aortic stenosis has been estimated at between 5–8 mm Hg per year for mean gradient, with a mean decline between 0.1–0.2 cm² per year in valve area.[14] However, it is very difficult to predict the progression of aortic stenosis in any given patient. Valve replacement in a patient who has previously undergone CABG can be technically complex and associated with an increased mortality.[15] The possible evolution of moderate aortic stenosis and the risk of subsequent surgery leads to AVR, associated with CABG, being recommended in patients who have moderate aortic stenosis associated with coronary lesions requiring surgery. Valve replacement should be performed if valve area is below 1 cm² and considered if between 1–1.5 cm², and/or if mean aortic gradient is between 30–50 mm Hg.[1]

Choice of prosthesis

The major determinant of the choice between a mechanical prosthesis and a bioprosthesis is the comparison between the presumed life expectancy of the patient and the duration of the prosthesis. Bioprostheses are clearly recommended for patients over 80 years old, while mechanical prostheses are generally preferred in patients aged < 70 years. The choice may be difficult between 70 and 80 years. Coronary disease is frequently associated in this age group and can be considered as a promoting factor for a mechanical prosthesis, though this point is controversial.[16] Patients undergoing combined aortic and coronary surgery may have a life expectancy that will expose them to primary degeneration of the bioprosthesis. The risk of reoperation, which is still high in the elderly, is even more increased in patients who have previously undergone combined aortic and coronary surgery.

Medical treatment after combined aortic and coronary surgery

Patients who have undergone AVR with a mechanical prosthesis can benefit from moderate anticoagulation (target international normalised ratio 2–3), provided their thromboembolic risk is low—that is, patients in sinus rhythm, without previous embolism and with no severe enlargement of the left atrium.[17] Moderate anticoagulation ensures an efficient protection against embolic events at a lower haemorrhagic risk. This point is particularly important after combined aortic and coronary surgery because patients should also be treated with aspirin. The combination of anticoagulants and aspirin is not recommended in all patients with prosthetic heart valves, but its use is supported by the results of clinical trials in patients who have mechanical heart valves associated with atherosclerotic disease.

Patients with CABG particularly benefit from treatment with statins. It is logical to consider prescribing a statin in most, if not all, patients who have undergone combined aortic and coronary surgery. The choice of the type of statin must take into account the possibility of drug interaction with oral anticoagulant treatment.

> **Combined aortic valve replacement and coronary artery bypass grafting (CABG)**
>
> - CABG should be conducted in association with aortic valve replacement, when possible, for all coronary arteries with significant stenosis.
>
> - In patients who have significant, non-bypassable coronary artery stenosis, aortic valve replacement, if otherwise indicated, should not be contraindicated on the basis of coronary status.
>
> - The progression of aortic stenosis and the problems related to valve replacement after previous coronary surgery support wide indications for aortic valve replacement in patients who have moderate aortic stenosis and in whom CABG is indicated.

Coronary artery disease associated with other valve diseases

Aortic regurgitation

Left ventricular ejection fraction is clearly an important parameter to be taken into account in the decision to operate on a patient with severe aortic regurgitation, particularly in the absence of symptoms. In the case of significant coronary artery disease, the respective roles of aortic regurgitation and coronary disease in ventricular dysfunction can be debated. However, there are no grounds for using different thresholds in patients with or without coronary artery disease.

Just as in other valve diseases, degenerative lesions are a growing cause of aortic regurgitation. Degenerative aortic regurgitation may be associated with an aneurysm of the ascending aorta, thereby requiring not only valve replacement but a composite replacement with an aortic tube and a prosthesis associated with reimplantation of the coronary arteries. If the patient also requires CABG, mammary artery grafts should be used if possible to avoid the anastomosis of the grafts on the pathological ascending thoracic aorta.

Mitral stenosis

The frequency of coronary artery disease is low among patients with mitral stenosis because this rheumatic disease is predominantly found in young patients. In older patients the diagnosis and therapeutic management of coronary artery disease does not differ from other valve diseases. Angina pectoris can occur in patients with mitral stenosis and normal coronary arteries, and it could be related to ischaemia of the right ventricle. The only other unique feature of coronary disease in patients with mitral stenosis is the possibility of coronary embolism.

Mitral regurgitation

The association of mitral regurgitation and coronary artery disease differs from the associ-ation of other valve diseases with coronary atherosclerosis. As in other cases, this can be the conjunction of two different pathologies, but also a unique pathology, coronary artery disease being the only cause in the case of ischaemic mitral regurgitation.

Coronary artery disease associated with non-ischaemic mitral regurgitation
On this topic there are less data in the literature, compared with the association of aortic valve and coronary diseases, and most series concern mitral valve replacement associated with CABG. Combined valvar and coronary surgery is associated with a trend towards a higher perioperative mortality, but patients with associated coronary artery disease are also at higher risk than patients with isolated mitral valve disease and normal coronary arteries.[18] [19]

However, with the evolution of the epidemi-ology of heart valve disease and the improve-ment in techniques of valve repair, combined surgery performed in patients with mitral regurgitation in western countries most fre-quently associates mitral valve repair and CABG. The advantages of valve repair over valve replacement—that is, lower perioperative mortality and improved event-free late outcome—should be taken into account when associating valve repair with CABG, particu-larly in patients who have a preoperative impairment of left ventricular function. The advantages of an early operation in patients with severe mitral regurgitation are even more pronounced in patients who have concomitant coronary artery disease.[20] The association of coronary lesions with severe mitral regurgita-tion should therefore be an incentive to consider an early valve repair.

Ischaemic mitral regurgitation
Tackling the subject of mitral regurgitation in depth is beyond the scope of this paper, because it should not be considered as an interface between valvar and coronary disease, but only as an ischaemic disease.

Acute ischaemic mitral regurgitation is caused by rupture of the papillary muscle occurring at the acute phase of myocardial inf-arction, generally with an inferior location. Despite the high risk, urgent surgery is manda-tory because of the catastrophic prognosis.

Most problems in managing ischaemic mitral regurgitation are encountered in pa-tients with chronic ischaemic mitral regurgita-tion. Such patients have normal leaflets and the regurgitation is caused by modifications of the geometry and kinetics of the subvalvar appara-tus, as a consequence of the abnormalities of local myocardial contraction. Quantification of the regurgitation may be difficult, particularly because of the possibility of variations in the grade of mitral regurgitation according to the ischaemia.

There is a consensus for performing com-bined mitral and coronary surgery in the case of severe ischaemic mitral regurgitation (grade 3 or 4), although the operative risk is generally higher than in the case of non-ischaemic mitral regurgitation associated with coronary disease.

> ## Mitral regurgitation associated with coronary artery disease
>
> - The mechanism of mitral regurgitation should be carefully assessed in the preoperative evaluation:
>   - to differentiate ischaemic mitral regurgitation from non-ischaemic regurgitation associated with coronary disease;
>   - to evaluate the possibility of valve repair.
>
> - Valve repair should be considered early—that is, in NYHA class I or II—in patients who have severe mitral regurgitation associated with coronary artery disease.

Valve repair gives good immediate and mid term results in such patients, but we only have a few series with limited follow up.

The treatment of moderate ischaemic mitral regurgitation (grade 2) is a matter of debate. Moderate regurgitation is traditionally not corrected at the time of CABG. However, a subgroup analysis of the SAVE (survival and ventricular enlargement) study suggests that moderate mitral regurgitation has a negative prognostic value on the outcome of patients following myocardial infarction. Whether the correction of moderate ischaemic mitral regurgitation by valve repair will improve the outcome of such patients remains to be determined by further studies.

1. **ACC/AHA Guidelines for the Management of Patients with Valvular Heart Disease.** A report of the American College of Cardiology/American Heart Association task force on practice guidelines. *J Am Coll Cardiol* 1998;**32**:1486–88.
   - *These recent guidelines summarise most aspects of the management of valvar diseases, in particular as regards paraclinic assessment and indications for surgery. Recommendations are given regarding indications for coronary angiography in patients with valvar disease and for aortic valve replacement in patients undergoing coronary surgery.*

2. **Kvidal P, Bergström R, Hörte LG,** et al. Observed and relative survival after aortic valve replacement. *J Am Coll Cardiol* 2000;**35**:747–56.
   - *This large series with a long term follow up is particularly interesting owing to its analysis not only of absolute survival, but also relative survival as compared with a standard population. This provides useful information on predictive factors of late results of aortic valve replacement, in particular in patients aged over 70 years.*

3. **Akins CW, Daggett WM, Vlahakes GJ,** et al. Cardiac operations in patients 80 years old and older. *Ann Thorac Surg* 1997;**64**:606–15.

4. **Gilbert T, Orr W, Banning AP.** Surgery for aortic stenosis in severely symptomatic patients older than 80 years: experience in a single UK centre. *Heart* 1999;**82**:138–42.

5. **Stewart BF, Siscovick D, Lind BK,** et al. Clinical factors associated with calcific aortic valve disease. Cardiovascular health study. *J Am Coll Cardiol* 1997;**29**:630–4.
   - *A large population based study which enables the frequency of different degrees of aortic stenosis to be assessed. The analysis of predictive factors suggests the possibility of common factors in the pathogenesis of atherosclerosis and degenerative aortic stenosis.*

6. **Lund O, Flo C, Jensen FT,** et al. Left ventricular systolic and diastolic function in aortic stenosis. Prognostic value after valve replacement and underlying mechanisms. *Eur Heart J* 1997;**18**:1977–87.

7. **Mullany CJ, Elveback LR, Frye RL,** et al. Coronary artery disease and its management: influence on survival in patients undergoing aortic valve replacement. *J Am Coll Cardiol* 1987;**10**: 66–72.
   - *A comparative study of patients undergoing isolated aortic valve replacement with or without coronary disease and patients undergoing combined aortic and coronary surgery over two time periods. The results support a wide use of preoperative coronary angiography and the association of bypass grafting with aortic valve replacement.*

8. **Lytle BW, Cosgrove DM, Gill CC.** Aortic valve replacement combined with myocardial revascularization. *J Thorac Cardiovasc Surg* 1988;**95**:402–14.
   - *A study of 500 patients treated by combined aortic valve replacement and coronary surgery, with a 10 year follow up and an analysis of the predictive factors of late results.*

9. **Czer LS, Gray RJ, Stewart ME,** et al. Reduction in sudden late death by concomitant revascularization with aortic valve replacement. *J Thorac Cardiovasc Surg* 1988;**95**:390–401.
   - *This comparative study comprises 474 patients operated on for aortic valve replacement with or without bypass grafting. Despite differences in patient characteristics, long term results (up to 12 years) suggest a benefit of associating coronary and aortic surgery.*

10. **Lund O, Nielsen TT, Pilegaard HK,** et al. The influence of coronary artery disease and bypass grafting on early and late survival after valve replacement for aortic stenosis. *J Thorac Cardiovasc Surg* 1990;**100**:327–37.

11. **Iung B, Drissi MF, Michel PL,** et al. Prognosis of valve replacement for aortic stenosis with or without coexisting coronary heart disease: a comparative study. *J Heart Valve Dis* 1993;**2**:259–266.
    - *This study compared 144 patients treated by combined aortic and coronary surgery with 144 other patients operated on for aortic stenosis with normal coronary arteries, and who were matched for the main predictors of immediate and late results. There is a trend toward a higher operative mortality but not towards late death in the patients who had combined surgery.*

12. **Flameng WJ, Herijgers P, Szecsi J,** et al. Determinants of early and late results of combined valve operations and coronary artery bypass grafting. *Ann Thorac Surg* 1996;**61**:621–8.

13. **Bonow RO, Kent KM, Rosing D,** et al. Aortic valve replacement without myocardial revascularization in patients with combined aortic valvular and coronary artery disease. *Circulation* 1981;**63**:243–51.
    - *This comparative study reports good results of isolated aortic valve replacement in patients with aortic stenosis and coronary artery disease. However, the low severity of coronary lesions (18% of three vessel disease) and the follow up of only four years limit the relevance of the findings.*

14. **Brener SJ, Duffy CI, Thomas JD,** et al. Progression of aortic stenosis in 394 patients: relation to changes in myocardial and mitral valve dysfunction. *J Am Coll Cardiol* 1995;**25**:305–10.

15. **Odell JA, Mullany CJ, Schaff HV,** et al. Aortic valve replacement after previous coronary artery bypass grafting. *Ann Thorac Surg* 1996;**62**:1424–30.
    - *This series includes 145 patients operated on for aortic valve replacement after a previous coronary bypass grafting. It shows an increased operative morbidity and mortality, and generally recommends valve replacement in patients with moderate aortic stenosis who need coronary surgery.*

16. **Jones EL, Weintraub WS, Craver JM,** et al. Interaction of age and coronary disease after valve replacement: implications for valve selection. *Ann Thorac Surg* 1994;**58**:378–85.

17. **Acar J, Iung B, Boissel JP,** et al. AREVA: multicenter randomized comparison of low-dose vs. standard dose anticoagulation in patients with mechanical prosthetic heart valves. *Circulation* 1996;**94**:2107–12.
    - *This prospective, randomised trial concludes that there is a benefit from using moderate anticoagulation in selected patients after aortic valve replacement with a mechanical prosthesis. This is associated with a lower rate of bleeding without increasing the thromboembolic risk.*

18. **Lytle BW, Cosgrove DM, Gill CC,** et al. Mitral valve replacement combined with myocardial revascularization: early and late results for 300 patients, 1970 to 1983. *Circulation* 1985;**71**:1179–90.

19. **He GW, Hughes CF, McCaughan B,** et al. Mitral valve replacement combined with coronary artery operation: determinants of early and late results. *Ann Thorac Surg* 1991;**51**:916–23.

20. **Triboulloy C, Enriquez-Sarano M, Schaff HV,** et al. Impact of preoperative symptoms on survival after surgical correction of organic mitral regurgitation. Rationale for optimizing surgical indications. *Circulation* 1999;**99**:400–5.

20 Clinical anatomy of the aortic root

Robert H Anderson

The aortic valve, and its supporting ventricular structures, form the centrepiece of the heart. All chambers of the heart are related directly to the valve, and its leaflets are incorporated directly into the cardiac skeleton. As such, the valve is the focus for the echocardiographer. Yet still the precise structure of its component parts remains controversial, with persisting disagreements relating largely to the enigmatic "annulus". Indeed, it is difficult to find an unequivocal definition of the annulus, a structure appearing most frequently in the context of cardiac surgery.[1]

This review describes the arrangement of the aortic root in terms of the attachment of the aortic valvar leaflets, and their relations to the aorta and its ventricular support.[2] Recognising that these parts will still be considered to represent an annulus, I will try to show that the ring like structure thus described has considerable length, encompassing the entirety of the semilunar attachments of the leaflets. It is the recognition of the relation of these attachments to the anatomic and haemodynamic ventriculo-arterial junctions which is the key to understanding.[3]

Location of the aortic root

Although forming the outlet from the left ventricle, when viewed in the context of the heart

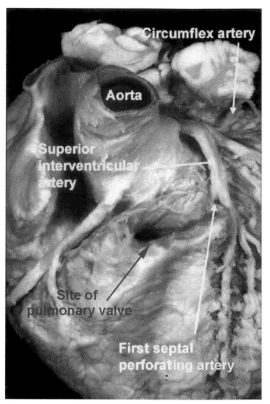

Figure 20.1. In this normal human heart, viewed in attitudinally correct orientation, the subpulmonary infundibulum has been transected, and the pulmonary valve removed, showing the central position of the aortic root within the cardiac short axis.

as it lies within the chest ("attitudinally correct orientation"[4]), the aortic root is positioned to the right and posterior relative to the subpulmonary infundibulum (fig 20.1). The subpulmonary infundibulum is a complete muscular funnel which supports in uniform fashion the leaflets of the pulmonary valve.[5] In contrast, the leaflets of the aortic valve are attached only in part to the muscular walls of the left ventricle. This is because the aortic and mitral valvar orifices are fitted alongside each other within the circular short axis profile of the left ventricle, as compared to the tricuspid and pulmonary valves which occupy opposite ends of the banana shaped right ventricle (fig 20.2). When the posterior margins of the aortic root are examined, then the valvar leaflets are seen to be wedged between the orifices of the two atrioventricular valves (fig 20.3). Sections in long axis of the left ventricle then reveal the full extent of the root, which is from the proximal attachment of the valvar leaflets within the left ventricle to their distal attachments at the junction between the sinusal and tubular parts of the aorta (fig 20.4).

How can we describe the aortic root?

Forming the outflow tract from the left ventricle, the aortic root functions as the supporting structure for the aortic valve. As such, it forms a bridge between the left ventricle and the ascending aorta. The anatomic boundary between the left ventricle and the aorta, however, is found at the point where the

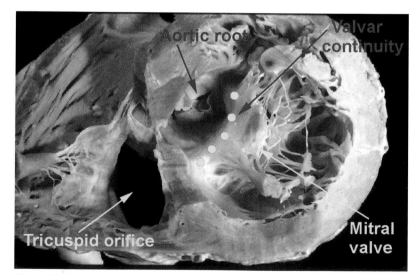

Figure 20.2. The ventricular apexes have been amputated from this ventricular mass, and the base of the heart is shown from beneath in left anterior oblique orientation. Note the central location of the aortic valve, which is overlapped by the mitral valve within the short axis of the left ventricle. The tricuspid and pulmonary valves are separated by the supraventricular crest in the roof of the right ventricle. The dotted line shows the area of fibrous continuity between the leaflets of the aortic and mitral valves.

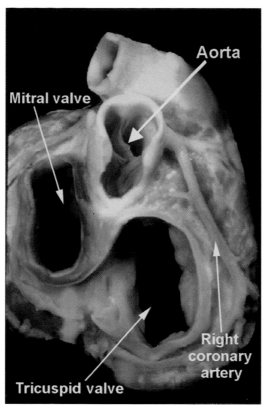

Figure 20.3. The short axis of the heart is photographed from above and from the right, producing a right posterior oblique orientation. Note that the aortic root is deeply wedged between the orifices of the mitral and tricuspid valves. Note also the origins of the coronary arteries from the sinuses of the aortic valve adjacent to the pulmonary trunk.

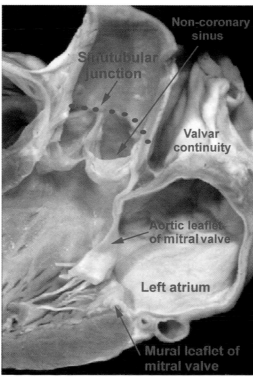

Figure 20.4. This is a close up of the aortic root, having sectioned the left ventricle along its own long axis. Note the length of the root between the basal attachments of the valvar leaflets and the sinutubular junction. Note also the thin areas of aortic wall which separate the left ventricular cavity from the pericardial space just below the level of the sinutubular junction.

ventricular structures change to the fibroelastic wall of the arterial trunk. This locus is not coincident with the attachment of the leaflets of the aortic valve. As shown in fig 20.4, the leaflets are attached within a cylinder extending to the sinutubular junction of the aorta. The semilunar attachments of the leaflets themselves form the haemodynamic junction between left ventricle and aorta. All structures distal to these attachments are subject to arterial pressures, whereas all parts proximal to the attachments are subjected to ventricular pressures.

Opening out the aortic root shows the complexities of these relations (fig 20.5). The structures distal to the semilunar attachments are the valvar sinuses, into which the semilunar leaflets themselves open during ventricular systole. Two of these valvar sinuses give rise to the coronary arteries, usually at or below the level of the sinutubular junction (figs 20.3 and 20.4). The arrangement of the coronary arteries permits these two sinuses to be called the right and left coronary aortic sinuses. When their structure is examined, it can then be seen that, for the greater part, the sinuses are made up of the wall of the aorta. At the base of each of these coronary sinuses, however, a crescent of ventricular musculature is incorporated as part of the arterial segment (fig 20.6). This does not happen within the third, non-coronary, sinus. This is because the base of this sinus is exclusively fibrous in consequence of the continuity between the leaflets of the aortic and mitral valves (fig 20.5).

Examination of the area of the root proximal to the attachment of the valvar leaflets also reveals unexpected findings. Because of the semilunar nature of the attachments, there are three triangular extensions of the left ventricular outflow tract which reach to the level of the sinutubular junction. These extensions, however, are bounded not by ventricular musculature, but by the thinned fibrous walls of the aorta between the expanded sinuses. Each of these triangular extensions places the most distal parts of the left ventricle in potential communication with the pericardial space or, in the case of the triangle between the two coronary aortic valvar sinuses, with the tissue plane between the back of the subpulmonary infundibulum and the front of the aorta (fig 20.4). The triangle between the left coronary and the non-coronary aortic valvar sinuses forms part of the aortic-mitral valvar curtain, with the apex of the triangle bounding the transverse pericardial sinus (fig 20.4). The triangle between the non-coronary and the right coronary aortic valvar sinuses incorporates within it the membranous part of the septum. This fibrous part of the septum is crossed on its right side by the hinge of the tricuspid valve, which divides the septum into atrioventricular and interventricular components. The apex of the triangle, however, continuous with the atrioventricular part of the septum, separates the left ventricular outflow tract from the right side of the transverse pericardial sinus, extending above the attachment of the supraventricular crest of the right ventricle.

When considered as a whole, therefore, the aortic root is divided by the semilunar attachment of the leaflets into supravalvar and subvalvar components.[1] The supravalvar components, in essence, are the aortic sinuses, but they contain at their base structures of ventricular origin. The supporting subvalvar parts are primarily ventricular, but extend as three triangles to the level of the sinutubular junction. Stenosis at the level of the sinutubular junction is usually described as being "supravalvar". In that the peripheral attachments of the leaflets are found at this level, the junction is also an integral part of the valvar mechanism.[6] Indeed, stretching of the sinutubular junction is one of the cardinal causes of valvar incompetence.

Does the aortic valve have an annulus?

As with so many disputes, the answer to this ongoing conundrum resides in the definition of an "annulus". In the strictest sense, an annulus is no more than a ring. In this respect, the entirety of the aortic root can be removed from the heart, and slipped on the finger in the form of a ring. Within the ring as thus removed, however, the leaflets themselves are not supported in ring-like, but rather in crown-like fashion. The answer regarding the presence or absence of an annulus, therefore, is very much in the eyes of the beholder. Some have argued that fibrous thickenings attach the leaflets within the root, and point to these supposed thickenings as the "annulus".[1] I find this confusing, since the purported thickenings are not universally present. Even when found, if removed they would constitute a crown-like circlet rather than a true ring. It is my own belief that the aortic root would be best understood if divorced from the concept of the "annulus". This is unlikely to happen. Suffice it to say, therefore, that the "ring" takes the form of the cylindrical aortic root in which the valvar leaflets are supported in crown-like fashion (fig 20.7).

Clinical implications

There are several inferences from the complex interplay of ventricular and arterial structures which make up the aortic root which are important in the clinical context. When seen in long axis section, the diameter of the root varies greatly through its short length. The root is much wider at the midpoint of the sinuses than at either the sinutubular junction or at the basal attachment of the leaflets. This becomes of significance when considering measurements of the "annulus" since, as discussed, the hinges of the leaflets extend through all these three levels. Proper values can only be provided when measurements are made at the bottom of the valvar attachments, at the widest point of the sinuses, and at the sinutubular junction. Similarly, if measurements were taken from the basal attachment of one leaflet to the compara-

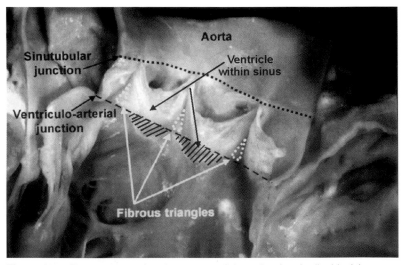

Figure 20.5. The aortic root has been opened through a longitudinal incision across the area of aortic-mitral valvar continuity, and spread open to show the semilunar attachments of the valvar leaflets. Note the interleaflet triangles extending to the sinutubular junction, and the crescents of myocardium at the base of the two coronary aortic sinuses.

ble point of an adjacent leaflet, as is frequently shown in diagrams, this would not measure the full diameter of the outflow tract, but rather a tangent across the root. These considerations are also important in a surgical context. The native valvar leaflets are obviously removed during the procedure of valvar replacement. The prostheses used for the purposes of replacement most usually have a truly circular sewing ring. Should the stitches used for securing this ring be placed within the semilunar remnants of the removed valvar leaflets, then there will be some distortion when the valve is

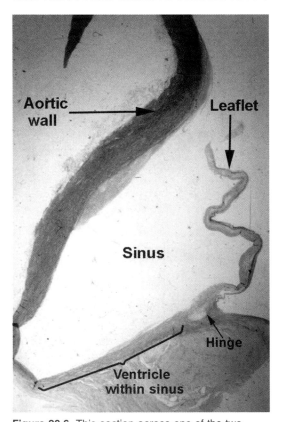

Figure 20.6. This section across one of the two coronary sinuses of the aortic valve shows how the hinge of the valvar leaflet is attached to the ventricular myocardium well proximal to the anatomic ventriculo-arterial junction (see fig 5 also).

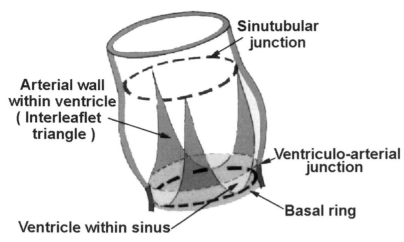

Figure 20.7. A diagrammatic representation of the aortic root shows its considerable length. The leaflets are attached within the cylinder of the root in the form of a coronet.

"seated", albeit that this does not usually compromise its subsequent function. When necropsied hearts are examined subsequent to valvar replacement, the circular sewing ring is usually found to be located at the anatomic ventriculo-arterial junction.[2] It is the normal discrepancy between this junction and the haemodynamic junction which is the key to understanding the clinical anatomy of the aortic root.

I am indebted to Dr Siew Yen Ho for her help in the preparation of this review, and to Karen McCarthy and Vi Hue Tran for help in preparing the illustrations. The work itself was supported by the British Heart Foundation together with the Joseph Levy Foundation.

1. **Yacoub MH, Kilner PJ, Birks EJ,** et al. The aortic outflow tract and root: a tale of dynamism and crosstalk. *Ann Thorac Surg* 1999;**68**(suppl):S37–43.

• A review of a lifetime's experience of surgery to the aortic root. Like many surgeons, however, Sir Magdi views the aortic valvar leaflets as though supported by an "annulus". Included in the review is a picture demonstrating the so-called "annulus", but this is taken at a single level across the semilunar hinge line of the leaflet. No consideration is given to the length of the root, nor the semilunar arrangement of the leaflets. Sir Magdi's picture should be compared with fig 6 as shown in this review.

2. **Sutton JPIII, Ho SY, Anderson RH.** The forgotten interleaflet triangles: a review of the surgical anatomy of the aortic valve. *Ann Thorac Surg* 1995;**59**: 419–27.
• An alternative account of the surgical anatomy of the aortic valve, taking cognisance of the semilunar arrangement of the leaflets, and the interdigitations thus produced between the aortic valvar sinuses and the fibrous extensions of the suboartic outflow tract.

3. **Anderson RH.** Editorial note: the anatomy of arterial valvar stenosis. *Int J Cardiol* 1990;**26**:355–60.
• A short note which emphasised the discrepancy between the anatomic and haemodynamic ventriculo-arterial junctions. It is appreciation of this discrepancy which is the key to understanding of the clinical anatomy.

4. **McAlpine WA.** Heart and coronary arteries. An anatomical atlas for clinical diagnosis, radiological investigation, and surgical treatment. Berlin: Springer-Verlag, 1995.
• This atlas was produced long before it was ready to be appreciated. The work is a true thing of beauty, and the gems to be found within its pages are manifold. It is not easy to understand, but the effort needed to extract the salient clinical material is well worth it.

5. **Stamm C, Anderson RH, Ho SY.** Clinical anatomy of the normal pulmonary root compared with that in isolated pulmonary valvular stenosis. *J Am Coll Cardiol* 1998;**31**:1420–5.
• An analysis of the normal pulmonary valve is used as the foundation for understanding the malformations which produce valvar stenosis. The key, once more, is to appreciate the semilunar arrangement of the leaflets. The essence of valvar stenosis is progressive fusion of the zones of apposition between the valvar leaflets.

6. **Stamm C, Li J, Ho SY,** et al. The aortic root in supravalvular stenosis: the potential surgical relevance of morphologic findings. *J Thorac Cardiovasc Surg* 1997;**114**:16–24.
• This analysis is concerned with so-called "supravalvar" stenosis. As is shown, the level of narrowing in this entity is almost always found at the sinutubular junction, and involves additionally the valvar leaflets.

21 Cardiovascular surgery for Marfan syndrome

Tom Treasure

In 1896 Antoine Marfan, a French paediatrician, presented a 5 year old girl to the Medical Society of the Paris Hospitals. She had striking abnormalities in her skeletal system with elongation of her long bones and fingers. Association of arachnodactyly with dislocated lenses was described in 1914 and the adoption of this as a syndrome was based upon these characteristic phenotypic appearances. Autosomal dominant inheritance was recognised in 1931. The first descriptions of a dilated aortic root and of dissection were in 1943.

The main cause of premature death in those with Marfan syndrome is dissection of the ascending aorta resulting in tamponade, left ventricular failure caused by aortic regurgitation, myocardial ischaemia from disruption of the coronary orifices, and stroke if the arch vessels are involved. Reports vary but a life expectancy of between 30–40 years of age was typical in the era before root replacement, with most of these premature deaths being attributable to aortic disease.[1][2] Avoidable deaths in the teens and 20s are not rare. There is a great clinical variability so the pool of patients, and hence the denominator against which the death rate is calculated, depends upon the clinical discipline of those collecting the cases and whether the emphasis is on lethal aortic manifestations, or on abnormalities of the eyes, or on spinal deformity. Neonatal Marfan syndrome has an extremely poor prognosis. Those who have survived to present in mature adult life are a favourable subset of the total spectrum of cases. Different clinics collect rather different sets of people with Marfan syndrome, but for those with an abnormal aorta the expectation of life is greatly improved by aortic root replacement.[3][4]

Diagnosing Marfan syndrome

Diagnosis by nosology

The *Berlin Nosology of Heritable Disorders of Connective Tissue* was published in 1986.[5] Under the headings skeletal, ocular, cardiovascular, pulmonary, skin, and central nervous system it lists four major manifestations—ectopia lentis, aortic dissection, dilatation of the ascending aorta, and dural ectasia—and a host of minor manifestations including arrhythmia and endocarditis. These last items indicate the arbitrariness of a nosology based on clinical features. The Berlin nosology has been replaced by the Gent criteria[6] that include the same major cardiovascular manifestations.

Genetic diagnosis

Although Marfan syndrome was clearly recognised as a disorder of connective tissue from the 1950s, the responsible component of the extracellular matrix was variously believed to be collagen, elastin, and hyaluronic acid. In the late 1980s fibrillin abnormalities were reproducibly identified by immunohistochemistry. The gene was found on chromosome 15. It appeared that there would be one absolute criterion for the diagnosis—did the individual carry the abnormal fibrillin gene or not? Unfortunately it turned out to be not nearly so simple. Nearly all the mutations have been family specific. More than 50 causative mutations have been found—nearly as many as families studied—explaining the variability on the clinical manifestations across the spectrum of Marfan syndrome, but not the relative consistency within families. Increasing knowledge of genotype has not allowed prediction of phenotype and therefore risk of aortic dissection for the individual.

We already knew that about 25% of cases have no family history and must be caused by sporadic mutations. It would not be too surprising to find that these individuals are statistically more likely to dissect, for in order to feature in a family tree the gene must be compatible with survival at least into adult life. Thus, even if we think we are being very scientific in making the diagnosis on a genetic or a molecular basis, the diagnostic group includes considerable variability from one case to another, not only clinically[7][8] but in terms of the ultrastructural and the exact chromosomal abnormality.

Diagnosis by gross morphology

The normal aorta has three gentle bulges, the aortic sinuses, just distal to the semilunar attachments of the three leaflets of the aortic valve. The cross sectional diameter of the aorta at the nadir of the leaflet attachment where the aorta and ventricular muscle meet, and at the upper limit of the attachment at the sinutubular junction, are very similar, with the leaflets supported with a spatial relation as if to the sides of a cylinder. The diameter of the more distal circle at the sinutubular junction is, if anything, slightly smaller than the left ventricular outflow. This relation is lost in the Marfan syndrome. The aortic root becomes bulbous and the attachments of the leaflets are splayed out. The commissures are attached to an aorta of much greater circumference than at the nadir of leaflet attachment, the leaflets no longer co-apt, and the valve leaks centrally. The widest part of the aorta is in the sinuses of Valsalva where the echocardiographer picks up the very tips of the leaflets as the valve opens. The coronary orifices are displaced upwards as the aortic wall proximal to them dilates.

Now that we know that there are nearly as many molecular subsets of the disease as there are families, several earlier conundrums become clear. One is the occurrence of inherited aortic dilatation with a propensity for dissection in people who are skeletally unremarkable

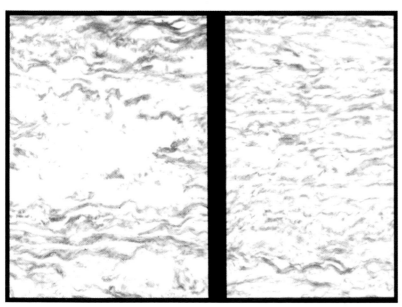

Figure 21.1. Histological appearance of a Marfan aorta. On the left is the severe form of medial degeneration called "cystic medial necrosis".

The term *form fruste* was used for the situation in which the aortic root is characteristic of Marfan syndrome but other features were absent. With the new knowledge about the variation in the genetic abnormality from one family to another, it begins to make sense that there is clinical variability between families. There appear to be those at risk of dissecting an aorta with Marfan morphology but who look normal. On the contrary there are Marfan families with severely affected skeletons whose aortas are not particularly large and who do not dissect. A distinction must be made, however, between the very characteristic morphology of Marfan syndrome and the more funnel shaped aortic dilatation seen in hypertension and post-stenotic dilatation associated with bicuspid valves.

Framing disease

The concept of "framing disease" emphasises that our view of diagnostic categories changes with the scientific and clinical information that we use and may change with time, and is to a variable degree arbitrary. Thus in Marfan syndrome we could make the diagnosis purely by a particular bodily habitus or we could define the disease by an abnormality of fibrillin. The two diagnostic frames will not encompass identical patient groups.

A way of framing the disease[9] that concentrated the attention on the aortic root while accepting that other features might or might not be present was to group Marfan cases within a diagnostic heading of annulo-aortic ectasia.[10] It is probably a term best avoided. Anderson teaches us that the term "annulus" is incorrect in the case of the aortic valve because there is no ring (see accompanying article).[11] There is another problem and that is that the measured diameter at the nadir of attachment of the aortic valve leaflets (the point loosely called the annulus) is characteristically normal in the presence of a very dilated Marfan aorta, even with severe regurgitation. It is the aortic sinuses that bear the brunt of the dilating process.

Should we make the morphological and histological abnormalities of the aorta our diagnostic criterion, since this is the focus of our surveillance and treatment, and not be distracted by a gallimaufry of clinical signs by which we decide whether the patient should or should not be included in the Marfan frame? Even here there is a problem because the degenerative change in the aortic media (loosely called cystic medial necrosis although not cystic and not necrotic) is the common end point of a number of aortic pathologies and is found both in hypertension and in the aortic wall beyond a bicuspid valve (fig 21.1).

Now that we know something of the gene involved in its inheritance, and of the structural and biochemical abnormalities that cause the collection of clinical features, need we carry on using the eponym, and indeed should we abandon the word syndrome?[12] "Dominantly inherited fibrillin abnormality" might be a better diagnostic frame.

The cardiovascular manifestations of Marfan syndrome can be viewed within any of these diagnostic frames, but in pragmatic terms cardiac surgical management is based on the morphology and size of the aortic root, the severity of aortic regurgitation, and its consequences for left ventricular function. The same is largely true of mitral valve disease associated with Marfan syndrome and with other abnormalities of the aorta. This diagnostic frame is the most appropriate in surgical decision making. This should come as no surprise. It is true of a number of other conditions that we treat. We treat aortic stenosis on its haemodynamic consequences almost independent of its aetiology, as we do most other examples of gross structural heart disease, congenital and acquired. Similarly, by the time a patient has end stage renal failure the management comprises renal replacement.[9] The original causal factor is of diminishing importance.

Indications for operating on the aorta in Marfan syndrome

Emergency surgery

Dissection involving the ascending aorta is an absolute indication for operation to replace the aortic root in Marfan syndrome. It is said that at surgery there may be evidence of previous healed dissections, suggesting previous episodes of dissection have been survived. Indeed, there may be scars and stretch marks on the intima of the very attenuated sinuses of a Marfan aorta, but I do not believe that aortic dissection of the type we diagnose characteristically in these patients (figs 21.2 and 21.3) heals back to a subtle intimal lesion.

In Marfan syndrome replacement of the sinuses of Valsalva and as much of the ascending aorta as possible (or is practical) is the standard operation. In dissection caused by hypertension, or from unknown causes, the standard operation is repair of the dissection with a more conservative replacement of only as much of the aorta as seems necessary (fig 21.4A, B).

Dissection of the descending aorta is managed as for any other aetiology with conservative hypotensive management and consideration of aortic replacement if there is ongoing expansion[13][14] or leaking.

Elective root replacement

Elective replacement of the aortic root involves replacement of the sinuses, the entire aorta up to the innominate artery, and reimplantation of the coronaries. Bentall devised this operation in the 1960s when he incorporated a Starr-Edwards valve, hand sewn into a tube graft.[15] Complete replacement of the ascending aorta was an impressive undertaking 30 years ago. Bentall's operation was used in its original form for some years with enface anastomosis of the coronary ostia to the graft and incorporation of the redundant aorta around the graft to contain bleeding from the multiple suture lines. While effective in containing what was a life threatening difficulty with the operation, this left the possibility of false aneurysm due to bleeding contained within the sack and a continued communication. The standard operation remains replacement of the root with a valved conduit but now most surgeons make neat button anastomoses of the coronary arteries, and resect the excess aorta and gain meticulous haemostasis under direct vision (fig 21.4C).

The most frequently used prosthesis incorporates a St Jude bileaflet pyrolytic carbon valve. These are factory produced, and the tube graft is impregnated with gelatin to prevent leakage.

There is growing popularity for valve conserving operations as promulgated by Yacoub and David (fig 21.4D).[16] In this operation the aortic sinuses are resected down to a couple of millimetres above the attachment of the aortic leaflets. The tube graft is scalloped to match and the leaflets are functional within an aortic tube graft. The operation is based upon the belief that the leaflets themselves will not stretch and result in regurgitation. This may be true but the leaflets themselves are not free of histological abnormality.

The key question is one of timing of the operation in the life of the Marfan patient. Leaving aside the question of aortic valvar regurgitation, the purpose in operating is to pre-empt dissection. The ideal time to replace the ascending aorta would be one or two months before it dissects. The problem is that we cannot predict with any confidence when an aorta will dissect. There really are no premonitory symptoms or signs of any value. We rely on measurement.

Aortic root measurements are made according to strict protocol (fig 21.5). The measurement at the level of the tip of the valve leaflets, carefully made to reflect a true diameter, is the measurement on which we base our decisions.

We know that the larger the aorta the higher the risk. There is a general rule that an aneurysm larger than 6 cm has a greater than 10% chance of rupture within the next year irrespective of site and aetiology, and if that risk is higher than that of planned surgery, surgery is the safer course. In Marfan syndrome where

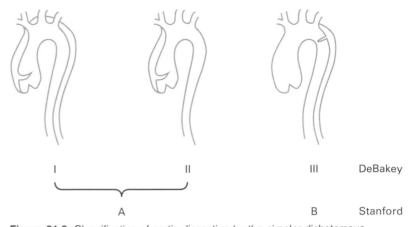

Figure 21.2. Classification of aortic dissection by the simpler dichotomous Stanford classification (ascending involved or not) and the older DeBakey system.

experienced surgeons can perform operations at low risk, planned replacement of the ascending aorta was advocated at 5.5 cm and has now come down to 5 cm in some units. Advocates of early surgery must be mindful of two things. One is that zero mortality is an illusion in a small series. Nine in a row without a death (0%) suddenly becomes 10% if the next patient dies. The other is that operative mortality may be low but deaths in subsequent years from infection, false aneurysm formation, coronary anastomotic problems, anticoagulant related bleeding, and valve thrombosis have to go into the head count if we are to advise patients wisely. We continue to watch some patients indefinitely. Older patients with stable aortic dimensions may have declared themselves outside of the risk group for aortic dissection (fig 21.6).

Another factor in making the decision to perform elective root replacement is the rate of change. Progressive enlargement of the aorta from one clinic visit to the next is an ominous sign. It is difficult to make a rule but, as an example, if the aortic dimension changed from 4.3 cm to 4.6 cm then to 4.9 cm at six monthly visits, we would advise surgery based on the rate of change without waiting for the size to reach 5 or 5.5 cm.[17]

A family history of dissection influences the decision towards operation. Tendency for the aorta to dissect runs in families and the genetic evidence that there are differences between families and similarities within them lends extra weight to this view.

Finally we take into account aortic regurgitation. The criteria for valve replacement in aor-

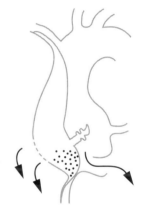

Figure 21.3. The typical form of lethal dissection, which is the most common cause of death in Marfan syndrome.

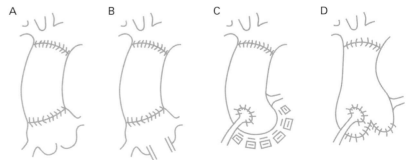

Figure 21.4. Operations for aortic dissection or ascending aortic replacement. (A) Simple tube replacement of the aorta for the sinotubular junction to the brachiocephalic origin. (B) Tube graft replacement and aortic valve replacement as separate components of the operation. (C) Composite graft replacement. (D) Leaflet sparing aortic root replacement.

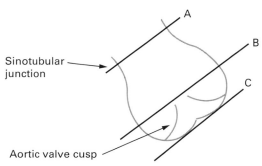

Figure 21.5. Points of echo measurement for surveillance of the aortic root. The diameter of the aortic root can be measured at three different levels. In Marfan syndrome level B is critical.

tic regurgitation are now well established.[18] If there are symptoms attributable to regurgitation and/or evidence of an increase in left ventricular end systolic dimension, then valve replacement is indicated to protect the left ventricle and the patient's prognosis. These rules apply equally in Marfan patients. If surgery is indicated to correct aortic regurgitation it is likely that the aortic dimensions are at or near the accepted criteria and root replacement should be performed. In any case, if the patient merits valve replacement, it would be extremely unwise to simply replace the valve and leave a Marfan aorta. If the morphology is that of a Marfan aorta and there are no particular reasons to preclude it, we would replace the root under these circumstances.

Throughout I have placed emphasis on the importance of replacing the sinuses. However, there are occasions when there is aortic regurgitation and an enlarged ascending aorta. There may be doubt about the morphology of the aorta. If the dilation of the aorta is above the coronary orifices and is not of Marfan type, replacement of the aortic valve and ascending aorta separately (fig 21.4B) is an alternative. There is a surgical rule of thumb. If the distance between the attachment of the aortic valve leaflets (that is, the suture line for a prosthetic valve or valved conduit) and the coronary orifices is so small as to make composite root replacement difficult, it is unlike a Marfan aorta. Then the ascending aorta and the valve can be considered separately and the sinuses left with the coronary orifices. Characteristically the sinuses have grown so large in Marfan's that the coronary ostia are displaced upwards making re-implantation relatively easy, at least in so far as the length of the coronary arteries is concerned.

Descending aortic replacement

Elective replacement of the dilated but undissected descending aorta is uncommon but should be seriously considered if the dilated segment is 6 cm or if the aorta of the patient under surveillance is enlarging and reaches 5 or 5.5 cm. These are difficult decisions and should be made by a surgeon familiar with the problem and confident in operating in this area. If the aorta is generally enlarged and extensive surgery would be required for relatively small gain, it may be wiser to continue surveillance and hope to be able to deal with problems as they present. The chances of coming alive to urgent surgery are better in the descending aorta that in the ascending aorta. Conversely if there is a severe but localised dilatation or dissection, in a patient who is otherwise doing well, the benefits may greatly exceed the risks entailed.[13 14]

There are also those who have chronic descending dissection. These include the many who have been operated on for ascending dissection in whom residual dissection in the arch and descending aorta remains. There are also those who had an acute descending dissection (type B) who should remain under surveillance.

As more patients who have had a replacement for ascending aortic dilation become long term survivors, it is likely that we will see progressive dilatation in the descending aorta as years go by. The follow up of these patients should be in expert hands, either under an aortic surgeon or a cardiologist committed to the practice. A succession of different doctors staffing or training in the cardiological clinic cannot be expected to understand the issues.

We are now using endoluminal grafts (also know to cardiologists as "covered stents") for a variety of aortic diseases. These will be considered in suitable Marfan cases.

Risk of paraplegia

In the best hands there is substantial risk of paraplegia at the time of surgery on the descending aorta. This ranges from a risk of under 5% for a localised resection of a saccular aneurysm to about 20% for extensive surgery to replace the thoraco-abdominal aorta.

The risks can be considered under two categories.

There is the *anatomical risk*. The extent to which the blood supply of the spinal cord is collateralised varies and is not predictable with

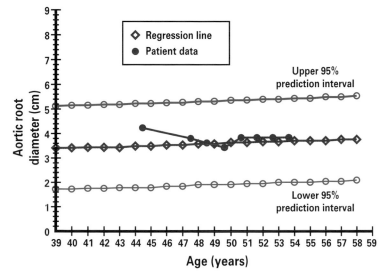

Figure 21.6. A patient who showed no increase in aorta size from the age of 44 to 54 years and an aortic dimension of around 40 mm. This patient does not reach any of our current criteria for root replacement.

142

any present techniques. In some there are very definite watershed zones. Paraplegia can result from the division of a single critical intercostal artery which gives rise to a key spinal artery. Of course, the longer the resected aorta the more likely that the blood supply of the cord will be anatomically compromised.

There is also a time related risk of infarction of the cord if its blood supply is interrupted by aortic cross clamping. This time related risk can be considered to be a *physiological risk*. To minimise this risk we use some form of bypass to the lower half of the body and keep periods of ischaemia as short as possible. The options for providing a blood supply to the lower half of the body during cross clamping are partial bypass (return to the femoral artery) or a heparinised (Gott) shunt from the arch to the femoral artery or, if the problem is localised, the descending thoracic aorta.

Mitral valve prolapse

Mitral valve prolapse should be assessed and treated as for any other cause of mitral regurgitation. If it is associated with aortic valve or root disease, the decision about timing and procedure is made more difficult. If there is mitral regurgitation meriting surgical correction and there is a margin of negotiation in its timing, it would be best if it could be done at the same time as the aortic surgery.

Valve conservation has the same advantages as for any other patient. However, these patients have many problems in their lives. My preference is towards mechanical valve replacement, particularly if surgery is being performed or has already been performed on the root and aortic valve. An opposite point of view would be biological solutions to spare anticoagulation throughout, in case the patient later needs multiple eye or spine operations.

The decisions about when to operate, what operative strategy to adopt, and the implication for anticoagulation are ones which I always share most fully with the patient and the family, including a written summary of the issues.[19] Thinking time is essential.

There is reasonable evidence that β blockers slow the rate of dilatation and reduce the number of events.[20] I suggest their use routinely. However, once the ascending aorta is replaced, if the remainder of the aorta appears stable the requirement for β blockers can be reconsidered. In the interest of the aorta, I advise against isometric forms of exercise.

Summary

- Aortic dissection is the most common cause of early death in Marfan patients
- Dissection can be averted by composite root replacement
- Aortic dimension, rate of increase, and family history are the best predictors
- Echocardiography is the best means of surveillance
- Root replacement is a serious undertaking with continuing risk of complications

6. **De Paepe A, Devereux RB, Dietz HC,** *et al.* Revised diagnostic criteria for the Marfan syndrome. *Am J Med Genet* 1996;**62**:417–26.

7. **Lipscomb KJ.** A clinical study of Marfan syndrome. MD thesis, University of London, 1999.

8. **Lipscombe KJ, Clayton-Smith J, Harris R.** Evolving phenotype of Marfan's syndrome. *Arch Dis Child* 1997;**76**:41–6.

9. **Rosenberg CE, Golden J, eds.** *Framing disease.* New Brunswick: Rutgers University Press, 1992.
- *Anyone who wants an interesting read, and does not mind doctors and medicine being scrutinised by outsiders with a social historical perspective, should dip into this book.*

10. **Ross DN, Frazier TG, Gonzalez-Lavin L.** Surgery of Marfan's syndrome and related conditions of the aortic root. *Thorax* 1972;**27**:52.
- *Donald Ross is a very important contributor in the development of surgical solutions for aortic valve and aortic root disease. Here under the heading of "annulo-aortic ectasia" he grouped 14 patients. Five patients had bicuspid aortic valves. All had "cystic medial necrosis", a histological finding which I would now regard as non-specific. It is a common end point whether the aorta is structurally vulnerable (Marfan), subject to a lifetime of a jet effect and turbulence (bicuspid valve) or years of hypertension. It may well be that there is also a unified need for surgical management of the aortic root. However, the special vulnerability of the aortic sinuses in Marfan mandates total root replacement while ascending aortic replacement may well suffice in other conditions.*

11. **Anderson RH.** Clinical anatomy of the aortic root. *Heart* 2000;**84**:670–3.

12. **Anderson JB.** The language of eponyms. *J R Coll Phys* 1996;**30**:174–7.

13. **Juvonen T, MA Ergin, JD Galla,** *et al.* Prospective study of the natural history of thoracic aortic aneurysms. *Ann Thorac Surg* 1997;**63**:1533–45.

14. **Coady MA, JA Rizzo, GL Hammond,** *et al.* What is the appropriate size criterion for resection of thoracic aortic aneurysms? *J Thorac Cardiovasc Surg* 1997;**113**:476–91.

15. **Bentall H, De Bono A.** A technique for complete replacement of the ascending aorta. *Thorax* 1967;**23**:338–9.
- *This is a remarkable contribution, now a classic "first".*

16. **Underwood MJ, El Khoury G, Deronck D,** *et al.* The aortic root: structure, function, and surgical reconstruction. *Heart* 2000;**83**:376–80.

17. **Treasure T, Reynolds C, Valencia O,** *et al.* The timing of aortic root replacement in the Marfan syndrome: computerised decision support. In: Enker J, ed. *Cardiac surgery and concomitant disease.* Berlin: Springer, 1999.

18. **Treasure T.** When to operate in chronic aortic valvar regurgitation. *Br J Hosp Med* 1993;**49**:613–29.
- *Not an original article but there are still plenty of our juniors who are not sure how the decision is made, and some senior physicians who wait too long!*

19. **Hankney GJ.** "You need an operation". *Lancet* 1999;**353** (surgery suppl):SI35–6.
- *A compelling article from the patient's respective written by a consultant neurologist faced with the decision to have elective aortic root replacement for an ascending aorta measuring 5.8 cm.*

20. **Shores J , Berger KR, Murphy EA,** *et al.* Progression of aortic dilatation and the benefit of long term β adrenergic blockage in Marfan syndrome. *N Engl J Med* 1994;**330**:1384–5.
- *A prospective open label trial which is the evidence base for the routine prescription of β blockers for Marfan patients with dilated aortas.*

1. **Hirst AE, Johns VJ, Kime SW.** Dissecting aneurysms of the aorta; a review of 505 cases. *Medicine* 1958;**37**:217.

2. **Murdoch JL, Walker BA, Halpern BL,** *et al.* Life expectancy and causes of death in the Marfan syndrome. *N Engl J Med* 1972;**286**:804–8.

3. **Finkbohner R, Johnston D, Crawford S,** *et al.* Marfan syndrome: long-term survival and complications after aortic aneurysm repair. *Circulation* 1995;**91**:728–33.

4. **Silverman DI, Burton KJ, Gray J,** *et al.* Life expectancy in the Marfan syndrome. *Am J Cardiol* 1995;**75**:157–60.

5. **Beighton P, de Paepe A, Danks D,** *et al.* International nosology of heritable disorders of connective tissue. *Am J Med Genet* 1988;**29**:581–94.

SECTION V: ELECTROPHYSIOLOGY

22 Temporary cardiac pacing

Michael D Gammage

Paul Zoll first applied clinically effective temporary cardiac pacing in 1952 using a pulsating current applied through two electrodes attached via hypodermic needles to the chest wall in two patients with ventricular standstill.[1] Although this technique was uncomfortable for the patients it was effective for 25 minutes in one patient and nearly five days in the second; this report heralded the ability to provide temporary ventricular rate support for patients with clinically significant bradycardia. Subsequent technological developments have provided endocardial, epicardial, and gastrooesophageal approaches to temporary cardiac pacing in addition to the refinement of external pacing. All approaches, however, are based on the provision of rate support from an external pulse generator via an electrode or electrodes which can be removed easily after a short period of pacing, as many of the situations requiring temporary pacing are transient and resolve spontaneously or have a correctable underlying cause. In a selected group of patients, permanent pacing treatment will need to be instigated before removal of the temporary system.

Indications for temporary pacing

The indications for temporary pacing can be considered in two broad categories: emergency (usually associated with acute myocardial infarction) or elective. There is, however, no clear consensus on indications for temporary pacing with most recommendations coming from clinical experience rather than scientific trials.[2] For many patients presenting with bradycardia, however, conservative therapy and treatment of the underlying problem is the most appropriate management strategy. As a general rule, patients who may need to go on to permanent pacing should only have a temporary transvenous pacing wire placed if they have suffered syncope at rest, are haemodynamically compromised by the bradycardia or have ventricular tachyarrhythmias in response to bradycardia. In particular, patients presenting with sinus node disease rarely need temporary pacing, and the risks of infection and compromise of subsequent venous access for permanent pacing usually outweigh the benefits in these patients. In patients requiring permanent pacing, prompt transfer for the procedure is appropriate but consideration of rate support to cover transfer to another hospital (where necessary) may occasionally require provision for temporary pacing, preferably transcutaneous.

Emergency temporary pacing

Any patient with acute haemodynamic compromise caused by bradycardia and/or episodes of asystole should be considered for temporary cardiac pacing. For the majority of patients, this is likely to occur in the setting of acute myocardial infarction; complete heart block with anterior infarction usually indicates a poor prognosis and a need for pacing whereas complete heart block with inferior infarction is usually reversible, associated with a narrow QRS, and responds to atropine. The American College of Cardiology/American Heart Association (ACC/AHA) guidelines for the management of acute myocardial infarction provide indications graded according to weight of evidence for benefit of pacing rather than site of infarction (table 22.1).[3] Table 22.2 gives the indications for temporary transvenous pacing, table 22.3 details situations where temporary pacing may offer benefit after acute myocardial infarction, and table 22.4 indicates those patients where temporary pacing is not indicated.

In the era of thrombolytic treatment, the occurrence of bradycardia often presents a dilemma for the admitting junior doctor. Should thrombolytic treatment precede or follow temporary pacing? There is a very clear pathway of management under these circumstances; thrombolysis is the priority and should not be delayed by temporary transvenous endocardial pacing. If the bradycardia is unresponsive to medical treatment (for example, atropine, isoprenaline), temporary external pacing should be instituted while the thrombolytic treatment is being prepared. If haemodynamically significant bradycardia continues after institution of thrombolytic treatment, a transvenous temporary pacing electrode should be placed by experienced staff from the external jugular, brachial or femoral route.[4]

Although temporary pacing is clearly indicated in patients suffering episodes of asystole, there is little evidence for haemodynamic benefit of temporary ventricular pacing over spontaneous rhythm in patients with bradycardia following acute myocardial infarction, although temporary dual chamber (atrioventricular synchronous) pacing has been shown to be beneficial.[5] There have been studies, however, suggesting prognostic benefit of continuous pacing in patients with transient high degree heart block following myocardial infarction,

Table 22.1 ACC/AHA classification of indications for pacing[3]

Class I	Conditions for which there is evidence and/or general agreement that a given procedure or treatment is beneficial, useful and effective
Class II	Conditions for which there is conflicting evidence and/or a divergence of opinion about the usefulness/efficacy of a procedure or treatment
Class IIa	Weight of evidence/opinion is in favour of usefulness/efficacy
Class IIb	Usefulness/efficacy is less well established by evidence/opinion
Class III	Conditions for which there is evidence and/or general agreement that a procedure/treatment is not useful/effective and in some cases may be harmful

Practice point

- Always institute thrombolytic treatment before considering transvenous temporary pacing in the bradycardic patient with an acute myocardial infarction.

although the role of subsequent permanent pacing remains unproven in this group.[6] [7]

Patients presenting with bradycardia outside the setting of acute myocardial infarction less frequently need to be considered for temporary pacing; in particular, those with indications for subsequent permanent pacing (for example, high degree heart block, sinus node disease) are often better managed without temporary pacing to reduce the risk of infection and to prevent compromise of subsequent venous access sites. Temporary pacing may, however, need to be considered if the patient has episodes of asystole, is haemodynamically compromised or develops tachyarrhythmias in response to bradycardia (for example, ventricular tachycardia or fibrillation). These tachyarrhythmias may occur as escape rhythms, either spontaneously or following ventricular ectopic beats.

Elective temporary pacing

This is generally undertaken in the setting of surgical or other intervention; either the patient has the potential for transient bradycardia as a result of their underlying pathology or the procedure to be undertaken is likely to produce transient or permanent bradycardia. Many authors continue to recommend temporary pacing to cover general anaesthesia in the presence of bifascicular block and first degree heart block, although there is little evidence to support the need for this approach.[8] Temporary transvenous pacing may also be used to terminate tachycardia through overdrive pacing (table 22.2).

Approaches to temporary pacing

Transvenous, endocardial pacing

There are arguments in favour of and against all the major venous access sites (internal and external jugular, subclavian, brachial, femoral); each is associated with particular problems including lead stability, infection, haemorrhage, pneumothorax, patient discomfort, etc. As this procedure is often performed in emergency/acute situations by relatively junior staff, the choice of route is often dictated by individual experience. Other considerations should include length of time that the temporary wire is anticipated to need to stay in situ; femoral placement probably offers the least stable wire position and limits patient mobility more than other routes. Current guidelines from the British Cardiac Society recommend the right internal jugular route as most suitable for the inexperienced operator; this offers the most direct route to the right ventricle, and is associated with the highest success rate and

Table 22.2 Indications for temporary transvenous cardiac pacing

Emergency/acute

Acute myocardial infarction: (Class I: ACC/AHA)[3]
- Asystole
- Symptomatic bradycardia (sinus bradycardia with hypotension and type I 2nd degree AV block with hypotension not responsive to atropine)
- Bilateral bundle branch block (alternating BBB or RBBB with alternating LAHB/LPHB)
- New or indeterminate age bifascicular block with first degree AV block
- Mobitz type II second degree AV block

Bradycardia not associated with acute myocardial infarction
- Asystole
- 2nd or 3rd degree AV block with haemodynamic compromise or syncope at rest
- Ventricular tachyarrhythmias secondary to bradycardia

Elective
- Support for procedures that may promote bradycardia
- General anaesthesia with:
  2nd or 3rd degree AV block
  Intermittent AV block
  1st degree AV block with bifascicular block
  1st degree AV block and LBBB
- Cardiac surgery
  Aortic surgery
  Tricuspid surgery
  Ventricular septal defect closure
  Ostium primum repair
Rarely considered for coronary angioplasty (usually to right coronary artery)

Overdrive suppression of tachyarrhythmias

fewest complications.[4] This was also the recommendation of Hynes and colleagues as a result of five years of temporary pacing experience in a coronary care unit setting.[9] In patients receiving or likely to receive thrombolytic treatment, the femoral, brachial or external jugular are the routes of choice. It is also generally best to avoid the left subclavian approach if permanent pacing may be required, as this is the most popular site for permanent pacing. Some permanent implanters prefer the right side, however, and establishing a relationship with the physician or surgeon responsible for permanent pacing is important. Many implanters also prefer to use the non-dominant side; assessing the patient's dominant hand is, therefore, appropriate.

Positioning the temporary pacing wire requires the combination of satisfactory anatomical and electrical data. Different venous approaches will require different techniques; probably the most important difference will be the result of approaching the right atrium from below (femoral route) or above (all other routes). The procedure needs appropriate instruments, a sterile environment, trained support staff, and good quality fluoroscopy equipment.[2]

Table 22.3 Situations where temporary pacing may offer benefit after acute myocardial infarction; placement of transcutaneous electrodes may be more appropriate than transvenous pacing (class II ACC/AHA)[3]

Class IIa	RBBB with LAFB or LPFB (new or indeterminate)
	RBBB with 1st degree AV block
	LBBB (new or indeterminate)
	Recurrent sinus pauses (> 3 seconds) not responsive to atropine
	Incessant VT, for atrial or ventricular overdrive pacing (transvenous pacing required)
Class IIb	Bifascicular block of indeterminate age
	New or age indeterminate isolated RBBB

Table 22.4   Situations where temporary pacing is not indicated

Acute myocardial infarction (Class III ACC/AHA)[3]
- First degree heart block
- Type I 2nd degree heart block (Wenckebach) with normal haemodynamics
- Accelerated idioventricular rhythm
- Bundle branch block or fascicular block known to exist before acute MI

Bradycardia not associated with acute myocardial infarction
- Sinus node disease without haemodynamic compromise or syncope at rest
- Type II 2nd degree or 3rd degree heart block (constant or intermittent) without haemodynamic compromise, syncope or associated ventricular tachyarrhythmias at rest

Temporary transvenous ventricular pacing

The lead must be advanced to the right atrium and then across the tricuspid valve. With a temporary wire, crossing the tricuspid valve is often performed most easily by pointing the lead tip downwards and towards to the left cardiac border and advancing across the valve. The lead is then advanced to a position at the right ventricular apex. If difficulty is experienced with this technique, an alternative is to create a loop in the right atrium by pointing the lead tip to the right cardiac border and then prolapsing the loop across the valve by rotating the lead. The lead tip may then require manipulation to the apex; this is often performed most easily by passing the lead tip to the right ventricular outflow tract, gently withdrawing the lead, and allowing the tip to drop down into the apex.

Temporary transvenous atrial pacing

Temporary atrial pacing leads have a preshaped J curve to enable positioning in the right atrial appendage. This necessitates approach from a superior vein and positioning is greatly assisted by a lateral screening facility on fluoroscopy. The tip of the lead should point forward with the J shape slightly opened out when slight traction is applied; unless this is achieved it is unlikely that the lead will be stable.

Following positioning of either or both leads, the leads must be secured to the skin to prevent displacement by movement or traction.

The majority of current temporary transvenous electrodes have a smooth, isodiametric profile with no fixation mechanism; this is to enable easy removal but does tend to make displacement more likely. Newer active fixation temporary leads are available with a fixation screw; these are small diameter (3.5 French), catheter delivered leads which remain easy to remove after 1–2 weeks. The active fixation mechanism improves lead stability and may improve the ease and acceptability of more physiological atrial based pacing in the temporary setting.

Epicardial pacing

This route is used following cardiac surgical procedures as it requires direct access to the external surface of the myocardium. Fine wire electrodes are placed within the myocardium from the epicardial surface and the connectors emerge through the skin. These electrodes can be removed with gentle traction when no longer required; their electrical performance tends to deteriorate quite rapidly with time, however, and reliable sensing/pacing capability is often lost within 5–10 days, especially when used in the atrium.

External (transcutaneous) pacing

This is a development of the original temporary pacing technique described by Zoll in 1952,[1] but has been refined to make it more clinically acceptable and easier to institute (fig 22.1); such devices should now be available in all coronary care units and accident and emergency units. The UK Resuscitation Council, as part of advanced life support, currently recommends this approach as pacing can be achieved rapidly with very little training and without the need to move the patient. Clinical studies have demonstrated the efficacy of the Zoll type non-invasive temporary pacemaker[10 11] for periods of up to 14 hours of continuous pacing with success rates of 78–94%, although many patients require sedation if conscious.[11] This approach certainly offers a "bridge" to transvenous approach for circumstances where the patient cannot be moved or staff with transvenous pacing experience are not immediately available. Positioning of the transcutaneous pacing electrodes is usually in an anteroposterior configuration (fig 22.2), but if this is unsuccessful, if external defibrillation is likely to be needed or if electrodes are placed during a cardiac arrest situation, the anterior-lateral configuration should be considered (fig 22.3).

Transoesophageal pacing

The oesophageal or gastro-oesophageal approach has been advocated for emergency ventricular pacing as it may be better tolerated than external pacing in the conscious patient.[12] Success rates of around 90% are claimed for ventricular stimulation using a flexible electrode positioned in the fundus of the stomach and pacing through the diaphragm. Transoesophageal atrial pacing (performed by placing the electrode in the mid to lower oesophagus to obtain atrial capture) is also well described,[13 14] but this approach is rarely used

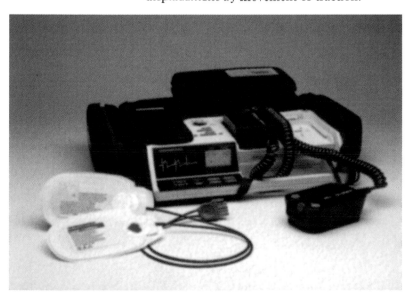

Figure 22.1. A modern monitor/external pacemaker/defibrillator.

148

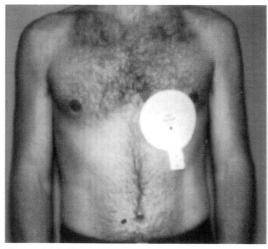
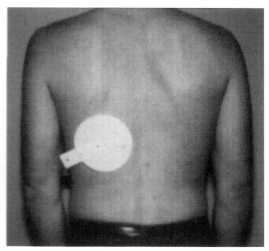

Figure 22.2. Typical anteroposterior positioning of transcutaneous pacing electrodes.

in the acute setting as electrode stability can be difficult to achieve and there is no protection against atrioventricular conduction disturbance.

Complications of temporary pacing

Complications may relate to the venous access, mechanical effects of the lead within the heart, the electrical performance of the pacemaker lead, or infection or thromboembolism caused by the presence of a foreign body. Complications can be expected in around 14–20% of patients[8][15] and the majority of these will be manifest as development of a pericardial rub, ventricular arrhythmias produced during electrode positioning, or infection.

Venous access
Apart from failure to gain venous access, pneumothorax or haemothorax relating to subclavian puncture are the most common problems, particularly in inexperienced hands. These can be avoided most easily by choosing another route; the anatomy of the subclavian vessels is very variable and there is no guaranteed method for avoiding pneumothorax or accidental puncture of the artery.

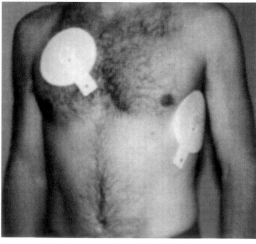

Figure 22.3. The anterolateral position for transcutaneous pacing electrodes.

Mechanical effects of the lead
In many patients, particularly after acute myocardial infarction, placing a pacing lead within the right ventricle will promote ventricular ectopic activity and occasionally prolonged ventricular arrhythmias.[15] These will usually resolve once manipulation of the lead has ceased but will occasionally require removal of the lead or repositioning. More frequently, patients become dependent on pacing immediately after placing the lead, making repositioning difficult. The temporary pacing lead is relatively stiff and of small diameter (usually 5–6 French); it is not unusual for these leads to penetrate and occasionally perforate the right ventricular wall. This is usually manifest by raised pacing thresholds and occasionally by pericarditic pain and a pericardial friction rub.[9] The lead can usually be withdrawn back into the ventricle and repositioned without problem; rarely this will result in cardiac tamponade caused by haemorrhage and will require appropriate urgent treatment. Echocardiographic assessment is recommended after repositioning under these circumstances.

Electrical performance of the lead
Pacing thresholds will vary according to the underlying pathology for which the patient is paced, and these can be affected further by concomitant drug treatment. Initial thresholds should be recorded and then checked and recorded at least once daily thereafter by competent staff. The patient should be paced with an output of at least twice voltage or current threshold; if pacing output needs to exceed 5.0 volts or 10.0 milliamps, repositioning of the lead should be considered. If pacing fails suddenly, always check connections to the external generator, generator batteries, and possible oversensing (go to VOO, fixed rate pacing). If pacing spikes can be seen but no capture occurs, increase output and consider repositioning or replacing the electrode.[2] The connectors on temporary epicardial wires are particularly fragile and prone to fracture. In one series of 113 temporary transvenous pacemakers, failure to sense or capture was seen in 37% of patients and was more common after 48 hours.[15]

Practice point

- Temporary pacemakers must be checked by competent staff *at least once daily* for pacing thresholds, evidence of infections around venous access sites, integrity of connections, and battery status of the external generator. Underlying rhythm should also be assessed and recorded at these checks.

Abbreviations
ACC/AHA: American College of Cardiology/American Heart Association
AV: atrioventricular
BBB: bundle branch block
DDD: dual chamber pacing
LBBB: left bundle branch block
LAHB: left anterior hemiblock
LPHB: left posterior hemiblock
RBBB: right bundle branch block
VOO: fixed rate, non-sensing ventricular pacing

Infection and thromboembolism

With careful attention to wound cleanliness, routine antibiotic treatment is not required but any sign of infection indicates the need to change the wire. In patients with prolonged temporary transvenous pacing from most routes (> 7 days) or when the wire is introduced via the femoral route, antibiotic prophylaxis should be considered. Most infections are caused by *Staphylococcus epidermidis*,[2] but coliforms should be considered when the femoral route is used; this route is probably best avoided in immunocompromised patients.[15] Thromboembolism is probably more common when the femoral route is used, with 5/25 patients in one series suffering deep venous thrombosis.[16] This route may be valuable following administration of thrombolytic treatment but should probably be avoided for prolonged use or in patients with increased thromboembolic risks.

The external generator

The generator allows adjustment of pacing output (voltage and/or current, and with newer devices also pulse width), pacing rate, pacing mode, and sensitivity to intrinsic activity. Dual chamber generators will allow greater flexibility in pacing mode and will offer adjustment of atrioventricular delay and refractory periods. Generators may be small enough to allow the patient to be ambulant or need to be placed at the bedside. The generator batteries must be checked at least daily and the generator sited so that it cannot fall and exert traction on the pacing lead.

Some generators may also offer high rate pacing (usually three times normal upper pacing rate) to allow overdrive pacing of tachyarrhythmias. Activation of this function is usually locked by a key or requires a sliding cover to be removed.

Newer digital temporary generators are usually locked after checking and adjustment to prevent inadvertent changes in programming.

Functional effects of pacing mode

Most temporary transvenous pacing involves stimulating from the right ventricular apex. This is associated with detrimental effects on cardiac function and, associated with loss of atrioventricular synchrony, results in a reduced cardiac output when compared with normal sinus rhythm at a similar rate. This was demonstrated by Murphy and colleague in 1992[5] who showed that temporary ventricular pacing at 80 beats per minute was no better than spontaneous bradycardia (10 had heart block, two had junctional bradycardia), whereas physiological dual chamber (DDD) pacing resulted in improved cardiac output, blood pressure, and falls in pulmonary wedge pressure and right atrial pressure. This would suggest that the majority of temporary pacing should be AV synchronous in the presence of normal sinus node activity but, despite this, the more complex procedure associated with temporary transvenous dual chamber has led to the continued routine use of ventricular pacing in the temporary setting. In the emergency/acute situation, the use of higher pacing rates can partially compensate for this,[5] but restoration and maintenance of AV synchrony should be considered in any patient remaining hypotensive after temporary ventricular pacing. Atrioventricular synchrony may be of particular value in optimising cardiac performance and reducing atrial fibrillation in the postcardiac surgical patient; careful attention should be paid to the electrical performance of the atrial epicardial leads as sensing characteristics often deteriorate after 4–5 days.

1. **Zoll PM.** Resuscitation of the heart in ventricular standstill by external electrical stimulation. *N Eng J Med* 1952; **247**:768–71.
- *The first description of temporary ventricular rate support using an external pacing device.*

2. **Fitzpatrick A, Sutton R.** A guide to temporary pacing. *BMJ* 1992;**304**:365–9.
- *An excellent and comprehensive guide to all aspects of temporary transvenous pacing. Includes guidelines for atrial lead positioning, advice about "troubleshooting" and when to stop temporary pacing.*

3. **Ryan TJ,** *et al.* ACC/AHA guidelines for the management of patients with acute myocardial infarction. *J Am Coll Cardiol* 1996;**28**:1328–428.
- *Task force statement giving precise guidelines regarding need for both temporary and permanent pacemakers after acute myocardial infarction.*

4. **Parker J, Cleland JGF.** Choice of route for insertion of temporary pacing wires: recommendations of the medical practice committee and council of the British Cardiac Society. *Br Heart J* 1993;**70**:294–6.
- *Statement on recommended clinical practice in the UK.*

5. **Murphy P, Morton P, Murtagh JG,** *et al.* Haemodynamic effects of different temporary pacing modes for the management of bradycardias complicating acute myocardial infarction. *Pacing Clin Electrophysiol* 1992;**15**:391–6.
- *An important study evaluating the haemodynamic effects of ventricular versus atrioventricular synchronous pacing which demonstrates the need to consider the haemodynamic consequences of treating and electrical conduction problem.*

6. **Hindman MC, Wagner GS, JaRo M,** *et al.* The clinical significance of bundle branch block complicating acute myocardial infarction. 2. Indications for temporary pacemaker insertion. *Circulation* 1978;**58**:689–99.

150

• A study demonstrating the poor prognostic implications of heart block following anterior myocardial infarction. It also details the prognostic implications of transient, high degree heart block following myocardial infarction and demonstrates the benefits of continuous pacing during hospital admission and continuing with permanent pacing for those with bundle branch block and transient high degree heart block.

7. **Ginks W, Sutton R, Oh W,** *et al.* Long-term prognosis after acute anterior infarction with atrio-ventricular block. *Br Heart J* 1977;**196**:189–92.
• A smaller study with follow up data for up to 84 months indicating no benefit to pacing in patients with anterior infarction, bundle branch block, and high degree atrioventricular block.

8. **Mikell FL, Weir EK, Chesler E.** Perioperative risk of heart block in patients with bifascicular block and prolonged PR interval. *Thorax* 1981;**36**:14–7.
• A small study (76 patients) suggesting that the presence of first degree heart block and bifascicular block may not carry the perioperative risk of higher degree heart block that many physicians assume (see recommendations from reference 2).

9. **Hynes JK, Holmes DR, Harrison CE.** Five-year experience with temporary pacemaker therapy in the coronary care unit. *Mayo Clin Proc* 1983;**58**:122–6.
• Paper detailing a large experience (1022 patients) of temporary transvenous pacing in a busy coronary care unit setting. This scale of experience will probably not be available in the thrombolytic era.

10. **Zoll PM, Zoll RH, Falk RH,** *et al.* External noninvasive temporary cardiac pacing: clinical trials. *Circulation* 1985;**71**:937–44.

11. **Madsen JK, Meibom J, Videbak R,** *et al.* Transcutaneous pacing: experience with the Zoll noninvasive temporary pacemaker. *Am Heart J* 1988;**116**:7–10.

12. **McEneaney DJ, Cochrane DJ, Anderson JA,** *et al.* Ventricular pacing with a novel gastroesophageal electrode: a comparison with external pacing. *Am Heart J* 1997;**133**:67–80.

13. **Santini M, Ansalone G, Cacciatore G,** *et al.* Transoesophageal pacing. *Pacing Clin Electrophysiol* 1990;**13**:1298–323.

14. **Benson DW, Sanford M, Dunnigan A,** *et al.* Transesophageal atrial pacing threshold: role of interelectrode spacing, pulse width and catheter insertion depth. *Am J Cardiol* 1984;**53**:63–7.

15. **Austin JL, Preis LK, Crampton RS,** *et al.* Analysis of pacemaker malfunction and complications of temporary pacing in the coronary care unit. *Am J Cardiol* 1982;**49**:301–6.
• Retrospective survey of problems associated with 113 temporary pacemakers in 100 patients showing that 37% developed evidence of pacing and/or sensing failure within 48 hours. Twenty percent suffered some form of complication; sepsis and thromboembolism were particularly likely with the femoral approach.

16. **Pandian NG, Kosowsky BD, Gurewich V.** Transfemoral temporary pacing and deep vein thrombosis. *Am Heart J* 1980;**100**:847–51.
• Paper showing 20% (5 of 25 patients) thromboembolic complication rate with femoral vein approach to temporary pacing.

23 Antiarrhythmic drugs: from mechanisms to clinical practice

Dan M Roden

All drugs currently marketed for the treatment of arrhythmias were developed in the absence of knowledge of the specific molecules the drugs target to achieve their therapeutic and adverse effects. Nevertheless, combining the characterisation of drug effects in vitro and in whole animal models with medicinal chemistry approaches to modify existing molecules has led to new compounds with related pharmacologic actions derived from older drugs (for example, procainamide begat flecainide). It has thus been natural to group drugs with common mechanisms of action. This approach can be useful for the clinician to the extent it allows prediction of a patient's response to a given drug. One widely used scheme is that popularised by Vaughan Williams in which drugs are subdivided into four broad "classes".[1] The Vaughan Williams classification has been criticised because many drugs fall into multiple classes (table 23.1): quinidine both blocks sodium channels and prolongs action potentials (class I + III), while amiodarone blocks sodium channels, exerts antiadrenergic actions, prolongs action potentials and QT intervals by blocking potassium channels, and blocks calcium channels (classes I + II + III + IV, respectively).[2][3] Moreover, both compounds exert other important pharmacologic actions, such as inhibition of specific pathways of drug elimination (both), α blockade with vasodilation (quinidine), and inter-

action with nuclear thyroid hormone receptors (amiodarone). These actions probably contribute to some of the effects observed during treatment with these compounds.

A virtue of the Vaughan Williams' approach to classification is that drugs of a common "class" frequently exhibit similar toxicities, notably proarrhythmia. This likely reflects the fact, discussed below and elsewhere in this series, that while the mechanisms whereby drugs suppress arrhythmias are incompletely defined and likely highly variable from patient to patient, the mechanisms underlying proarrhythmia are better understood and less variable among patients. Thus, for example, sodium channel blocking drugs with slow onset and offset kinetics of block (the "class Ic" (and to a lesser extent "Ia") effect, seen with flecainide) are likely to produce conduction slowing at normal rates and the stereotypical set of toxicities, described below (proarrhythmia: sodium channel block). As our understanding of the molecular basis of these and other proarrhythmia syndromes (and indeed arrhythmias in general) evolves, it seems likely that drugs exerting antiarrhythmic effects yet lacking the potential to cause serious toxicity may be developed.

The "Sicilian Gambit" proposed an alternate approach to classifying antiarrhythmic drug actions.[2] In this scheme, the arrhythmia mechanism assumes primacy, and antiarrhythmic drugs (or other treatments) are then classified by the way in which they interact with arrhythmogenic triggers or substrates to suppress arrhythmias. A near trivial example is macroreentry based on the presence of a bypass tract. Understanding this mechanism then allows the clinician to select drugs that target the portion of the circuit at which pharmacologic interruption is most likely (the AV node) or target the circuit by ablation of the accessory pathway. The identification of such a "vulnerable parameter" in an arrhythmia mechanism should, in theory, allow development of entirely new approaches to treatment.

Table 23.1 Antiarrhythmic drugs exert a multiplicity of electrophysiologic actions

	Na⁺ channel block (I*)		K⁺ channel block (III)		Ca²⁺ channel block (IV)	β-blockade (II)	Other clinically important autonomic or electrophysiologic actions (all ✓✓)
	At all rates	Predominantly at fast rates	I_{Kr}	Other K⁺ channels			
Adenosine					✓?		I_{K-ACh} activation
Amiodarone	✓✓		✓	✓	✓✓		Reduction of β receptor number (non-competitive β blockade), also a "class II" effect
β Blockers						✓✓	
Bretylium			✓?	✓?			Inhibition of norepinephrine (noradrenaline) reuptake
Calcium channel blockers (verapamil, diltiazem)			✓		✓✓		
Digitalis							Na⁺-K⁺ ATPase inhibition; vagotonic actions
Disopyramide	✓✓		✓	✓?			anticholinergic effects
Dofetilide			✓✓				
Flecainide	✓✓		✓	✓			
Ibutilide			✓✓				Na⁺ channel activation (also →↑QT)
Lidocaine		✓✓					
Mexiletine		✓✓					
Moricizine	✓✓						
Procainamide	✓✓		✓	✓?			Ganglionic blockade
Propafenone	✓✓		✓	✓		✓	
Quinidine	✓✓		✓✓	✓			α blockade; vagolytic
Sotalol			✓✓	✓		✓✓	
Tocainide		✓✓					

✓✓ clinically important drug action.
✓ reported drug action that may contribute to clinical effects.
*Roman numerals refer to the Vaughan Williams classification.

Table 23.2 Important side effects of antiarrhythmic drugs

	Mortality post-MI	Exacerbation of sustained VT	Atrial flutter with 1:1 AV conduction	Torsades de pointes	Brady-arrhythmia	Exacerbation of heart failure	Other clinically important adverse effects
Adenosine					✓ (transient)		
Amiodarone	↓			Rare	✓		Pulmonary fibrosis Photosensitivity Corneal microdeposits Cirrhosis Neuropathy Hypotension (IV)
β Blockers	↓↓				✓✓	✓ (acute)	Bronchospasm Altered response to hypoglycaemia
Bretylium							Hypotension
Calcium channel blockers (verapamil, diltiazem)	↔				✓	✓	Constipation (verapamil)
Digitalis	↔				✓		Arrhythmias Altered mentation, vision Nausea
Disopyramide				✓		✓	Constipation Urinary retention Glaucoma Dry mouth
Dofetilide	↔			✓			
Flecainide	↑↑	✓	✓	✓		✓	
Ibutilide				✓			
Lidocaine							Altered mentation Seizures
Mexiletine	↑						Nausea Tremor
Moricizine	↑↑						
Procainamide	↑			✓			Drug induced lupus (arthritis, rash, occasional pericarditis) Nausea Hypotension (IV) Marrow aplasia
Propafenone			✓		Occasional	✓	Bronchospasm (especially in PMs)
Quinidine	↑	✓	✓	✓	✓		Diarrhea Nausea
Sotalol	↔			✓		✓	Bronchospasm
Tocainide							Nausea Marrow aplasia

PM, poor metabolisers. IV, intravenous.

For example, it is increasingly recognised that altered intracellular calcium homeostasis may play an important role in arrhythmias in settings such as heart failure. Drugs targeting the molecular events that make altered intracellular calcium homeostasis arrhythmogenic might therefore attack the "vulnerable parameter" in this situation.

Differential drug effects in atrial flutter versus atrial fibrillation was an interesting (and it turns out incorrect) prediction of the initial publication of the Sicilian Gambit. It was postulated that atrial fibrillation should respond particularly well to drugs that prolong atrial refractoriness, while atrial flutter would respond especially well to drugs that slow conduction. In fact, clinical studies have demonstrated that the exact opposite occurs. Drugs with predominant QT prolonging effects (dofetilide, ibutilide) are more effective in atrial flutter than in atrial fibrillation, whereas drugs with predominant sodium channel blocking effects (flecainide) are more effective in fibrillation than flutter. It seems likely that QT prolonging agents are especially effective because they prolong refractoriness in an especially vulnerable portion of the circuit to terminate flutter (or that they affect the boundaries of the circuit). Thus, this interesting exception to the initial prediction of the Sicilian Gambit merely serves to reinforce the underlying concept, that a full understanding of arrhythmia mechanisms is desirable to use available treatments rationally and to develop new ones.

Pharmacology

A contemporary view is that all drugs exert their desirable and undesirable effects by interacting with specific molecular targets.[2 3] A common set of targets for antiarrhythmic drugs are ion channels, the pore forming protein structures that underlie ionic currents flowing during the action potential. Specificity of drug action is achieved by drugs that target only a single population of ion channels. The virtue of this approach is that side effects (caused by interaction with other targets) are rare. Unfortunately, as discussed below, targeting individual cardiac ion channels may result in significant proarrhythmia. Amiodarone is an example of a drug with multiple ion channel and other target molecules, and it seems likely that the low incidence of proarrhythmia during amiodarone treatment reflects the fact that "antidotes" to specific proarrhythmia syndromes are built into the drug's mechanism of action. On the other hand, extracardiac side effects are particularly common during amiodarone treatment, again reflecting this multiplicity of pharmacologic targets. A detailed discussion of all the pharmacologic actions of all available antiarrhythmics is beyond the scope of this review. Nevertheless, it is useful to consider widely used drugs with respect to pharmacologic actions that assume special

Table 23.3   Clinically important pharmacokinetic characteristics of antiarrhythmic drugs

	Elimination half life					Bio-availability <100%	Active metabolite(s)	Major route(s) of metabolism			
	sec	<60 min	2–12 hr	>12 hr	IV use			CYP3A4	CYP2D6	Renal excretion	Other
Adenosine	✓				✓						Cellular adenosine reuptake
Amiodarone				✓	✓	✓	✓	✓			
β Blockers		✓	✓		✓	✓	some				
Bretylium			✓		✓					✓	
Calcium channel blockers (verapamil, diltiazem)			✓		✓	✓	✓	✓			
Digoxin				✓	✓	✓					P-glycoprotein
Disopyramide			✓		✓ (not US)		✓	✓			
Dofetilide			✓					(minor)		✓	
Flecainide				✓	✓ (not US)				✓	✓	
Ibutilide			✓		✓						
Lidocaine		✓			✓		✓	✓			
Mexiletine			✓				✓	✓			
Moricizine			✓				✓				
Procainamide			✓		✓		✓				N-acetylation
Propafenone			✓		✓ (not US)		✓		✓		
Quinidine			✓		✓ (rarely used)		✓	✓			
Sotalol			✓		✓ (not US)					✓	
Tocainide			✓							✓	

relevance in clinical management. These include proarrhythmia syndromes discussed below and other important adverse effects presented in table 23.2 as well as pharmacokinetic properties presented in table 23.3.

Proarrhythmia: torsades de pointes

Torsades de pointes is estimated to occur in 1–8% of patients exposed to QT prolonging antiarrhythmics: sotalol, quinidine, dofetilide, and ibutilide fall into this category. While this reaction is generally viewed as "unpredictable", certain risk factors can be identified: female sex, underlying heart disease (particularly congestive heart failure or cardiac hypertrophy), hypokalaemia, and hypomagnesaemia. In patients receiving these drugs for atrial fibrillation (the majority in contemporary practice), the reaction is quite uncommon when the underlying rhythm is actually atrial fibrillation but tends to occur shortly after conversion to sinus rhythm; ibutilide may be an exception.[4] The clinical parallels between torsades de pointes in drug associated cases and in the congenital long QT syndromes has suggested the possibility that some patients displaying apparently "idiopathic" responses to drugs may in fact harbour subclinical congenital long QT syndrome mutations. With the identification of the disease genes in the congenital form of the syndrome has come the possibility of testing this idea, an area of very active research.[5]

Most drugs that cause torsades de pointes have as a major pharmacologic action block of a specific repolarising potassium current, I_{Kr}. Thus, patients are thought to develop drug induced torsades de pointes either because the channels underlying I_{Kr} are unusually sensitive to drug block (which is now recognised with hypokalaemia and with some mutations) or because they harbour subclinical mutations in other repolarising channels. In the latter case, baseline QT intervals can be normal because of a robust I_{Kr}, but block of the current produces exaggerated QT prolongation.

The management of torsades de pointes includes recognition, withdrawal of any offending agents, empiric administration of magnesium regardless of serum magnesium, correction of serum potassium to 4.5–5 mEq/l, and manoeuvres to increase heart rate (isoprenaline (isoproterenol) or pacing) if necessary. Long term management of patients with QT prolongation on a congenital or even acquired basis usually relies on β blockers, although in some cases pacemakers or implantable cardioverter defibrillators (ICDs) are advocated.

Proarrhythmia: sodium channel block

The first drugs used to suppress cardiac arrhythmias were quinidine, procainamide, and lidocaine, which share the common property of sodium channel block. Modifications in these chemical structures led to compounds with more potent sodium channel blocking capability. Indeed agents with this property (flecainide, propafenone) are very effective in suppressing isolated ectopic beats and are among the drugs of choice for treatment of re-entrant supraventricular tachycardia in patients with no underlying structural heart disease. However, extensive clinical studies with these agents, and drugs that are no longer available but that exerted very similar pharmacologic properties, have identified a number of serious liabilities of sodium channel block.

First, in patients with a history of sustained ventricular tachycardia related to a remote myocardial infarction, exacerbation of ventricular tachycardia is common. Such exacerbation presents as a pronounced increase in frequency of episodes, which are often slower than pre-drug, but less organised and more difficult to cardiovert. Treatment of this arrhythmia by additional sodium channel block is undesirable; β blockers or sodium infusion have been found effective in anecdotes. Deaths have been reported. The mechanism of ventricular tacchyarrhythmia (VT) in these cases is thought to relate to slow conduction in border zone tissue, and the conduction slowing caused by sodium channel blockers tends to further exacerbate the clinical arrhythmia.

Second, the rate of atrial flutter, a macro-reentrant arrhythmia occurring in the right atrium, is usually slowed by sodium channel block. When this occurs, the patient who pre-drug had atrial flutter at 300/min and 2:1 atrioventricular (AV) transmission with narrow complexes at 150/min may present with wide complex tachycardia at 200/min, representing a slowing of atrial flutter to 200/minute and 1:1 AV transmission. QRS widening often accompanies this fast rate since sodium channel block is enhanced at fast rates.[6] The management of this entity requires recognition, withdrawal of offending agents, and AV nodal blocking drugs. This reaction can occur not only in patients being treated with flecainide, propafenone, or quinidine for atrial flutter (where, as described above, sodium channel blockers may not be especially effective) but also in patients whose presenting arrhythmia is atrial fibrillation and is "converted" by drug to atrial flutter. Many experts would not prescribe these drugs to patients with atrial fibrillation or flutter without co-administering an AV nodal blocking drug.

Third, sodium channel block increases threshold for pacing and defibrillation.

Fourth, the use of the sodium channel blockers flecainide or encainide to suppress ventricular extrasystoles in patients convalescing from myocardial infarction was found in the cardiac arrhythmia suppression trial (CAST) to increase mortality.[7] While the mechanism underlying this effect is not known, a synergistic action of sodium channel block and recurrent transient myocardial ischemia to provoke ventricular tachycardia or ventricular fibrillation is strongly suspected from clinical and animal model studies. The clinical implication of CAST for contemporary antiarrhythmic treatment and antiarrhythmic drug development cannot be underestimated. As a result of this landmark trial:

- non-sustained ventricular arrhythmias are generally not treated (or treated with antiadrenergic agents);
- we recognise increasingly that the risk of adverse reactions to antiarrhythmic drugs is driven by an interaction between the drug and an abnormal electrophysiologic substrate;
- drug development moved away from drugs with prominent sodium channel blocking properties to drugs with more prominent effects to prolong action potentials[8];
- and non-pharmacologic therapy has emerged as a major mode of treatment.[9]
- Most importantly, CAST demonstrated the power of the controlled clinical trial to evaluate treatments for any disease and the dangers of relying on surrogate end points (such as extrasystoles) to guide drug therapy.

Effect of drugs on long term arrhythmia mortality

A number of other studies have also supported a detrimental effect of sodium channel blockers in the post-myocardial infarction population. Early trials with disopyramide and mexiletine both showed trends to increased mortality. In CAST-II, moricizine was found to increase mortality notably in the two weeks following the institution of treatment, although the effect long term was less striking than with flecainide and encainide. A meta-analysis[10] and a non-randomised post-hoc analysis[11] suggested that quinidine or procainamide treatment in patients with atrial fibrillation was associated with a higher mortality than among patients not receiving these agents. The role of antiarrhythmic drugs to maintain sinus rhythm versus AV nodal blocking drugs or other treatment to control rate in atrial fibrillation is being studied in AFFIRM, whose results should be available in the next 2–3 years.

One consequence of CAST was a general consensus, on the part of clinical investigators and regulatory authorities, that licensing new antiarrhythmic drugs might well require demonstration that those drugs did not increase mortality. Two large mortality trials have been conducted with "pure" I_{Kr} blocking compounds: SWORD tested the dextro-rotary (non-β blocking) isomer of sotalol, and DIAMOND tested dofetilide. In SWORD, d-sotalol increased mortality,[12] whereas in DIAMOND, dofetilide produced no effect on mortality.[13] These differences likely arose from differences in trial design, and in particular efforts to minimise the possibility of torsades de pointes during long term treatment in DIAMOND. Amiodarone has been tested in a CAST-like population and been found to exert a modest effect to decrease mortality,[14] an effect that may be potentiated by co-administration of β blockers.[15] Despite numerous attempts, calcium channel blockers have not been shown to exert a major effect to reduce mortality following myocardial infarction. ALIVE is testing a new potassium channel blocking agent (azimilide). At this point, the mainstay of drug treatment to reduce mortality following myocardial infarction remains therapies directed at maintaining a normal cardiovascular "substrate", such as β blockers, angiotensin converting enzyme (ACE) inhibitors, HMG-CoA reductase inhibitors (statins), and aspirin.

Drug interactions

Because antiarrhythmic drugs often have narrow margins between the doses or plasma concentrations required to achieve a desired therapeutic effect and those associated with toxicity, drug interactions tend to be especially prominent. This difficulty is exacerbated by the fact that most patients receiving antiarrhythmic drugs receive other treatments as well. Conceptually, drug interactions arise from two distinct mechanisms, pharmacokinetic and pharmacodynamic. Pharmacokinetic drug interactions arise when one drug modifies the absorption, distribution, metabolism, or elimination of a second. Pharmacodynamic interactions arise because of interactions that blunt or exaggerate pharmacologic effects without altering plasma drug concentrations.

The greatest likelihood of important pharmacokinetic drug interactions arises when a

Table 23.4 A molecular view of drug metabolism

	CYP3A4	CYP2D6	CYP2C9	P-glycoprotein
• Substrates	Amiodarone Quinidine Many HMG CoA reductase inhibitors (statins) Terfenadine, astemizole Cisapride Many calcium channel blockers Lidocaine, mexiletine Cyclosporine Many HIV protease inhibitors Sildenafil	Propafenone Flecainide Codeine Timolol Metoprolol Popranolol	Warfarin	Digoxin Many antineoplastic agents
• Inhibitors	Amiodarone Verapamil Cyclosporine, erythromycin, clarithromycin Ketaconazole, itraconazole Mibefradil, other calcium channel blockers Ritonavir	Quinidine Propafenone TCAs Fluoxetine	Amiodarone	Quinidine Amiodarone Verapamil Cyclosporine Erythromycin Ketaconazole Itraconazole
• Inducers	Rifampin Phenytoin Phenobarbital			

TCAs, tricyclic antidepressants.

drug is eliminated by a single pathway and a second drug is administered that modifies the activity of that pathway. Identification of specific genes whose expression results in the enzymes or transport systems mediating drug disposition has led to the realisation that, in some patients, mutations in these genes can result in abnormal drug disposition even in the absence of interacting drugs. Thus, the field of drug interactions and of genetically determined drug disposition are closely linked. The clinical consequences of modulating a drug disposition pathway depend on the pharmacologic effects produced by altered parent drug concentrations and/or altered concentrations of active metabolites whose generation depends on the pathway targeted. These general principles are best understood by considering specific examples (table 23.4).

CYP3A4

More drugs are metabolised by this enzyme than by any other. CYP3A4 is expressed not only in the liver, but also in the intestine and other sites, such as kidney. Presystemic drug metabolism by CYP3A4 in the intestine and the liver is one common mechanism whereby some drugs have a very limited systemic availability. The activity of CYP3A4 varies widely among individuals, although there is no genetically determined polymorphism yet described. As shown in table 23.4, many widely used cardioactive agents are substrates for CYP3A4 and inhibition or induction of CYP3A4 activity can lead to important drug interactions.

Perhaps the most spectacular example of a CYP3A4 mediated drug interaction was that between terfenadine and the CYP3A4 inhibitors erythromycin or ketaconazole.[16] Terfenadine is a very potent I_{Kr} blocker in vitro but is ordinarily almost completely (> 98%) metabolised by CYP3A4 before entry into the systemic circulation. With co-administration of CYP3A4 inhibitors, this presystemic metabolism is inhibited, terfenadine plasma concentrations rise > 100 fold, and torsades de pointes can ensue. A similar mechanism also explains torsades de pointes during treatment

with astemizole and cisapride, and has led to withdrawal or limitations of the drugs' use. CYP3A4 metabolism is induced by co-administration of drugs such as rifampin, phenytoin, and phenobarbital. In this circumstance, concentrations of CYP3A4 substrates may fall, with attendant loss of pharmacologic effect. This has been well documented with quinidine and mexiletine.

CYP2D6

This enzyme is expressed in the liver and is responsible for biotransformation of many β blockers (timolol, metoprolol, propranolol), propafenone, and codeine. CYP2D6 "poor metabolisers" are deficient in CPY2D6 activity, on a genetic basis; 7% of whites and African Americans (but very few Asians) are poor metabolisers. Quinidine and a number of antidepressants (both tricyclics and selective serotonin reuptake inhibitors such as fluoxetine) are potent CYP2D6 inhibitors. When these inhibitors are given to patients receiving β blockers or propafenone (which has weak β blocking activity), or such substrate drugs are administered to patients who are poor metabolisers, exaggerated β blockade occurs. Indeed, clinical data strongly support the idea that absence of CYP2D6 activity increases the likelihood of side effects during propafenone treatment.[17] On the other hand, absence of CYP2D6 activity in a patient receiving codeine results in failure of biotransformation to a more active metabolite (morphine). Thus, in this situation, inhibition of drug metabolism actually leads to a ("paradoxical") decrease in pharmacologic effect.

P-glycoprotein

Movement of drugs across cell membranes is increasingly recognised as a process dependent on normal expression and function of specific "transport" molecules. The most widely studied of these is P-glycoprotein, expressed on the luminal aspect of enterocytes, on the biliary canalicular aspect of hepatocytes, and the capillaries of the blood–brain barrier. Many widely used drugs are P-glycoprotein substrates, although the functional consequences of

Table 23.5   Clinical conditions modifying choice of antiarrhythmic agents

Clinical condition	Treatments to consider	Contraindicated or undesirable treatments
Arrhythmias		
Torsades de pointes	*Acute:* Magnesium Isoproterenol Pacing Raise serum K+ *Chronic QT prolongation:* β Blockers Pacing	*QT prolonging drugs:* Quinidine Procainamide Disopyramide Sotalol Ibutilide Dofetilide ???Amiodarone
Polymorphic VT with short QT intervals	Anti-ischaemic intervention Intravenous amiodarone	Lidocaine, procainamide (ineffective)
Sustained monomorphic VT	IV procainamide or sotalol	Lidocaine (ineffective)
RV outflow tract VT, fascicular VT	Verapamil β Blocker Adenosine (acutely)	
QT interval prolongation	Flecainide Propafenone Lidocaine Mexiletine ???Amiodarone	Quinidine Orocainamide Disopyramide Sotalol Ibutilide Dofetilide ???Amiodarone
Atrial fibrillation + structural heart disease		Flecainide
Atrial fibrillation with rapid ventricular rate and pre-excitation	IV procainamide cardioversion	Verapamil Adenosine Digitalis
Other concomitant conditions		
Heart failure	Digitalis *Also acceptable:* Amiodarone Dofetilide Quinidine	Diltiazem, verapamil β Blockers if severe Flecainide Disopyramide
Sinus/AV nodal disease		All drugs discussed have the potential to worsen bradyarrhythmias, particularly: Diltiazem, verapamil β Blockers Digitalis Amiodarone
Diffuse conduction system disease		Above + most other antiarrhythmics
Chronic lung disease		Amiodarone
Inflammatory arthritis		Procainamide
Chronic bowel disease		Quinidine (exacerbates diarrhoea) Verapamil, disopyramide (exacerbate constipation)
Asthma		β Blockers Propafenone
Tremor		Lidocaine Mexiletine

This table is not meant to supplant discussions of treatments of choice for various arrhythmia syndromes outlined in other parts of this series. Rather, specific clinical conditions which may dictate an unusual or specific choice of drugs are presented.
IV, intravenous.

P-glycoprotein inhibition are small because most drugs have other pathways for their elimination. Clinically, the most important P-glycoprotein substrate in cardiovascular use is digoxin, which does not undergo extensive metabolism by enzymes such as *CYP3A4* or *CYP2D6*. Rather, its bioavailability is limited by re-excretion by P-glycoprotein into the intestinal lumen, and its elimination is accomplished by excretion by P-glycoprotein and possibly other transporters in liver and kidney. The effect of multiple, structurally unrelated drugs such as quinidine, verapamil, amiodarone, cyclosporine, erythromycin, and itraconazole to increase digoxin concentrations likely has the common mechanism of P-glycoprotein inhibition.[18]

Pharmacodynamic drug interactions

Pharmacodynamic interactions tend to manifest primarily in patients with underlying heart disease. Thus, when β blockers and calcium channel blockers are co-administered, pronounced bradycardia or heart block occurs primarily in patients with underlying conduction system disturbances. Similarly, exacerbation of heart failure is more of a problem when multiple drugs with cardiodepressant actions (including, prominently, antiarrhythmics) are co-administered to patients with underlying heart disease.

Putting it all together: matching the patient, the drug, and the arrhythmia

Decades of clinical investigation and, more recently, whole animal, cellular, molecular, and genetic studies, have now positioned clinicians to more rationally prescribe and monitor treatment with drugs designed to treat cardiac arrhythmias. A number of very important principles can be enunciated based on these data.

Establish a firm diagnosis

The treatment of ventricular tachycardia as aberrantly conducted supraventricular tachycardia not only exposes patients to risk, but delays appropriate therapy. Other diagnostic issues that may impact on choice of treatments include recognition of specific arrhythmias "syndromes", such as torsades de pointes, "idiopathic" ventricular tachycardia arising in the right ventricular outflow tract or the conducting system, polymorphic ventricular tachycardia with a short QT interval arising in a patient with acute ischaemia, and pre-excitation, particularly in a patient with atrial fibrillation (table 23.5). Each of these syndromes has a specific identified mechanism, and specific treatments that are indicated and contraindicated, based on mechanistic principles.

Anticipate side effects

Unfortunately, the choice of specific agents to be used in common arrhythmia syndromes is often driven more by the clinician's estimate of a likely adverse effect rather than a clear understanding of mechanism or that one drug demonstrates efficacy that is superior to another. Thus, sodium channel blocking agents such as flecainide or propafenone are highly inappropriate to use in treating patients with atrial fibrillation in patients with ischaemic cardiomyopathy, yet are among the drugs of choice in patients with no structural heart disease.[19] Disopyramide is a reasonable option for some patients with atrial fibrillation, but should not be used in patients with glaucoma or prostatism because of the likelihood of precipitating extracardiac adverse effects. Patients with borderline long QT intervals may be at increased risk for torsades de pointes during QT prolonging treatments such as sotalol or dofetilide.

Another variation of this consideration is the presence of chronic non-cardiac disease (table 23.5). Thus, amiodarone may be relatively contraindicated in a patient with advanced lung disease for two reasons. First, some data suggest such patients may be at increased risk for amiodarone mediated pulmonary toxicity. The second, more important, difficulty with amiodarone from a practical point of view is the likelihood that the patient will present at some point in the future with an exacerbation of dyspnoea, and it will be very difficult, if not impossible, to sort out whether the drug or the underlying disease is responsible. Similarly, drug induced lupus is sufficiently common during long term treatment with procainamide that this drug is especially difficult to use in patients with diseases such as rheumatoid arthritis.

Consider polypharmacy

Many patients for whom antiarrhythmic drug treatment is prescribed are receiving other drugs for cardiac or non-cardiac indications. The prescribing physician should therefore be particularly vigilant when new drugs are added to or removed from a complex regimen in a patient with advanced heart disease, as the

Trial acronyms
AFFIRM: Atrial Fibrillation Follow-up Investigation of Rhythm Management
ALIVE: Azimilide post-Infarct Survival Evaluation
CAMIAT: Canadian Amiodarone Myocardial Infarction Arrhythmia Trial
CAST: Cardiac Arrhythmia Suppression Trial
DIAMOND: Danish Investigation of Arrhythmia and Mortality on Dofetilide
EMIAT: European Myocardial Infarction Amiodarone Trial
IMPACT: International Mexiletine and Placebo Antiarrhythmic Coronary Trial
SPAF: Stroke Prevention in Atrial Fibrillation
SWORD: Survival With Oral d-sotalol

likelihood of unanticipated drug actions is high. Drugs that call for special vigilance are those known to be inhibitors of specific metabolic pathways (table 23.4).

Approach to evaluation of treatment

General principles of rational drug use apply especially to narrow therapeutic index agents such as antiarrhythmics. The baseline arrhythmia should be qualified (for example, do episodes of atrial fibrillation occur daily or monthly?).[19] Low drug doses that produce efficacy are more desirable than higher ones. Plasma concentration monitoring, ECG evaluation, and interval history should be evaluated during treatment to detect or anticipate potential toxicity. Therapeutic goals should be defined as therapy starts: Get rid of all atrial fibrillation? All symptoms? Should the patient with cardiac arrest survive to get to the hospital, or be discharged from the hospital?[20] Drugs should not be declared ineffective unless those goals are met in a compliant patient receiving doses just below those that produce, or are likely to produce, toxicity.

Finally, patients never "fail" drugs—drugs fail patients.

1. **Vaughan Williams EM.** Classification of antiarrhythmic action. *Handbook of Experimental Pharmacology* 1989;**89**:45–62.
* *The Vaughan Williams approach to classification, developed in the late 1960s, remains widely used by clinical cardiologists, primarily because of its ability to predict antiarrhythmic drug toxicity.*

2. **Task Force of the Working Group on Arrhythmias of the European Society of Cardiology.** The Sicilian Gambit: a new approach to the classification of antiarrhythmic drugs based on their actions on arrhythmogenic mechanisms. *Circulation* 1991;**84**:1831–51
* *The "Sicilian Gambit" proposed that definition of arrhythmia mechanisms would allow identification of specific "vulnerable parameters" that available or new drugs could target to best suppress arrhythmias.*

3. **Priori SG, Barhanin J, Hauer RN,** *et al.* Genetic and molecular basis of cardiac arrhythmias; impact on clinical management. Study group on molecular basis of arrhythmias of the working group on arrhythmias of the European Society of Cardiology. *Eur Heart J* 1999;**20**:174–95 (also published in *Circulation* 1999;**99**:518–528, 674–81)
* *An in-depth summary of current thinking on the molecular and genetic basis of arrhythmias and how these might form the basis for new treatments.*

4. **Stambler BS, Wood MA, Ellenbogen KA,** *et al*, **the Ibutilide Repeat Dose Study Investigators.** Efficacy and safety of repeated intravenous doses of ibutilide for rapid conversion of atrial flutter or fibrillation. *Circulation* 1996;**94**:1613–21.

158

5. **Roden DM, Lazzara R, Rosen MR,** *et al*, **the SADS Foundation Task Force on LQTS.** Multiple mechanisms in the long QT syndrome: current knowledge, gaps, and future directions. *Circulation* 1996;**94**:1996–2012.

6. **Crijns HJ, van Gelder IS, Lie KI.** Supraventricular tachycardia mimicking ventricular tachycardia during flecainide treatment. *Am J Cardiol* 1988;**62**:1303–6.

7. **CAST Investigators.** Preliminary report: effect of encainide and flecainide on mortality in a randomized trial of arrhythmia suppression after myocardial infarction. *N Engl J Med* 1989;**321**:406–12.
• *The cardiac arrhythmia suppression trial (CAST) was a landmark study that defined the phenomenon of increased mortality during long term antiarrhythmic drug treatment. CAST has had huge implications for use of available drugs, development of new drugs, and the use of the large randomised placebo controlled trial to evaluate "hard end points" (such as mortality) during drug treatment, rather than relying on drug effects on surrogates such as extrasystole suppression.*

8. **Hondeghem LM, Snyders DJ.** Class III antiarrhythmic agents have a lot of potential, but a long way to go: reduced effectiveness and dangers of reverse use-dependence. *Circulation* 1990;**81**:686–90.

9. **Buxton AE, Lee KL, Fisher JD,** *et al.* A randomized study of the prevention of sudden death in patients with coronary artery disease. Multicenter unsustained tachycardia trial investigators. *N Engl J Med* 1999;**341**:1882–90.

10. **Coplen SE, Antman EM, Berlin JA,** *et al.* Efficacy and safety of quinidine therapy for maintenance of sinus rhythm after cardioversion. *Circulation* 1990;**82**:1106–16.
• *This meta-analysis indicated that while quinidine appears more effective than placebo in maintaining sinus rhythm, it is associated with a > 3 fold increase in mortality. While the study has been criticised because many of the original reports were published before concentration monitoring or awareness of the digoxin–quinidine interaction, and because some of the excess quinidine deaths were non-cardiac (malignancy, suicide), it nevertheless highlighted the problem further examined prospectively, with variable outcomes, in studies such as CAST, CAST-II, IMPACT, EMIAT, CAMIAT, SWORD, and DIAMOND.*

11. **Flaker GC, Blackshear JL, McBride R,** *et al.* Antiarrhythmic drug therapy and cardiac mortality in atrial fibrillation. *J Am Coll Cardiol* 1992;**20**:527–32.
• *A retrospective analysis of antiarrhythmic drug treatment in 1330 patients enrolled in the SPAF study indicated > 2.5 fold increased mortality in those receiving antiarrhythmic drugs (primarily quinidine and procainamide), especially in the presence of heart failure.*

12. **Waldo AL, Camm AJ, DeRuyter H,** *et al.* Effect of d-sotalol on mortality in patients with left ventricular dysfunction after recent and remote myocardial infarction. *Lancet* 1996;**348**:7–12.

13. **Torp-Pedersen C, Moller M, Bloch-Thomsen PE,** *et al.* Dofetilide in patients with congestive heart failure and left ventricular dysfunction. Danish investigations of arrhythmia and mortality on dofetilide study group. *N Engl J Med* 1999;**341**:857–65.

14. **Connolly SJ, Cairns J, Gent M,** *et al.* Effect of prophylactic amiodarone on mortality after acute myocardial infarction and in congestive heart failure—meta-analysis of individual data from 6500 patients in randomised trials. *Lancet* 1997;**350**:1417–24.
• *A meta-analysis of EMIAT, CAMIAT, and other post-MI studies with amiodarone indicating a modest but demonstrable effect of the drug to reduce mortality.*

15. **Boutitie F, Boissel JP, Connolly SJ** *et al.* Amiodarone interaction with beta-blockers : analysis of the merged EMIAT (European myocardial infarct amiodarone trial) and CAMIAT (Canadian amiodarone myocardial infarction trial) databases. *Circulation* 1999;**99**:2268–75.

16. **Woosley RL, Chen Y, Freiman JP,** *et al.* Mechanism of the cardiotoxic actions of terfenadine. *JAMA* 1993;**269**:1532–6.
• *Terfenadine was found to be a potent I_{Kr} blocker and elevated plasma terfenadine concentrations resulting from inhibition of the drug's CYP3A4-mediated metabolism were thereby mechanistically linked to torsades de pointes.*

17. **Lee JT, Kroemer HK, Silberstein DJ,** *et al.* The role of genetically determined polymorphic drug metabolism in the beta-blockade produced by propafenone. *N Engl J Med* 1990;**322**:1764–8.
• *This study demonstrated that a pharmacological response during drug treatment (β blockade with propafenone) is tightly linked to CYP 2D6 phenotype, with poor metaboliser subjects developing higher concentrations, and greater β blockade.*

18. **Fromm MF, Kim RB, Stein CM,** *et al.* Inhibition of P-glycoprotein-mediated drug transport: a unifying mechanism to explain the interaction between digoxin and quinidine. *Circulation* 1999;**99**:552–7.
• *This study used combined experiments in in vitro models and in genetically modified mice to implicate quinidine inhibition of digoxin transport by P-glycoprotein as a major mechanism underlying the effect of quinidine to elevate serum digoxin, recognised 20 years previously.*

19. **Anderson JL, Gilbert EM, Alpert BL,** *et al.* Prevention of symptomatic recurrences of paroxysmal atrial fibrillation in patients initially tolerating antiarrhythmic therapy: a multicenter, double-blind, crossover study of flecainide and placebo with transtelephonic monitoring. *Circulation* 1989;**80**:1557–70.

20. **Kudenchuk PJ, Cobb LA, Copass MK,** *et al.* Amiodarone for resuscitation after out-of-hospital cardiac arrest due to ventricular fibrillation. *N Engl J Med* 1999;**341**:871–8.

website
extra

Additional references appear on the Heart website

24 Treatment of atrial flutter

Albert L Waldo

After atrial fibrillation, atrial flutter is the most important and most common atrial tachyarrhythmia. Although it was first described 80 years ago, techniques for its diagnosis and management have changed little for decades. The diagnosis rested almost entirely with the 12 lead ECG, and treatment options included only the use of a digitalis compound to slow and control the ventricular response rate, and/or the use of either quinidine or procainamide in an attempt to convert the rhythm to sinus rhythm or to prevent recurrence of atrial flutter once sinus rhythm was established.

The past 25 years have produced major changes. A series of studies has advanced our understanding of the mechanism(s) of atrial flutter. Old techniques to diagnose atrial flutter have been significantly refined, and new diagnostic techniques have been developed. Beginning with the advent of DC cardioversion in the 1960s, major advances in the treatment of atrial flutter have occurred. β Blockers and calcium channel blockers are now available for use as an adjunct to or in lieu of digitalis treatment to control the ventricular response rate. New antiarrhythmic agents are available for use to suppress atrial flutter or convert it to sinus rhythm. Atrial pacing techniques to interrupt or suppress atrial flutter have evolved. Catheter ablation techniques either to cure atrial flutter or to control the ventricular response rate have been developed, and related surgical treatments are available. Even automatic low energy cardioversion of atrial flutter to sinus rhythm has been developed.

Mechanisms and classification of atrial flutter

Most of the advances in our understanding of atrial flutter have come from our understanding its mechanism. There is a long history, summarised recently,[1] of studies in animal models which have contributed to our understanding of atrial flutter. While those studies have been and continue to be most helpful, a series of studies in patients—principally using catheter electrode mapping and pacing techniques—has established that classical atrial flutter is caused by a re-entrant circuit confined to the right atrium in which the impulse travels up the atrial septum, with epicardial breakthrough superiorly in the right atrium where the impulse then travels inferiorly down the right atrial free wall to re-enter the atrial septum (fig 24.1).[2-7] When the circulating wave front re-enters the atrial septum, it travels through an isthmus bounded by the inferior vena cava, Eustachian ridge, the coronary sinus os on one side and the tricuspid valve annulus on the other side (the "atrial flutter isthmus"). Atrial flutter caused by this mechanism is called *typical atrial flutter*,[8] although it also has been called common atrial flutter and counterclockwise atrial flutter. A 12 lead ECG during typical atrial flutter with characteristic negative "sawtooth" atrial flutter waves in leads II, III, and aVF is shown in fig 24.2. It is also recognised that impulses can travel in this re-entrant circuit in the opposite direction, so that the impulse travels down the atrial septum and breaks through to the epicardium via the same atrial flutter isthmus to travel up the right atrial free wall and then re-enter the septum superiorly (fig 24.1).[3] This form of atrial flutter is called *reverse typical atrial flutter*,[8] although it has in the past been called atypical atrial flutter, clockwise atrial flutter, uncommon atrial flutter, and rare atrial flutter. A 12 lead ECG during reverse typical atrial flutter with characteristic positive flutter waves in leads II, III, and aVF is shown in fig 24.3.

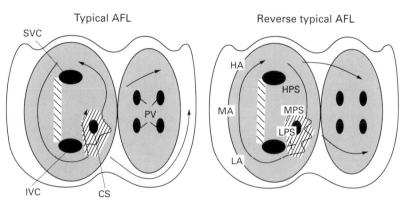

Figure 24.1. Left: atrial activation in typical atrial flutter (AFL). Right: activation in reverse typical AFL. The atria are represented schematically in a left anterior oblique view, from the tricuspid (left) and mitral rings. The endocardium is shaded and the openings of the superior (SVC) and inferior vena cava (IVC), coronary sinus (CS), and pulmonary veins (PV) are shown. The direction of activation is shown by arrows. Dashed areas mark approximate location of zones of slow conduction and block. Lettering on the right hand panel marks the low (LPS), mid (MPS), and high (HPS) posteroseptal wall, respectively. Modified after Cosío FG et al. J Cardiovasc Electrophysiol 1996;7:60–70.

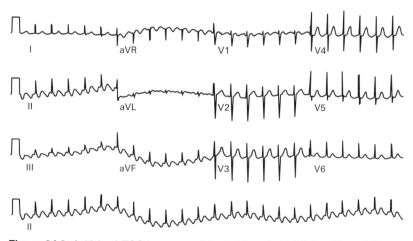

Figure 24.2. A 12 lead ECG in a case of typical type I atrial flutter. The atrial rate is 300 bpm and the ventricular rate is 150 bpm; 2:1 AV block is present. Note that the atrial activity is best seen in leads II, III, and aVF and is barely perceptible in lead I. Reproduced with permission from Waldo AL, Kastor JA: Atrial flutter. In: Kastor JA, ed. Arrhythmias. Philadelphia: WB Saunders Co, 1994:105–15.

Types of atrial flutter

- Typical atrial flutter

- Reverse typical atrial flutter

- Incisional atrial re-entry

- Left atrial flutter

- Atypical atrial flutter

Two other mechanisms of atrial flutter are now well recognised. One, *incisional atrial re-entry*,[8] is seen in patients after repair of congenital heart defects that involve one or more right atrial free wall incisions in which the re-entrant circuit travels around the line of block caused by the incision.[9] Interestingly, it has recently been shown[10] that when atrial flutter does occur chronically in patients following repair of congenital heart defects, it is usually caused by a re-entrant circuit that includes the atrial flutter isthmus. Additionally, *a left atrial flutter* is now recognised that is thought generally to circulate around one or more of the pulmonary veins or the mitral valve annulus, but this re-entrant mechanism has not been well characterised. And finally, there are some forms of atrial flutter which are quite unique, and have now been called truly atypical atrial flutter.[8]

All these types of atrial flutter fall under the category of type I atrial flutter as described by Wells and colleagues.[11] They are distinguished by the fact that they can always be interrupted by rapid atrial pacing, and have a rate range between 240–340 beats/min (bpm).[11] Type II atrial flutter[11] is a more rapid atrial flutter (rates > 340 bpm) which is still being characterised. It is presently thought to be caused by a re-entrant circuit with a very rapid rate which causes fibrillatory conduction to much or most of the atria, resulting in an atrial fibrillation pattern in the ECG.[12 13]

Epidemiology and clinical significance

Atrial flutter typically is paroxysmal, usually lasting seconds to hours, but on occasion lasting longer. Occasionally, it is a persistent rhythm. Atrial flutter as a stable, chronic rhythm is unusual, as it usually reverts either to sinus rhythm or to atrial fibrillation, either spontaneously or as a result of treatment. However, atrial flutter has been reported to be present for up to 20 years or more. It can occur in patients with ostensibly normal atria or with abnormal atria. Atrial flutter occurs commonly in patients in the first week after open heart surgery. Patients with atrial flutter not uncommonly demonstrate sinus bradycardia or other manifestations of sinus node dysfunction. Atrial flutter is also associated with chronic obstructive pulmonary disease, mitral or tricuspid valve disease, thyrotoxicosis, and surgical repair of certain congenital cardiac lesions which involve large incisions or suture lines in the atria.[10] It is also associated with enlargement of the atria for any reason, especially the right atrium.

Atrial flutter is most often a nuisance arrhythmia. Its clinical significance lies largely in its frequent association with atrial fibrillation, its previously little appreciated association with thromboembolism, especially stroke,[14 15] and its frequent association with a rapid ventricular response rate (fig 24.2). The association of atrial flutter with a rapid ventricular rate is important because the rapid ventricular rate is principally responsible for many of the associated symptoms. And, in the presence of the Wolff-Parkinson-White syndrome or a very short P-R interval (≤ 0.115 s) in the absence of a delta wave, it may be associated with 1:1 atrioventricular (AV) conduction, sometimes with dire consequences. Furthermore, if the duration of the rapid ventricular response rate is prolonged, it may result in ventricular dilatation and congestive heart failure.

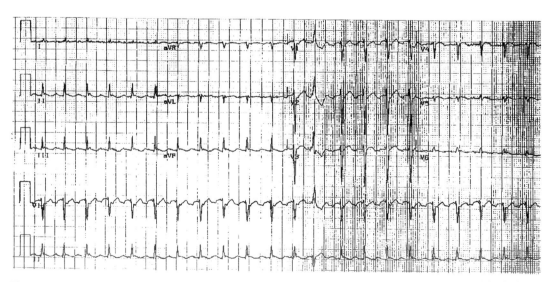

Figure 24.3. 12 lead ECG from a patient with reverse typical atrial flutter confirmed at electrophysiological study. The atrial rate is 266 bpm with 2:1 AV conduction. Note the positive flutter waves in leads II, III, and aVF, and the negative flutter waves in lead V₁. Reproduced courtesy of N Varma, MD.

Management of atrial flutter

Acute treatment

When atrial flutter is diagnosed, three options are available to restore sinus rhythm: (1) administer an antiarrhythmic drug; (2) initiate DC cardioversion; or (3) initiate rapid atrial pacing to terminate the atrial flutter (fig 4). Selection of acute treatment for atrial flutter with either DC cardioversion, atrial pacing or antiarrhythmic drug therapy will depend on the clinical presentation of the patient and both the clinical availability and ease of using these techniques. Since DC cardioversion requires administration of an anaesthetic agent, this may be undesirable in the patient who presents with atrial flutter having recently eaten or the patient who has severe chronic obstructive lung disease. Such patients are best treated with either antiarrhythmic drug therapy or rapid atrial pacing to terminate the atrial flutter, or with an AV nodal blocking drug to slow the ventricular response rate. When atrial flutter is associated with a situation requiring urgent restoration of sinus rhythm—for example, 1:1 AV conduction or hypotension—prompt DC cardioversion is the treatment of choice. For the patient who develops atrial flutter following open heart surgery, use of the temporary atrial epicardial wire electrodes to perform rapid atrial pacing to restore sinus rhythm is the treatment of choice (fig 24.4).

Whenever rapid control of the ventricular response rate to atrial flutter is desirable, use of either an intravenous calcium channel blocking agent (verapamil or diltiazem) or an intra-venous β blocking agent (usually esmolol, although propranolol or metoprolol can also be used) is usually effective. Aggressive administration of a digitalis preparation, usually intravenously, to control ventricular rate (it might also convert the atrial flutter either to atrial fibrillation with a controlled ventricular response rate or to sinus rhythm) is also acceptable, but generally is not the treatment of choice except in the presence of pronounced ventricular dysfunction. DC cardioversion of atrial flutter to sinus rhythm has a very high likelihood of success. When this mode of treatment is selected, it may require as little as 25 joules, although at least 50 joules is generally recommended because it is more often successful. Because 100 joules is virtually always successful and virtually never harmful, it should be considered as the initial shock strength.

Antiarrhythmic drug treatment can be used to convert atrial flutter to sinus rhythm. Three drugs—ibutilide, flecainide, and propafenone—have a reasonable expectation of accomplishing this. Ibutilide, which can only be used intravenously, is associated with a 60% likelihood of converting atrial flutter to sinus rhythm.[16] Because ibutilide dramatically prolongs ventricular repolarisation, and consequently the Q-T interval, there is a small incidence of torsades de pointes associated with its use.[17] However, these episodes, should they occur, are usually self limited, and because of the short half life of this drug, the period of such risk is quite brief, usually less than one hour. Nevertheless, one should be prepared to administer intravenous magnesium and even perform DC cardioversion to treat a prolonged episode of torsades de pointes should it occur when using ibutilide. Flecainide and propafenone, when used intravenously[18] or when used orally but in a single high dose (300 mg for flecainide or 600 mg for propafenone) also may be effective in cardioverting this rhythm to sinus. When using either of these drugs, the atrial rate may slow dramatically—for example, to 200 bpm. Therefore, it is best given with a calcium channel blocker or β blocker to prevent the possibility of 1:1 AV conduction of the significantly slowed atrial flutter rate. Antiarrhythmic drug treatment also may be used before performing either DC cardioversion or rapid atrial pacing: (1) to slow the ventricular response rate (with a β blocker, a calcium channel blocker, digoxin or some combination of these drugs); (2) to enhance the efficacy of rapid atrial pacing in restoring sinus rhythm (use of procainamide, disopyramide or ibutilide); or (3) to enhance the likelihood that sinus rhythm will be sustained following effective DC cardioversion (use of a class IA, class IC or class III antiarrhythmic agent).

Long term treatment of atrial flutter

Recent improvements in the efficacy of catheter ablation techniques and the long recognised difficulty in achieving adequate chronic suppression of atrial flutter with drug treatment have significantly affected the approach to long term treatment of atrial flutter. In short, if atrial flutter is an important clinical problem in any patient, characterisation of the mech-

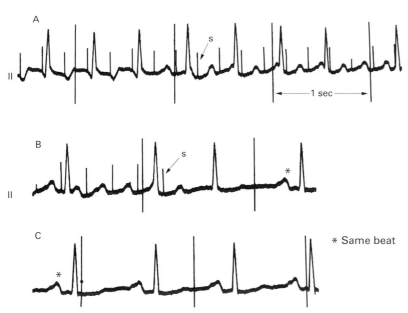

Figure 24.4. ECG lead II recorded from a patient with typical atrial flutter (spontaneous atrial cycle length of 204 ms). Rapid atrial pacing from a high right atrial site at a cycle length of 254 ms (not shown), at a cycle length of 242 ms (not shown), and at a cycle length of 232 ms (not shown) failed to terminate the atrial flutter. Panel A shows ECG lead II recorded during high right atrial pacing at a cycle length of 224 ms. Note that with the seventh atrial beat in this tracing, and after 22 seconds of atrial pacing at a constant rate, the atrial complexes suddenly became positive. Panel B shows ECG lead II recorded at the termination of atrial pacing in the same patient. Note that with abrupt termination of pacing, sinus rhythm occurs. In panel C, the first beat (asterisk) is identical to the last beat in panel B (asterisk). S, stimulus artifact. Time lines are at 1 second intervals. Modified from Waldo AL, et al. Circulation 1997;56:737–45.

Acute treatment of atrial flutter

- Depends on clinical presentation
  - need for prompt restoration of sinus rhythm: DC cardioversion
  - elective restoration of sinus rhythm: antiarrhythmic drug treatment (ibutilide or class IC agent), DC cardioversion or rapid atrial pacing
  - ventricular rate control: often required (β blocker or calcium channel blocker), especially with use of class IC antiarrhythmic agent

anism of atrial flutter followed by catheter ablation as treatment of choice (cure) is now recommended.

Catheter ablation treatment

Two types of catheter ablation are available for the treatment of chronic or recurrent atrial flutter, one curative and one palliative. Appropriate application of radiofrequency energy via an electrode catheter can be used to cure atrial flutter. Advances in both electrophysiologic mapping and radiofrequency catheter ablation techniques have improved the efficacy of this therapeutic approach to about a 95% cure rate for patients with typical or reverse typical atrial flutter,[7 19] making it the treatment of choice in most patients in whom the arrhythmia is clinically important. The technique involves electrophysiologic study of the atria during atrial flutter to identify the location of the re-entrant circuit and then to confirm that the re-entrant circuit includes a critical isthmus between the inferior vena cava–Eustachian ridge–coronary sinus ostium and the tricuspid valve (fig 24.5). When this latter area is identified, radiofre-

quency energy is delivered through the electrode catheter to create a bidirectional line of block across it. This isthmus may be difficult to ablate completely,[7 19] but combined entrainment pacing and mapping techniques have now evolved which permit both the reliable demonstration that this isthmus is a part of the re-entrant circuit, and that application of radiofrequency energy has produced complete bidirectional conduction block in this isthmus. When the latter is demonstrated, successful ablation of atrial flutter has been accomplished.

Similarly, when incisional re-entrant atrial flutter is identified by electrophysiological mapping techniques, a vulnerable isthmus usually can be identified and successfully ablated using radiofrequency catheter ablation techniques.[9] There is insufficient information available to discuss the likely efficacy of successful radiofrequency ablation techniques to cure left atrial flutter or atypical atrial flutter, although contemporary electrophysiological mapping techniques are capable of identifying the location of the re-entrant circuits associated with these types of atrial flutter, making effective ablation treatment a possibility.

AV nodal–His bundle ablation to create high degree AV block (generally third degree AV block) can be used palliatively to eliminate the rapid ventricular response rate to atrial flutter. It does not prevent the atrial flutter, and requires placement of a pacemaker system. For patients in whom catheter ablation of atrial flutter is unsuccessful and in whom antiarrhythmic drug treatment is either ineffective or is not tolerated, or in whom atrial flutter with a clinically unacceptable rapid ventricular response rate recurs despite drug treatment, producing third degree AV block or a high degree of AV block provides a successful form of therapy. Selection of a pacemaker in such circumstances should be tailored to the needs of the patient, and may include a single chamber, rate responsive, ventricular pacemaker or a dual chamber pacemaker with mode switching capability.

Antiarrhythmic drug treatment

Atrial flutter is quite difficult to suppress completely with drug treatment. In fact, based on available long term data, drug treatment offers a limited ability to maintain sinus rhythm without occasional to frequent recurrences of atrial flutter, even when multiple agents are used. This is among the reasons why this form of therapy is no longer the long term treatment of choice in most patients with atrial flutter. For patients in whom drug treatment is selected, an important measure of efficacy should be the frequency of recurrence of atrial flutter rather than a single recurrent episode. For instance, recurrence only at long intervals—for example, once or twice per year—probably should be classified as a treatment success rather than a failure.

In the past, standard antiarrhythmic drug treatment consisted of administration of a class IA agent (quinidine, procainamide, or disopyramide) in an effort to prevent recurrence. However, recent studies indicate that the type

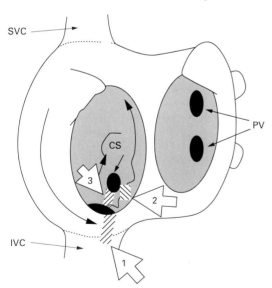

Figure 24.5. Targets for typical or reverse typical atrial flutter ablation. The schematic drawing shows the atria in an anterior view. The endocardium, inside the tricuspid (left) and mitral (right) rings, is shaded. The openings of the inferior vena cava (IVC), coronary sinus (CS), and left pulmonary veins (PV) are shown in black. Long arrows show activation sequence in common atrial flutter. The striped areas (large open arrows) mark ablation targets: 1, IVC–tricuspid valve isthmus; 2, CS–tricuspid valve isthmus; 3, CS–IVC isthmus. SVC, superior vena cava. Reproduced with permission from Cosío et al.[19]

IC antiarrhythmic agents flecainide and propafenone are as effective, if not more effective, are generally better tolerated, and have less organ toxicity than class IA agents. Principally because of their serious adverse effects demonstrated in the cardiac arrhythmia suppression trial (CAST I), it is widely accepted that class IC agents should not be used in the presence of underlying ischaemic heart disease. In fact, this approach has generally been extrapolated to include the presence of underlying structural heart disease. Nevertheless, class IC agents are recommended for long term suppression of atrial flutter in the absence of structural heart disease.

Moricizine, a class I drug with A, B, and C properties, also may be effective in the treatment of atrial flutter. The long term data from CAST II, in which moricizine and placebo were no different in terms of mortality, suggests that moricizine may be a good choice for patients with atrial flutter and coronary artery disease late (> 3 months) after a myocardial infarction. However, more data are required to establish moricizine's efficacy and safety in this clinical setting.

In addition, the class III antiarrhythmic agents amiodarone, sotalol, and dofetilide also may be quite effective. When using sotalol or dofetilide, care must be taken to avoid Q-T$_c$ interval prolongation much beyond 500 ms in order to avoid precipitation of torsades de pointes. Amiodarone appears to be quite effective, but its potential toxicity is a well recognised concern, making widespread use of this drug to treat atrial flutter problematic.[20] Thus, the use of amiodarone as the drug of first choice to treat atrial flutter probably should be limited to patients with notably depressed left ventricular function. Since atrial flutter tends to recur despite antiarrhythmic drug treatment, it is important to remember that on a class IA (quinidine, procainamide, disopyramide) or especially a class IC or IC-like (flecainide, propafenone, moricizine) agent, the atrial flutter rate may be much slower (for example, 180–220 bpm) than in the absence of one of these drugs. Therefore, it is very important that adequate block of AV nodal conduction be present, usually with concurrent use of a β blocker or a calcium channel blocker, alone or in combination with digoxin.

Anticoagulant treatment
Although one study found neither atrial clot formation nor stroke associated with atrial flutter in a relatively small cohort of patients after open heart surgery, the association of the potential risk of stroke with atrial flutter has now been established.[14 15] Other data support this association. Thus, atrial flutter and atrial fibrillation often co-exist in patients. Additionally, using transoesophageal echocardiography, a high incidence of spontaneous echo contrast and atrial thrombi have been documented, as were striking abnormalities in the left atrial appendage in patients with atrial flutter. In short, in patients with atrial flutter, daily warfarin treatment to achieve an international normalised ratio (INR) of 2 to 3 is recom-

---

Long term treatment of clinically important atrial flutter

- Treatment of choice: radiofrequency catheter ablation to achieve cure

- Alternative treatment (warfarin therapy usually required)
    - drug treatment (class IC, III or IA antiarrhythmics plus an AV nodal blocking drug)
    - device implantation (antitachycardia pacemaker or low energy atrial defibrillator)
    - His bundle ablation plus pacemaker implantation

---

mended using the same criteria as for atrial fibrillation. Also, the same criteria apply for cardioversion. Thus, if the patient has had atrial flutter for greater than 48 hours and the INR is not therapeutic (INR ≥ 2), warfarin treatment should be either initiated or adjusted, and after achieving a therapeutic INR for three consecutive weeks, cardioversion may be attempted. Following cardioversion, the patient should remain on warfarin with a therapeutic INR for four weeks.

Permanent antitachycardia pacemaker treatment
Although rarely used as treatment, in selected patients consideration should be given to implantation of a permanent antitachycardia pacemaker to interrupt recurrent atrial flutter and restore sinus rhythm. While there is only a small published series of patients treated with such devices, it nevertheless has been shown to be safe and effective. Since precipitation of atrial fibrillation is always a potential problem when using any form of pacing to treat atrial flutter, if any pacing induced episodes of atrial fibrillation are clinically unacceptable, placement of a permanent antitachycardia pacemaker to treat atrial flutter should be avoided. To decrease or eliminate an incidence of inadvertent precipitation of atrial fibrillation as well as to decrease the frequency of atrial flutter episodes, chronic use of an antiarrhythmic drug may be desirable.

Surgical treatment
Presently, there is little if any role for surgical ablation of the atrial flutter. Nevertheless, there is a limited experience. Klein, Guiraudon and colleagues have reported on three operated patients in whom cryoablation of the region between the coronary sinus orifice and the tricuspid annulus successfully prevented recurrent atrial flutter in two.[21 22] However, the third patient had subsequent symptomatic atrial fibrillation. Similarities between these surgical data and the catheter ablation data are apparent. Also, Canavan and colleagues reported the successful surgical interruption of the atrial flutter re-entrant circuit after intraoperative mapping in an adolescent who had an atrial septal defect repair as a child.[23] The atrial flutter re-entrant circuit was around the atriotomy.

164

Summary

Most atrial flutter is caused by re-entrant excitation in the right atrium. The 12 lead ECG remains the cornerstone for the clinical diagnosis. Acute treatment entails control of the ventricular response rate and restoration of sinus rhythm. Currently, radiofrequency catheter ablation treatment provides the expectation of cure, although atrial fibrillation may subsequently occur. Alternatively, antiarrhythmic drug treatment to suppress recurrent atrial flutter episodes may be useful, recognising that recurrences are common despite therapy. Use of an antitachycardia pacemaker may be helpful in selected patients to terminate atrial flutter, as may His bundle ablation with placement of an appropriate pacemaker system to control the ventricular response rate. Anticoagulation with warfarin in patients with recurrent or chronic atrial flutter is recommended using criteria applied to patients with atrial fibrillation.

Supported in part by grant RO1 HL38408 from the National Institutes of Health, National Heart, Lung, and Blood Institute, Bethesda, Maryland, USA.

1. **Waldo AL.** Pathogenesis of atrial flutter. *J Cardiovasc Electrophysiol* 1998;**9**:518–25.
• *Short review of the pathogenesis of atrial flutter.*

2. **Olshansky B, Okumura K, Hess PG,** *et al.* Demonstration of an area of slow conduction in human atrial flutter. *J Am Coll Cardiol* 1990;**16**:1639–48.
• *Mapping studies of typical atrial flutter.*

3. **Cosío FG, Goicolea A, Lopez-Gil M,** *et al.* Atrial endocardial mapping in the rare form of atrial flutter. *Am J Cardiol* 1990;**66**:715–20.
• *Mapping studies of reverse typical atrial flutter.*

4. **Olgin JE, Kalman JM, Fitzpatrick AP,** *et al.* Role of right atrial endocardial structures as barriers to conduction during human type I atrial flutter. Activation and entrainment mapping guided by intracardiac echocardiography. *Circulation* 1995;**92**:1839–48.
• *Studies defining the boundaries of the typical atrial flutter re-entrant circuit.*

5. **Kalman JM, Olgin JE, Saxon LA,** *et al.* Activation and entrainment mapping defines the tricuspid annulus as the anterior boundary in atrial flutter. *Circulation* 1996;**94**:398–406.
• *Studies defining the boundaries of the atrial flutter re-entrant circuit.*

6. **Nakagawa H, Lazzara R, Khastgir T,** *et al.* Role of the tricuspid annulus and the Eustachian valve/ridge on atrial flutter. Relevance to catheter ablation of the septal isthmus and a new technique for rapid identification of ablation success. *Circulation* 1996;**94**:407–24.
• *Studies defining the boundaries of the atrial flutter re-entrant circuit.*

7. **Cosio FG, Arribas F, Lopez-Gil M,** *et al.* Atrial flutter mapping and ablation. I. Studying atrial flutter mechanisms by mapping and entrainment. *PACE* 1996;**19**:841–53.
• *Electrode catheter mapping studies to identify the vulnerable part of the atrial flutter re-entrant circuit.*

8. **Saoudi N, Cosío F, Chen SA,** *et al.* A new classification of atrial tachycardias based on electrophysiologic mechanisms. *Eur J Cardiol* In press.
• *Explanation and examples of the new classification of atrial flutter.*

9. **Van Hare GF, Lesh MD, Ross BA,** *et al.* Mapping and radiofrequency ablation of intraatrial reentrant tachycardia after the Senning or Mustard procedure for transposition of the great arteries. *Am J Cardiol* 1996;**77**:985–91.
• *Studies of patients with chronic atrial flutter caused by incisional re-entry following surgical repair of a congenital heart lesion.*

10. **Chan DP, Van Hare GF, Mackall JA,** *et al.* Importance of the atrial flutter isthmus in post-operative intra-atrial reentrant tachycardia. *Circulation* In press.
• *Studies of patients with chronic atrial flutter following surgical repair of a congenital heart lesion demonstrating that in 75% of these patients, the atrial flutter re-entrant circuit utilises the atrial flutter isthmus.*

11. **Wells JL Jr, MacLean WAH, James TN,** *et al.* Characterization of atrial flutter. Studies in man after open heart surgery using fixed atrial electrodes. *Circulation* 1979;**60**:665–73.
• *Studies characterising type I and type II atrial flutter in patients.*

12. **Waldo AL, Cooper TB.** Spontaneous onset of type I atrial flutter in patients. *J Am Coll Cardiol* 1996;**28**:707–12.
• *Studies demonstrating that atrial fibrillation generally precedes the onset of atrial flutter.*

13. **Matsuo K, Tomita Y, Khrestian CM,** *et al.* A new mechanism of sustained atrial fibrillation: studies in the sterile pericarditis model [abstract]. *Circulation* 1998;**98**:I–209.
• *Demonstration of the nature of atrial fibrillation generated by a re-entrant circuit of very short cycle length (very rapid rate) which produces fibrillatory conduction.*

14. **Wood KA, Eisenberg SJ, Kalman JM,** *et al.* Risk of thromboembolism in chronic atrial flutter. *Am J Cardiol* 1997;**79**:1043–7.
• *Study demonstrating important risk of stroke or systemic embolism in the presence of atrial flutter but in the absence of anticoagulation treatment.*

15. **Seidl K, Haver B, Schwick NG,** *et al.* Risk of thromboembolic events in patients with atrial flutter. *Am J Cardiol* 1998;**82**:580–4.
• *Study demonstrating thromboembolic risk associated with atrial flutter.*

16. **Ellenbogen KA, Clemo HF, Stambler BS,** *et al.* Efficacy of ibutilide for termination of atrial fibrillation and flutter. *Am J Cardiol* 1996;**78**(suppl 8A):42–5.
• *Study showing efficacy of ibutilide in conversion of atrial flutter to sinus rhythm.*

17. **Stambler BS, Wood MA, Ellenbogen KA,** *et al.* Efficacy and safety of repeated intravenous doses of ibutilide for rapid conversion of atrial flutter or fibrillation. *Circulation* 1996;**94**:1613–21.
• *Study highlighting risks as well as efficacy of ibutilide therapy of atrial flutter.*

18. **Suttorp MJ, Kingma JH, Jessuren ER,** *et al.* The value of class IC antiarrhythmic drugs for acute conversion of paroxysmal atrial fibrillation or flutter to sinus rhythm. *J Am Coll Cardiol* 1990;**16**:1722–7.
• *Study showing efficacy of class IC agents in conversion of atrial flutter to sinus rhythm.*

19. **Cosío FG, Arribas F, Lopez-Gil M,** *et al.* Atrial flutter mapping and ablation. II. Radiofrequency ablation of atrial flutter circuits. *PACE* 1996;**19**:965–75.
• *Review of ablation techniques to cure atrial flutter.*

20. **Podrid PJ.** Amiodarone: reevaluation of an old drug. *Ann Int Med* 1995;**122**:689–700.
• *Good review of use of amiodarone for atrial flutter, including data on adverse effects of this drug.*

21. **Klein GJ, Guiraudon GM, Sharma AD,** *et al.* Demonstration of macroreentry and feasibility of operative therapy in the common type of atrial flutter. *Am J Cardiol* 1986;**57**:587–91.

22. **Guiraudon GM, Klein GJ, Sharma AD,** *et al.* Surgical alternatives for supraventricular tachycardias. *Am J Cardiol* 1989;**64**:92J–6J.

23. **Canavan TE, Schuessler RB, Cain ME,** *et al.* Computerized global electrophysiological mapping of the atrium in a patient with multiple supraventricular tachyarrhythmias. *Ann Thorac Surg* 1988;**46**:232–5.

25 Radiofrequency catheter ablation of ventricular tachycardia

William G Stevenson, Etienne Delacretaz

Management of patients with ventricular tachycardia (VT) is often difficult. Drug treatment is often ineffective. Implantable defibrillators terminate episodes but do not prevent them. Radiofrequency (RF) catheter ablation offers potential arrhythmia control without the adverse effects of antiarrhythmic treatment. However, the procedure is often challenging and efficacy is less than for ablation of supraventricular tachycardias. The efficacy and safety depend on the particular type of tachycardia and its likely origin. These factors can be predicted from the underlying heart disease and the electrocardiographic characteristics of the tachycardia.

VTs are either polymorphic or monomorphic. Polymorphic tachycardias have a continuously changing QRS morphology, indicating a variable sequence of ventricular activation and no single site of origin. The cause is often ischaemia or drug induced QT prolongation; ablation is not an option.

Monomorphic VT has a constant QRS morphology from beat to beat, indicating repetitive ventricular depolarisation in the same sequence. An arrhythmia focus or structural substrate is present that can be targeted for ablation. The QRS morphology often indicates the likely arrhythmogenic region. A left bundle branch block-like configuration in lead V1 indicates an origin in the right ventricle or the interventricular septum. A frontal plane axis that is directed inferiorly (dominant R waves in leads II, III, AVF) indicates an origin in the superior aspect of the ventricle, either the anterior wall of the left ventricle or the right ventricular outflow tract. A frontal plane axis directed superiorly indicates initial depolarisation of the inferior wall of the left or right ventricle. Dominant R waves in leads V3–V4 favour a location nearer the base of the heart than the apex. Dominant S waves in these leads favour a more apical location. The QRS morphology is an excellent guide to the arrhythmia origin when the ventricles are structurally normal, but less reliable when VT is caused by infarction or ventricular scar.

The underlying heart disease provides further important information. VT in patients without identifiable structural heart disease is referred to as "idiopathic". These tachycardias usually occur in specific locations and have specific QRS morphologies. Tachycardias associated with scar, such as prior myocardial infarction, have a QRS morphology that tends to indicate the location of the scar. Patients with non-ischaemic cardiomyopathies, including valvar heart disease, have an increased incidence of bundle branch re-entry tachycardia (see below), although other mechanisms are frequent in these patients as well.

Idiopathic VT

VT in patients without structural heart disease is uncommon.[1-3] Most originate from a small focus, making them susceptible to ablation. The prognosis is good; sudden death rarely if ever occurs unless some other form of heart disease is present, but tachycardia can be sufficiently rapid to cause syncope or severe symptoms. Rarely, VT is incessant and causes heart failure with depressed ventricular function that resolves with control of the arrhythmia. Although the focus can be anywhere in the ventricles, the vast majority originate from one of two locations.

Idiopathic right ventricular outflow tract tachycardia

The most common idiopathic VT originates from a focus in the outflow tract of the right ventricle (fig 25.1).[1 2] The mechanism is most likely triggered automaticity.[4] VT has a left bundle branch block configuration in ECG lead V1 with a frontal plane axis that is directed inferiorly or inferiorly and to the right. Premature ventricular contractions with an identical morphology are often present during sinus rhythm. Tachycardia may occur in repetitive bursts (referred to as repetitive monomorphic VT). In some patients non-sustained VT and frequent premature beats are severely symptomatic and warrant treatment. Although echocardiogram, ECG, and angiography are generally normal, cardiac magnetic resonance imaging may identify areas of focal thinning, hypokinesis or fatty infiltration. The major diagnostic consideration is that of arrhythmogenic right ventricular dysplasia (see below).

In contrast to scar related re-entry (see below) the automaticity that causes these tachycardias is often provoked by adrenergic stimulation and appears to be sensitive to increases in intracellular calcium. Treatment with calcium channel blockers (verapamil and diltiazem), which is contraindicated in most other types of VT, often suppresses the arrhythmia. β Adrenergic blockers are also often effective, particularly if the arrhythmias are provoked by exercise. Catheter ablation is a reasonable consideration when pharmacologic treatment is not effective or tolerated. It can be considered for patients with sustained VT, non-sustained bursts of VT, or frequent symptomatic ventricular premature beats. The focus is located by finding the earliest site of activation during tachycardia (activation sequence mapping) (fig 25.1), or by finding the site where pacing exactly reproduces the QRS

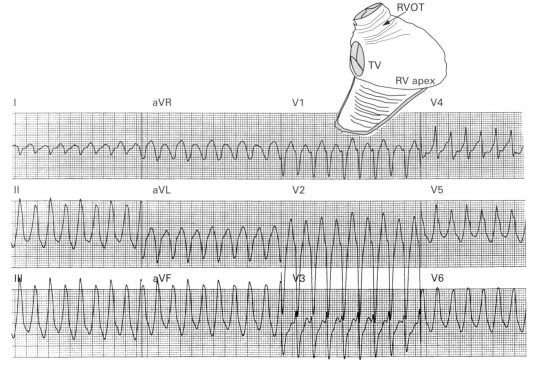

Figure 25.1. Idiopathic right ventricular outflow tract tachycardia. The 12 lead ECG shows tachycardia with a left bundle branch block, configuration and frontal plane axis directed inferiorly. The schematic at the upper right shows the right ventricle viewed from the right anterior oblique position with the free wall of the ventricle folded down. The location of the tachycardia in the right ventricular outflow tract (RVOT) is indicated with an arrow. TV, tricuspid valve; RV, right ventricle.

morphology of the tachycardia (pace mapping). Ablation is successful in approximately 85% of patients.[1] Failures are caused either by an inability to induce the arrhythmia in the laboratory, preventing adequate mapping, or by the location of the focus deep within the septum or in the epicardium over the septum, beyond the reach of endocardial RF ablation lesions. Occasionally ablation from the left side of the interventricular septum is required. Complications are infrequent, but cardiac perforation and coronary artery occlusion during ablation in the left ventricular outflow tract have occurred.[2]

Idiopathic left ventricular, verapamil sensitive tachycardia

The most common idiopathic left VT has a right bundle branch block configuration with a frontal plane axis that is directed superiorly, or rarely inferiorly and to the right.[1 3] Administration of intravenous verapamil terminates tachycardia suggesting that slow calcium channel dependent tissue is involved. The mechanism appears to be re-entry involving the distal fascicles of the left bundle branch. Re-entry involving Purkinje tissue in or adjacent to a left ventricular false tendon, which is present in more than 90% of patients, has also been suggested.

When treatment with β adrenergic blockers and/or calcium channel blockers is ineffective or not tolerated catheter ablation is a reasonable alternative. Mapping for ablation seeks sites where a discrete Purkinje potential precedes the QRS complex during tachycardia.[3] Ablation is successful in approximately 90% of patients. Failures are sometimes caused

by catheter induced trauma to the arrhythmia focus (or possibly the false tendon) which then prevents initiation, precluding mapping. Complications are infrequent but damage to the aortic or mitral valve apparatus from catheter manipulation can occur.

VT related to regions of scar

The majority of sustained monomorphic VTs are caused by re-entry involving a region of ventricular scar. The scar is most commonly caused by an old myocardial infarction, but arrhythmogenic right ventricular dysplasia, sarcoidosis, Chagas' disease, other non-ischaemic cardiomyopathies and surgical ventricular incisions for repair of tetralogy of Fallot, other congenital heart diseases, or ventricular volume reduction surgery (Batista procedure) can also cause scar related re-entry. Dense fibrotic scar creates areas of anatomic conduction block. Secondly, fibrosis between surviving myocyte bundles decreases cell to cell coupling, and distorts the path of propagation causing slow conduction, which promotes re-entry (fig 25.2).[5] These re-entry circuits often contain a narrow isthmus of abnormal conduction. Depolarisation of the small mass of tissue in the isthmus is not detectable in the body surface ECG. The QRS complex is caused by propagation of the wavefront from the exit of the circuit to the surrounding myocardium (fig 25.2). After leaving the exit of the isthmus, the circulating re-entry wavefront may propagate through a broad path along the border of the scar (loop), back to the entrance of the isthmus. A variety of different circuit

Bipolar voltage

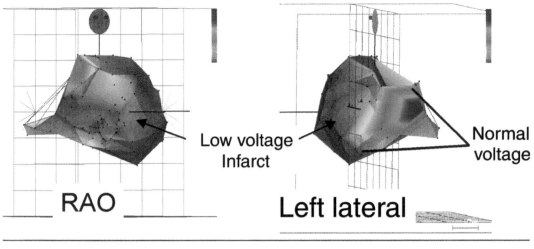

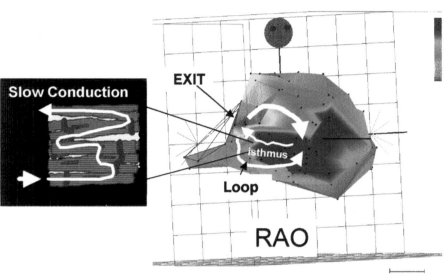

Figure 25.2. The mapping data are from a patient with VT late after anterior wall myocardial infarction. Mapping was performed using a system that plots the precise catheter position along with colour coded electrophysiologic information (CARTO Biosense Webster, Diamond Bar, California, USA). The top two panels show the left ventricle in right anterior oblique (RAO) and left lateral views. In this case, colours indicate the electrogram voltage, rather than timing. The lowest voltage regions are shown in red, progressing to greater voltage regions of yellow, green, blue, and purple. A large anteroapical infarction is indicated by the extensive low voltage, red region. The lower right panel shows the map of VT in the same patient. The ventricle is again shown in a right anterior oblique projection with the apex at the right and the base at the left hand side of the image. The colours indicate the activation sequence and arrows have been drawn to clarify the activation sequence of the circuit. The re-entry circuit is located in the septum. The wavefront starts at the red area (exit) near the base of the septum and splits into two loops that circle around the superior and inferior aspect of the septum toward the apex, re-entering an isthmus in the circuit that is proximal to the exit region. RF ablation in the isthmus abolished tachycardia. The mechanism of slow conduction through the infarct region that has been observed in previous histopathologic studies is illustrated schematically in the inset at lower left. Surviving myocyte bundles are separated by fibrous tissue that forces the wavefront to take a circuitous path through the region.

configurations are possible. Ablation lesions produced with standard RF ablation catheters are usually less than 8 mm in diameter, relatively small in relation to the entire re-entry circuit, and can be smaller than the width of the re-entry path at different points in the circuit. Successful ablation of a large circuit is achieved either by targeting an isthmus where the circuit can be interrupted with one or a small number of RF lesions, or by creating a line of RF lesions through a region containing the re-entry circuit.

Identification of critical isthmuses is often challenging. The abnormal area of scarring, where the isthmus is located, is often large and contains "false isthmuses" (bystanders) that

confuse mapping. In most cases a portion of an isthmus is located in the subendocardium where it can be ablated. However, in some cases the isthmuses or even the entire circuits are deep to the endocardium or even in the epicardium and cannot be identified or ablated from the endocardium.

The situation is further complicated by the frequent presence of multiple potential re-entry circuits, giving rise to multiple different monomorphic VTs in a single patient. Ablation in one area may abolish more than one VT, or leave VT circuits in other locations intact. The frequent presence of multiple VTs also complicates interpretation of outcomes. VTs that have been documented to occur spontaneously are referred to as "clinical tachycardias". Those that are induced in the electrophysiology laboratory, but have not been previously observed, are sometimes referred to as "non-clinical tachycardias". However, a "non-clinical VT" may occur later, after ablation of the "clinical VT". In addition the ECG of spontaneous VTs terminated by an implanted defibrillator or emergency medical technicians is often not available. Thus the distinction between "clinical" and "non-clinical" is often uncertain.

When VT is slow and haemodynamically tolerated a re-entry circuit isthmus can usually be found during catheter mapping (fig 25.2). Extensive mapping during VT is not possible when VT causes haemodynamic instability or the re-entry circuit is not stable, but repeatedly changes causing multiple different morphologies of monomorphic VT.

Ablation of VT after myocardial infarction

Most reported series included patients who had at least one mappable VT. Gonska and colleagues selected 72 patients who had a single clinical VT. RF ablation abolished the clinical VT in 74% of patients; 60% of the total group remained free of spontaneous VT recurrences during follow up.[6] Stevenson,[7] Rothman,[8] and Strickberger[9] and associates targeted multiple VTs for ablation in 108 patients with recurrent VT. An average of 3.6–4.7 different VTs were inducible per patient. All inducible monomorphic VTs were abolished in 33% of patients; in 22% of patients ablation had no effect. In the remaining 45% of patients the re-entry substrate was "modified"; the VTs targeted for ablation were rendered non-inducible, but other VTs remained. During mean follow ups ranging from 12–18 months, 66% of patients remained free of recurrent VT and 24% suffered recurrences. The incidence of sudden death was 2.8%, but most patients had an implanted defibrillator; the sudden death risk may be higher if ablation is used as sole treatment.

Saline irrigation of the ablation electrode (cooled RF ablation) may create larger lesions to reach deep portions of re-entry circuits by allowing current delivery without excessive heating at the surface of the tissue, which can cause formation of coagulum that prevents further energy application. A recent multicentre trial evaluated a saline irrigated RF ablation catheter (Cardiac Pathways Corp, Sunnyvale, California, USA) in 146 patients (prior myocardial infarction in 82%; average (SD) left ventricular ejection fraction 31 (13)%) who had an average of 25 (31) episodes of VT in the two months before ablation despite antiarrhythmic drug treatment.[10] All mappable VTs were eliminated in 75% of patients. During a follow up of 243 days 54% of patients remained free of spontaneous VT; 81% experienced a more than 75% reduction in the number of VT episodes in the two months after ablation, as compared to before ablation.

Patients with VT caused by prior infarction have depressed ventricular function and concomitant illnesses. Ablation is often a late attempt in controlling refractory arrhythmias, sometimes after significant haemodynamic compromise has developed. Significant complications of stroke, transient ischaemic attack, myocardial infarction, cardiac perforation requiring treatment, or heart block occur in approximately 5–8% of patients. Procedure related mortality is 1% in pooled data and 2.8% in the one reported multicentre trial of cooled RF ablation discussed above.

During follow up the largest source of mortality is death from heart failure, with an incidence of approximately 10% over the following 12–18 months.[6–10] This risk of death is not unexpected in this population. However, ablation injury to contracting myocardium outside the infarct or injury to the aortic or mitral valves during left ventricular catheter manipulation are procedural complications that could exacerbate heart failure. Restricting ablation lesions to areas of infarction, as identified from low amplitude electrograms in regions observed to have little contractility on echocardiogram or ventriculogram, is prudent.

Arrhythmogenic right ventricular dysplasia

Arrhythmogenic right ventricular dysplasia is associated with fibrous and fatty scar tissue in the right and often the left ventricles. VT typically has a left bundle branch block-like configuration in V1, consistent with a right ventricular origin. When right ventricular involvement is extensive, the success of ablation is variable.[11] Individual VTs can be ablated, but others may develop later possibly related to progression of the disease process. Ablation is reserved as a palliative treatment for frequent episodes. Although the right ventricle can be quite thinned, the risk of perforation during mapping does not seem to be substantially increased.

VT caused by non-ischaemic cardiomyopathy

The mechanisms of sustained monomorphic VT in non-ischaemic cardiomyopathies (including idiopathic cardiomyopathy and valvar heart disease) are diverse. In a series of 26 patients with monomorphic VT the causes were scar related re-entry circuits in 62% of patients, an ectopic focus in 27%, and bundle branch re-entry in 19%.[12] Ablation was successful for 60% of the scar related VTs and 86% of the VTs caused by focal automaticity. The difficulties in ablation of scar related VT are similar to those encountered in patients with prior myocardial infarction; multiple tachycardias are not uncommon, but reduction in the number of episodes and termination of incessant tachycardia can often be achieved. Successful ablation of scar related VTs in patients with sarcoidosis, scleroderma, Chagas' disease,[13] and late after repair of tetralogy of Fallot[14] have also been reported, although experience is limited.

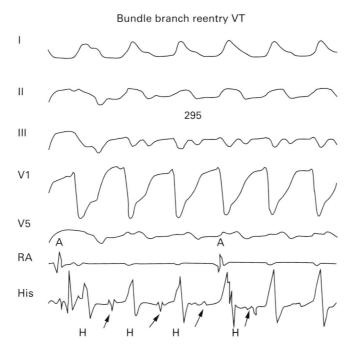

Bundle branch reentry VT

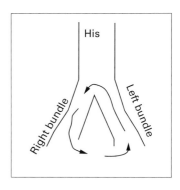

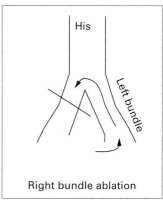

Right bundle ablation

Figure 25.3. Bundle branch re-entry tachycardia. The left hand panel shows bundle branch re-entry tachycardia initiated in the electrophysiology laboratory. From the top are surface ECG leads and intracardiac recordings from the right atrium (RA) and His bundle position (His). VT has a left bundle branch block configuration and cycle length of 295 ms. Atrioventricular dissociation is evident in the right atrial recording (RA). A His bundle deflection (arrows) precedes each QRS indicating that the His-Purkinje system is closely linked to the tachycardia. The schematic in the right hand panels illustrates the mechanism. The wavefront circulates down the right bundle, through the interventricular septum, and up the left bundle (top panel). Ablation of the right bundle branch interrupts the circuit (bottom panel).

> **Problems and emerging solutions for ablation of scar related tachycardias**

Intramural and epicardial circuits

Mapping arrhythmia foci or circuits that are deep within the myocardium or in the epicardium is being attempted in one of two ways. Small, 2 French electrode catheters can be introduced into the coronary sinus and advanced out into the cardiac veins. Epicardial circuits can sometimes be identified, but only when the vessel cannulated happens to be in the region of the circuit. Ablation through the vein may carry the risk of injury to adjacent coronary artery.

Sosa and colleagues have developed an epicardial approach inserting an introducer into the pericardial space in the manner used for pericardiocentesis.[13] Epicardial foci have been identified and ablated using this approach. The risk of damage to adjacent lung and epicardial vessels requires further evaluation.

The size of standard RF ablation lesions is limited by formation of a high resistance barrier of coagulated proteins on the ablation electrode when its temperature reaches 100°C. To increase current delivery without coagulum formation, the electrode can be cooled by irrigation with saline, or by using a larger tip electrode, which increases the surface area available for cooling by the circulating blood.[10] Ablation methods that increase lesion size

could increase the risk of myocardial damage that could further depress ventricular function. Careful assessment of risks are required with each advance.

Unstable monomorphic VT

Two approaches are being evaluated for ablation of scar related VT that is difficult to map with a roving catheter because of haemodynamic instability or instability of the re-entry circuit. One approach involves defining the area of scar from its low amplitude sinus rhythm electrograms (fig 25.2, top panels); then selecting portions of the scar likely to contain a part of the re-entry circuit based on the VT QRS morphology or pace mapping; and then placing a series of anatomically guided ablation lesions through the abnormal region.[15 16] Ellison and colleagues targeted the likely re-entry exit region in five patients with frequent unmappable VT. All three patients with prior myocardial infarction were free of recurrent VT during follow ups of 14–22 months. The procedure was not successful in the two with non-ischaemic cardiomyopathy.[15] Marchlinski and colleagues applied a more extensive series of RF ablation lines through regions of scar in 16 patients with recurrent unmappable VT (prior myocardial infarction in nine patients).[16] During a median follow up of eight months 75% remained free of VT recurrences. One patient suffered a stroke, emphasising the potential risk of placing extensive lesions in the left ventricle.

Table 25.1 Ventricular tachycardia mechanisms and ablation considerations

	Mechanism	Ablation efficacy	Complication risk
Idiopathic VT			
RV outflow tract	Automaticity	80–90%	Low, but rare fatalities
LV verapamil sensitive	Re-entry	90%	Low
Post-MI "mappable" VT	Re-entry		
Reduction in VT episodes		70–80%	5–10%
Prevention of all VT		50–67%	5–10%
Post-MI "unmappable"		?	?
Other scar related VTs	Re-entry		
RV dysplasia + RV dilation		Palliative	?
Non-ischaemic cardiomyopathy		~60%	Low
Bundle branch re-entry VT	Re-entry through bundle branches	100%	AV block

AV, atrioventricular; LV, left ventricular; RV, right ventricular; MI, myocardial infarction; VT, ventricular tachycardia.

VT that is unmappable with a single roving catheter may be mapped with a system that simultaneously records electrograms throughout the ventricle during one or a few beats of the unstable VT, following which the VT can be terminated to allow ablation during stable sinus rhythm. Multielectrode basket catheters have been successfully deployed through a long sheath into the ventricle, but have somewhat limited sampling.[17] An alternative system (Endocardial Solutions, St Paul, Minnesota, USA) records electrical potentials from an electrode grid array within the cavity of the ventricle. Electrical potentials at the endocardial surface some distance away are calculated. Sites of early endocardial activity, which are likely adjacent to re-entry circuit exits, are usually identifiable; in some cases, isthmuses have been identified.[18 19] Schilling and colleagues used this system to guide ablation in 24 patients (20 with prior infarction) and recurrent VT. During a mean follow up of 18 months, 64% were free of recurrent VT. In 15 patients Strickberger and associates achieved ablation of 15 of 19 (78%) VTs that were selected for ablation in 15 patients with prior infarction; 10 were free of recurrent VT during a short one month follow up. Major complications of stroke, perforation, and death from pump failure occurred in three patients. Further evaluation with regards to safety and efficacy are warranted.

Bundle branch re-entry VT

Bundle branch re-entry causes only 5% of all sustained monomorphic VTs in patients referred for electrophysiologic study, but is important to recognise because it is easily curable.[20] In its usual form the excitation wavefront circulates up the left bundle branch, down the right bundle branch, and then through the interventricular septum to re-enter the left bundle (fig 25.3), causing VT with a left bundle branch block configuration. Less commonly, the circuit revolves in the opposite direction. This VT occurs in patients who slowed conduction through the His Purkinje system and is usually associated with severe left ventricular dysfunction. The sinus rhythm ECG usually displays incomplete left bundle branch block. The VT is often rapid, commonly causing syncope or cardiac arrest. Ablation of the right bundle branch is relatively easy and effective. AV conduction is further impaired by ablation, necessitating implantation of a pacemaker or defibrillator with bradycardia pacing in 15–30% of patients. Bundle branch re-entry VT coexists with scar related VTs in some patients; implantation of a defibrillator is usually considered.

Current clinical application

Catheter ablation is a useful treatment for selected patients with VT. It should be considered for patients with recurrent, symptomatic idiopathic VT and is the first line treatment for bundle branch re-entry VT.

Catheter ablation offers improved arrhythmia control in two thirds of patients who have a mappable scar related VT (table 25.1). It can be lifesaving for patients with incessant VT, and can decrease frequent episodes of VT causing therapies from an implanted defibrillator. Before considering ablation possible aggravating factors should be addressed. Although myocardial ischaemia by itself does not generally cause recurrent monomorphic VT, it can be a trigger in patients with scar related re-entry circuits. Furthermore severe ischaemia during induced VT increases the risk of mapping and ablation procedures. An assessment of the potential for ischaemia is generally warranted in patients with coronary artery disease who are being considered for catheter ablation. Patients with left ventricular dysfunction should also have an echocardiogram to assess the possible presence of left ventricular thrombus that could be dislodged and embolise during catheter manipulation in the left ventricle.

The difficulty of the procedure increases when unmappable VTs are present. Many laboratories restrict ablation attempts to patients with mappable VTs. Current studies focusing on methods of ablation of unmappable VTs and epicardial and intramural arrhythmia foci are likely to increase efficacy and applicability. Scar related VTs are often associated with poor ventricular function and multiple inducible VTs. Most patients will remain candidates for an implanted defibrillator, with ablation used for control of symptoms caused by frequent arrhythmia recurrences.

1. Rodriguez LM, Smeets JL, Timmermans C, *et al*. Predictors for successful ablation of right- and left-sided idiopathic ventricular tachycardia. *Am J Cardiol* 1997;**79**:309–14.
- *Based on mapping and ablation of 35 right ventricular outflow tract VTs and 13 idiopathic left ventricular VTs, electrocardiogram patterns associated with lower efficacy are described.*

2. Coggins DL, Lee RJ, Sweeney J, *et al*. Radiofrequency catheter ablation as a cure for idiopathic tachycardia of both left and right ventricular origin. *J Am Coll Cardiol* 1994;**23**:1333–41.

3. Nakagawa H, Beckman KJ, McClelland JH, *et al*. Radiofrequency catheter ablation of idiopathic left ventricular tachycardia guided by a Purkinje potential. *Circulation* 1993;**88**:2607–17.
- *Evidence is presented that the Purkinje system is involved in idiopathic left ventricular tachycardia and can be targeted for ablation.*

4. Lerman BB, Stein K, Engelstein ED, *et al*. Mechanism of repetitive monomorphic ventricular tachycardia. *Circulation* 1995;**92**:421–9.

5. de Bakker JM, van Capelle FJ, Janse MJ, *et al*. Slow conduction in the infarcted human heart. 'Zigzag' course of activation. *Circulation* 1993;**88**:915–26.
- *The mechanism of slow conduction in scar is shown in detailed pathophysiologic study of explanted hearts. The authors' other classic papers are referenced.*

6. Gonska BD, Cao K, Schaumann A, *et al*. Catheter ablation of ventricular tachycardia in 136 patients with coronary artery disease: results and long-term follow-up. *J Am Coll Cardiol* 1994;**24**:1506–14.
- *This paper and the following three references are the largest series of catheter ablation for VT after infarction with follow up data.*

7. Stevenson WG, Friedman PL, Kocovic D, *et al*. Radiofrequency catheter ablation of ventricular tachycardia after myocardial infarction. *Circulation* 1998;**98**:308–14.

8. Rothman SA, Hsia HH, Cossu SF, *et al*. Radiofrequency catheter ablation of postinfarction ventricular tachycardia: long-term success and the significance of inducible nonclinical arrhythmias. *Circulation* 1997;**96**:3499–508.

9. Strickberger SA, Man KC, Daoud EG, *et al*. A prospective evaluation of catheter ablation of ventricular tachycardia as adjuvant therapy in patients with coronary artery disease and an implantable cardioverter-defibrillator [see comments]. *Circulation* 1997;**96**:1525–31.

10. Calkins H for the Cooled RF Multicenter Investigator Group. Catheter ablation of ventricular tachycardia in patients with structural heart disease using cooled RF energy: results of a prospective multicenter study. *J Am Coll Cardiol* 2000;**35**:1905–14..
- *The first large multicenter trial of catheter ablation for drug refractory VT defining efficacy and risks of a saline cooled RF ablation system.*

11. Ellison KE, Friedman PL, Ganz LI, *et al*. Entrainment mapping and radiofrequency catheter ablation of ventricular tachycardia in right ventricular dysplasia. *J Am Coll Cardiol* 1998;**32**:724–8.

12. Delacretaz E, Stevenson WG, Ellison KE, *et al*. Mapping and radiofrequency catheter ablation of the three types of sustained monomorphic ventricular tachycardia in nonischemic heart disease. *J Cardiovasc Electrophysiol* 2000;**11**:11–17.
- *Types of VT, mapping, and ablation approaches are described for patients with non-ischaemic cardiomyopathy (excluding right ventricular dysplasia) and monomorphic VT.*

13. Sosa E, Scanavacca M, D'Avila A, *et al*. Endocardial and epicardial ablation guided by nonsurgical transthoracic epicardial mapping to treat recurrent ventricular tachycardia. *J Cardiovasc Electrophysiol* 1998;**9**:229–39.
- *A description is provided of the technique for entry into the pericardial space and successful ablation of scar related VT in Chagas' disease.*

14. Stevenson WG, Delacretaz E, Friedman PL, *et al*. Identification and ablation of macroreentrant ventricular tachycardia with the CARTO electroanatomical mapping system. *Pacing Clin Electrophysiol* 1998;**21**:1448–56.

15. Ellison KE, Stevenson WG, Sweeney MO, *et al*. Catheter ablation for hemodynamically unstable monomorphic ventricular tachycardia. *J Cardiovasc Electrophysiol* 2000;**11**:41–4.

16. Marchlinski FE, Callans DJ, Gottlieb CD, *et al*. Linear ablation lesions for control of unmappable ventricular tachycardia in patients with ischemic and nonischemic cardiomyopathy. *Circulation* 2000;**101**:1288–96.
- *An extensive set of linear RF lesions successfully abolished all inducible VTs in 7 of 15 patients with unmappable VT. Reference values for electrogram voltage in areas of scar are also provided.*

17. Schalij MJ, van Rugge FP, Siezenga M, *et al*. Endocardial activation mapping of ventricular tachycardia in patients: first application of a 32-site bipolar mapping electrode catheter. *Circulation* 1998;**98**:2168–79.

18. Schilling RJ, Peters NS, Davies DW. Feasibility of a noncontact catheter for endocardial mapping of human ventricular tachycardia. *Circulation* 1999;**99**:2543–52.
- *Description of a novel "non-contact mapping system" for ablation of VT supports feasibility.*

19. Strickberger SA, Knight BP, Michaud GF, *et al*. Mapping and ablation of ventricular tachycardia guided by virtual electrograms using a noncontact, computerized mapping system. *J Am Coll Cardiol* 2000;**35**:414–21.

20. Blanck Z, Dhala A, Deshpande S, *et al*. Bundle branch reentrant ventricular tachycardia: cumulative experience in 48 patients. *J Cardiovasc Electrophysiol* 1993;**4**:253–62.

SECTION VI: CONGENITAL HEART DISEASE

26 Antenatal diagnosis of heart disease

Lindsey Allan

In 1980, several reports appeared almost simultaneously of the identification of normal cardiac anatomy in fetal life. The recognition of several different forms of structural cardiac anomaly followed soon after. At this time, cardiac evaluation was confined to pregnancies at increased risk of congenital heart disease (CHD), such as those with a family history of CHD or where extracardiac malformations had been detected. However, up to 90% of CHD occurs in pregnancies where there are no known high risk features. For this reason, in 1985 a group based in Paris put forward the idea of teaching the obstetrician to assess the heart in a simplified form during routine obstetric scanning, which was well established at that time in France. As a result, four chamber view scanning became an integral part of the fetal anatomical survey in many countries by the end of the 1980s. In the early 1990s, some authors suggested extending the cardiac assessment to include great artery scanning in order to detect a higher proportion of cases of major congenital heart disease.[1] If cardiac screening is confined to the four chamber view, about 2/1000 studies will be abnormal and would represent about 60% of the major heart disease seen in infants. If the great arteries are also examined, about 3/1000 cases would be abnormal, and over 90% of major heart disease would be detectable prenatally. Therefore, in ideal circumstances, the vast majority of serious heart malformations could be detected before 20 weeks' gestation. Unfortunately, the reality is far from this for several reasons:

- differing policies for obstetric scanning
- differing guidelines for scanning
- differing skill at scanning.

About 2% of live births have fetal structural malformations, the majority of which can be detected by ultrasound. About 25% of these malformations are cardiac in nature and about half of these are serious or life threatening. Despite these facts, and the opportunity during pregnancy for comprehensive evaluation of the fetal anatomy in fine detail, there is no universal agreement as to either the necessity for or the technique of fetal anatomical scanning. Some countries, such as Norway, France, and Germany, have instituted a government sponsored policy for routine anatomical screening by ultrasound. In the UK, routine screening is generally well accepted but not uniformly adopted or standardised in all parts of the country. In the USA, routine scanning is not recommended but is allowed only for specific indications, although these are fairly all encompassing. In practice, this leads to later scanning in the US and "targeted" scanning rather than a comprehensive anatomical survey.

Where an anatomical survey is performed, the timing of the scan varies—for example, in France it is usually between 20–22 weeks, in Norway 18 weeks. In general, the later in the mid-trimester that scanning is performed the more successful will be the detection of abnormalities, partly because scanning becomes easier and partly because some lesions become more evident as pregnancy advances. However, later detection of malformations will limit the options for interrupting the pregnancy or make it much more difficult both emotionally for the parents and technically for the obstetrician. Thus, the ideal policy would be a universal anatomical scan at a compromise time of between 18–20 weeks' gestation.

Although there are recommended guidelines for the technique of fetal scanning provided by the Royal College of Obstetricians and the American Colleges of Obstetrics and of Radiology, none are enforced and there is no standardisation of practice. This would be much easier in the UK than in the US and could be universally computerised to a standard format, but to my knowledge this is still not happening.

The skill involved in scanning is extremely variable for several reasons. A sonographer, whether a technician, an obstetrician, or a radiologist, needs:

- to train with a high volume of patients
- to maintain skills continuously with sufficient numbers of patients
- to be exposed continually to a critical number of abnormal fetuses
- to be provided with constant feedback and retraining.

In order to achieve and maintain a high level of expertise in scanning, the practitioner should be doing this as a full time or nearly full time commitment. Where ultrasound is performed in small numbers, the requisite practice necessary is quite unattainable. Nearly all scanning in the UK is hospital based, with delivery numbers usually over 2000 per year. Therfore, the necessary volume of patients is less of a problem in the UK than in the US, where scanning often takes place in private offices in small numbers.

As a result of the differing policies and standards in obstetric ultrasound, the results of the detection of all malformations in the screening setting varies with the organ involved, but is particularly poor in reference to the heart. During screening, reported detection rates vary between 4.5% and 96% for major CHD, with the most papers giving a rate of 15–20%.[2-6] This is consistent with recent experience in our referral centre for paediatric cardiology, when 18% of infants requiring cardiac surgery in the first year of life during 1998 were identified prenatally. The rate of detection of four chamber view anomalies prenatally is better, but averages only about 50%,[7 8] despite the fact that universally nearly all pregnancies are scanned at least once (figs 26.1, 26.2, and 26.3). Thus, the technology and personnel are in place in obstetric care, but they are not used to their maximum capability.

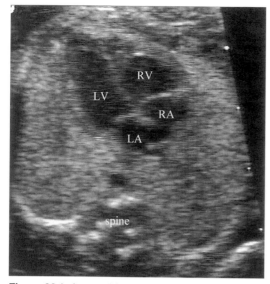

Figure 26.1. A normal four chamber view showing a heart of normal size (about one third of the thorax) in a normal position within the thorax (about 45° to the midline). There are two equally sized atria and two equally sized ventricles. In the moving image both atrioventricular valves would be seen to open equally. There is a "cross" at the crux of the heart, where the atrial and ventricular septum meet at the insertion of the two atrioventricular valves. LA, left atrium; RA, right atrium; LV, left ventricle; RV, right ventricle.

Cardiac evaluation at referral to paediatric cardiologists

A common misconception among paediatric cardiologists is that fetal cardiology is the same as paediatric echocardiography but a bit smaller. Therefore, nearly all paediatric echocardiographers in the US would not hesitate to offer fetal echocardiography as part of their practice. However, it is clear that quite a different spectrum of disease is seen prenatally,[9] and fetal heart scanning is quite a different skill. Success in accurate diagnosis will be

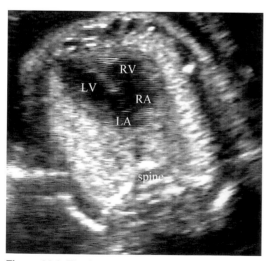

Figure 26.2. The fetal heart is oriented similarly to the normal example seen in fig 1. The most common anomaly detected prenatally is depicted. There is no "cross" appearance at the crux of the heart owing to a common atrioventricular junction and a complete atrioventricular septal defect. Despite the obvious difference between this and the four chamber view of the normal heart, only about 50% of cases are detected in fetal life.

partly dependent on technical skills, which again require training and practice. In the US, there are recommended guidelines for training, and a minimum number of scans in order to maintain skills, but these are not commonly known and certainly are not adhered to. Experience of fetal malformations therefore is so diluted that few practitioners have sufficient numbers to maintain a high standard of expertise. In addition, most paediatric cardiologists know little of fetal medicine and obstetric pathology, which have an important influence on fetal cardiac evaluation.

Although the majority of paediatric cardiology centres in the UK now offer fetal echocardiography, this is usually confined to one or two cardiologists and, theoretically, there should be sufficient numbers in each regional centre to provide adequate experience. However, there is no system of independent review or systematic quality control in place anywhere, to my knowledge. Indeed, in the US, pathological correlation after termination of pregnancy is quite rare for various reasons, not least being the difficulty in obtaining remuneration for pathological services, despite their vital role in quality control.

Problems and limitations

Limitations of fetal echocardiography are related to:
- image quality
- subtle lesions, such as small ventricular septal defects
- developing or progressive lesions
- lesions which are undetectable before birth.

Image quality is dependent on the skill and experience of scanning in addition to local factors such as gestational age, fetal position, and the thickness of the maternal abdomen. Maternal obesity is an increasing problem everywhere but particularly in the US, especially in the poorer states. This is the most important limitation to image quality, which in turn will limit confidence in excluding malformations in the fetus in any anatomical system. Even though the resolution of ultrasound equipment has improved vastly since the early 1980s, a great deal more detail is also expected during fetal scanning, and there are a significant proportion of patients where detail is just not possible because of the way scanning is presently organised. As up to 10% of adult Americans are said to be morbidly obese, this group should probably be managed with a different strategy, perhaps with early transvaginal scanning instead of transabdominal scans; to date this problem has not been addressed by the ultrasound community.

In a small proportion of fetuses, CHD becomes evident or more evident as pregnancy progresses.[3] Thus, the cardiac evaluation can be normal at 18 weeks although a significant malformation is found later or at birth. This is true of some cases of aortic or pulmonary stenosis, cardiac tumours, or cardiomyopathies. It is rare for a life threatening malformation to

Figure 26.3. This fetal heart is oriented similarly to the normal example shown in fig 1. The second most common anomaly detected prenatally is depicted. The left atrium is small. The left ventricle is hypoplastic with the right heart forming the apex. The mitral valve is not patent. This is mitral atresia, in its most frequent setting of the hypoplastic left heart syndrome. Again, this defect is only detected prenatally in just over half of cases.

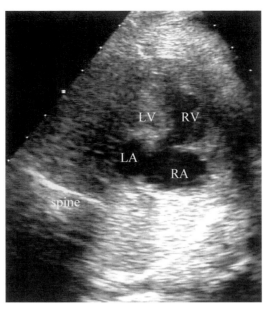

arise after 20 weeks' gestation, but it can occur. In addition, minor lesions can be overlooked because of the limits of ultrasound resolution, such as small ventricular septal defects; a persistent arterial duct and an atrial septal defect cannot be predicted prenatally as these communications are always present prenatally. Thus, there are confidence limits with even detailed fetal heart scanning. It is important to realise, however, that confidence limits may be much wider with poor image quality.

Latest technologies

By 14 weeks' gestation, the cardiac connections can be identified in many patients transabdominally. The connections can be seen in almost all patients at this stage transvaginally, however, and in much finer detail than on the transabdominal scan. Expertise with this technique is essential and the paediatric cardiologist should use the experienced gynaecological technician to display the fetal cardiac images, in a setting where transvaginal scanning is routine. At present, a cardiac scan at 14 weeks is confined to the high risk patient, such as those with a family history of CHD or those whose fetus has been found to have an increased nuchal fold.

The data concerning nuchal translucency in early pregnancy (10–12 weeks) are fascinating and intriguing.[10] When the translucent region at the back of the neck is increased in size, there is a high incidence of associated chromosomal anomalies, cardiac malformations, or both, with the incidence of heart disease increasing with increasing nuchal thickness. Conversely, 50% of fetuses subsequently found to have CHD had an abnormal nuchal fold measurement. This may reflect the "insult" which has caused the fetal heart malformation. Extension of the nuchal translucency screening program, which has received little attention in the US so far, is likely to have important implications for the improved detection of both chromosomal and cardiac malformations. In addition, the earlier the diagnosis of fetal malformation is

made in pregnancy, the more likely are parents to choose interruption. If a pregnancy with increased nuchal thickening is continuing, fetal echocardiography is recommended, ideally at 14 weeks, which is the earliest time a cardiac scan can be completely comprehensive.

Impact on paediatric cardiology

The impact on paediatric cardiology may include:

- reduced prevalence of CHD, especially complex forms
- improved morbidity after delivery and perioperatively
- improved perioperative mortality.

Decisions about termination of pregnancy are influenced by many different factors, including gestational age at diagnosis, social circumstances, and socioeconomic group. Generally speaking, however, if complex heart disease is detected in a pregnancy at less than 20 weeks' gestation, over half the parents will choose to interrupt the pregnancy. This is true in the UK and the US. Thus, about half of the complex forms of CHD which the paediatric cardiologist would expect to see and treat postnatally may only be seen once in prenatal life. As fetal cardiology preferentially detects the complex forms of heart disease which require long term cardiac care and follow up, this is bound to have an impact on paediatric cardiology in the future. As an example of this, termination of pregnancy has been shown to have lowered the prevalence of pulmonary atresia in England and Wales, compared with Scotland and Ireland where either the diagnosis was not made in the fetus or termination was not chosen.[11] The frequency of complex one ventricle type cardiac repairs may therefore become less common in the coming years.

Some forms of CHD are associated with early decompensation and even death of the infant before the malformation can be recognised and treated. This applies mainly to those where either the pulmonary or systemic circulation is dependent on the patency of the arterial duct, or the lesions which require "mixing" at an adequate atrial septal defect such as transposition of the great arteries or total anomalous pulmonary venous drainage. It appears intuitively obvious that if CHD is recognised prenatally and delivery takes place in or near a paediatric cardiology centre, thus avoiding delay in diagnosis and emergency transfer of a sick neonate, the morbidity for the infant will be minimised. This has been shown in several studies although improvement in mortality has been harder to prove, partly because fetal echocardiography preferentially detects more severe forms of CHD which have a higher mortality per se.[12 13] However, a recent study of infants with transposition of the great arteries, where there were adequate numbers to answer this question, showed conclusively that there was a much lower mortality in those cases prenatally diagnosed.[14] Thus, the impact on paediatric cardiology, if fetal heart scanning improved to the ideal level of expertise, would be a decrease in the number of complex malformations, but those patients with CHD who come to surgery would do so in optimum status without prior insult. This would have a potentially significant effect on saving of resources by reducing complex disease and improving both the cardiac and neurological outlook for the survivors of treatment.

Medico-legal aspects

Certainly in the US, and increasingly in the UK, one is continually aware of the fear of litigation. One would imagine that this would result in more rigid standards and codes of practice in the US, but in reality this does not appear to happen. Litigation is so sporadic, and frequently occurs in the most unexpected circumstances, that it does not seem to deter careless attention to training or practice guidelines. In the case of an obstetrician who misses a four chamber view anomaly on a prenatal scan, the parents can sue for wrongful life. To my knowledge there is no precedent for this in court, although out of court settlements have been made in such circumstances. However, the RADIUS study was a large multicentre scanning program based in the midwest and eastern US, where no cardiac malformation was detected outside tertiary centres, despite a supposedly uniform scanning format.[15] This publication gives the obstetrician a reasonable defence that such malformations are not detectable by the present general "standard of care". A little threat of litigation may be no bad thing if it encourages self regulation within the medical profession, uniform codes of practice, and quality control initiated by doctors themselves. However, an atmosphere of litigation, especially if the application and outcome of suits are extremely unpredictable, leads to bad clinical practice, with over investigation and over treatment.

Differences between the UK and the US

Some of the differences between the UK and the US in terms of the practice of fetal cardiology have been alluded to above. The most striking difference in medical practice is that in the UK there is, in general, an atmosphere of collective responsibility for the health service among doctors, and for the impact of care on society as a whole. Despite the dissatisfaction among the medical profession in the UK, which appears to have grown in the last 10 years, the organised nature of the UK National Health Service provides a unique opportunity for imposing and maintaining uniform standards of practice and for collecting data for quality control across the whole service. This would demand a willingness on the part of practitioners to be part of a drive to improve the quality of service and to confront the hazards of "audit", but such an effort would be applicable to many aspects of obstetric and paediatric cardiology practice.

1. **Achiron R, Glaser J, Gelernter I,** *et al.* Extended fetal echocardiographic examination for detecting cardiac malformations in low risk pregnancies. *BMJ* 1992;**304**:671–4.

2. **Sharland GK, Allan LD.** Screening for congenital heart disease prenatally. Results of a 2½ year study in the south east Thames region. *Br J Obstet Gynaecol* 1992;**99**:220–5.

3. **Yagel S, Weissman A, Rotstein Z,** *et al.* Congenital heart defects. Natural course and in utero development. *Circulation* 1997;**96**:550–5.
• *An impressive number of patients, more than 22 000, were screened between 1990 and 1994 for fetal anomalies, including cardiac malformations. Of 168 cases of CHD, 80% were diagnosed before 22 weeks' gestation. However, a small proportion of cases evolve or become evident only in the last trimester of pregnancy.*

4. **Buskens E, Grobbee DE, Frohn-Mulder IM,** *et al.* Efficacy of routine fetal ultrasound screening for congenital heart disease in normal pregnancy. *Circulation* 1996;**94**:67–72.

5. **Tegnander E, Eik-Nes SH, Johansen OJ,** *et al.* Prenatal detection of heart defects at the routine fetal examination at 18 weeks in a non-selected population. *Ultrasound Obstet Gynecol* 1995;**5**:372–80.

6. **Todros T, Faggiano F, Chiappa E,** *et al.* Accuracy of routine ultrasonography in screening heart disease prenatally. Gruppo Piemontese for prenatal screening of congenital heart disease. *Prenatal Diagn* 1997;**17**:901–6.

7. **Montana E, Khoury MJ, Cragan JD,** *et al.* Trends and outcomes of prenatal diagnosis of congenital cardiac malformations by fetal echocardiography in a well defined birth population, Atlanta, Georgia, 1990–1994. *J Am Coll Cardiol* 1996;**28**:1805–9.
• *A population based study which identified 1589 cases of CHD during the five year period from 1990 to 1994. Overall, 6% were identified prenatally, rising from 2.6% to 12.7% over time. Four chamber view anomalies, such as the hypoplastic left heart syndrome, increased to a 40% detection rate by the end of 1994.*

8. **Allan LD.** Atrioventricular septal defect in fetal life. *Am J Obstet Gynecol* In press.

9. **Allan LD, Sharland GK, Milburn A,** *et al.* Prospective diagnosis of 1,006 consecutive cases of congenital heart disease in the fetus. *J Am Coll Cardiol* 1994;**23**:1452–8.
• *A sufficiently large series of fetal CHD to allow meaningful comparison of the spectrum of disease seen prenatally with postnatal life. There is over representation of disease where the four chamber view is abnormal and a relative paucity of great artery anomalies. The method of selection of cases for fetal echocardiography also increases the rate of chromosomal and extracardiac anomalies.*

10. **Hyett J, Perdu M, Sharland G,** *et al.* Using fetal nuchal translucency to screen for major congenital cardiac defects at 10–14 weeks of gestation: population based cohort study. *BMJ* 1999;**318**:81–5.
• *In a series of over 29 000 chromosomally normal fetuses, where the nuchal fold was measured between 10–14 weeks' gestation, over 50% of those with congenital heart disease had values above the 95th centile. Thus, fetuses with nuchal thickening constitute a newly recognised but extremely important high risk group for referral for fetal echocardiography.*

11. **Daubeney PE, Sharland GK, Cook AC,** *et al.* Pulmonary atresia with intact ventricular septum: impact of fetal echocardiography on incidence at birth and postnatal outcome. UK and Eire collaborative study of pulmonary atresia with intact ventricular septum. *Circulation* 1998;**98**:562–6.
• *A large series of cases of pulmonary atresia with intact ventricular septum were identified in a multicentre study over a 4 year period. Of 83 cases recognised in fetal life, there was a high rate of termination of pregnancy. Of the continuing pregnancies who reached live birth (29), no difference in survival could be shown in those prenatally diagnosed. However, the worst end of the spectrum of disease was removed from the series as a result of termination. The high rate of detection coupled with the option of termination led to a reduced prevalence of live born infants with this lesion in England in comparison to other parts of the UK and Eire.*

12. **Chang AC, Huhta JC, Yoon GY,** *et al.* Diagnosis, transport, and outcome in fetuses with left ventricular outflow tract obstruction. *J Thorac Cardiovasc Surg* 1991;**102**:841–18.

13. **Copel JA, Tan AS, Kleinman CS.** Does a prenatal diagnosis of congenital heart disease alter short-term outcome? *Ultrasound Obstet Gynecol* 1997;**10**:237–41.

14. **Bonnet D, Coltri A, Butera G,** *et al.* Detection of transposition of the great arteries in fetuses reduces neonatal morbidity and mortality. *Circulation* 1999;**99**:916–18.
• *Of 318 neonates with transposition of the great arteries, 68 were recognised prenatally. There was improved morbidity before surgery in the prenatally diagnosed group and there was no mortality either before surgery or perioperatively. In contrast in the group diagnosed in postnatal life, 15 died before surgery and there were 20 perioperative deaths. This is the only study to date which has had the statistical power of numbers to answer this question meaningfully.*

15. **Ewigman BG, Crane JP, Frigoletto FD,** *et al.* Effect of prenatal ultrasound screening on perinatal outcome. *N Engl J Med* 1993;**329**:821–7.

27 Fetal and infant markers of adult heart diseases

Marjo-Riitta Järvelin

There is growing evidence of an increasingly complex and multifactorial aetiology of heart diseases.[1] [w1] It seems likely that the large geographic variations in cardiovascular disease (CVD) morbidity and mortality,[w2] even though at least partly genetic in origin, are influenced by factors acting prenatally and in early life, or by a combination of factors present throughout the life course. Changes in fetal growth pattern have been related to adult disease risk,[1] and there are many theories about the underlying mechanisms affecting cell division during critical periods of tissue development. The critical periods vary according to the tissue in question, and that is why there have been attempts to explore the timing of exposure in order to predict more specifically the adult disease risk.

This article examines: firstly the historical evolution of theories on childhood factors which have an influence in adulthood; secondly what is known today about the effect of early life factors on heart disease risk; and thirdly the specific problems in longitudinal studies which explore these factors and adult disease risk.

Dawn of the "hypothesis of the 20th century"

Biological programming: a new theoretical model about the aetiology of heart disease

The dawn of modern epidemiology came after the second world war, first with ecological studies comparing CVD incidence and mortality, and subsequently multicentre cross sectional and follow up studies on CVD.[w3] The studies showed that populations with high CVD mortality have high cholesterol and high blood pressure, and that smoking and obesity are common among these populations.[w4] This led to the *lifestyle model* in understanding the aetiology of chronic diseases, where the key issues are health behaviour and the interaction between genes and an adverse environment in adult life. This was consequently followed by intervention programmes, which have significantly improved heart disease risk status in many countries.[w3] However, lifestyle factors only explain part of the heart disease risk, which is why other reasons have been sought. For example, in the mid 1980s Rose pointed out that the well established risk factors for coronary heart disease (CHD)—cigarette smoking, high serum cholesterol, and high

blood pressure—have a limited ability to predict disease risk in adults.[w5] In the large international MONICA (monitoring trends and determinants in cardiovascular disease) project,[w2] [w4] only 25% of the variance in CHD mortality was explained by conventional risk factors. Could childhood influences explain this gap in our understanding of the aetiology of CVD?

In Norway in the 1970s, Forsdahl[2] put forward the hypothesis that the geographical differences in CVD mortality might not be related to the contemporary circumstances, but to poverty or deprivation in early life (table 27.1). However, the importance of fetal and early life circumstances for adult health had been suggested almost a century earlier by the chief medical officer to the Board of Education in Britain, who wrote: "recent progress has shown that the health of the adult is dependent upon the health of the child and that the health of the child is dependent upon the health of the infant and its mother".[w6]

A new hypothesis developed following observations in the 1980s by Barker and colleagues, in accordance with Forsdahl, based upon positive relations between the areas with the highest CVD and infant mortality rates,[3] and lower birth weight and increased risk of CVD mortality[4] (table 27.1). These historical cohort studies[3–5] [w7] [w8] and evidence from animal experiments[1] [w9] suggest that chronic diseases are biologically "programmed" in utero or in early infancy. Programming is the process where a stimulus or insult (for example, undernutrition, hormones, antigens, drugs or sensory stimuli) at a critical period of development induces long lasting changes in cells which in turn changes the structure or function of organs, tissues or body systems.[w7] [w10] In the case of heart disease, it is hypothesised that fetal undernutrition during middle gestation in particular raises the risk of later disease by the programming of blood pressure, cholesterol metabolism, blood coagulation, and hormonal settings.[5] Consequently, it was suggested that the lifestyle model in the evolution of adult degenerative diseases needs to be replaced by a new model, the central feature of which is the concept *of biological programming in fetal and infant life.* This revolutionary model of the 20th century has received both an enthusiastic and sceptical response. Critical testing of this model is warranted owing to inevitable biases related to historical studies.

Social programming and adult diseases

During the past 10 years sociomedical research has pointed out the importance of social differences between countries and populations in explaining differences in health. This ideology has created *a social programming model* in parallel to the biological programming model.[6] Social programming means that the effect of the early social environment on health is mediated by the social environment and school achievement during growth, and by employment opportunities, living conditions, and lifestyle factors. The social programming model is supported by various studies showing an independent effect of childhood social circumstances on adult health.[7] [w11]

Evidence for an association between childhood factors and heart disease risk

Heart disease morbidity and mortality

The first studies reporting an association between birth weight and CHD came from Hertfordshire and Sheffield study populations.[4] [8] Both in men and women—even though the relation was weaker in women[9]—CHD mortality decreased progressively with increasing birth weight. Since then there have been several, mainly retrospective cohort studies which have replicated these observations and also demonstrated the association between size at birth and non-fatal CHD.[w12] [w13] To date, there have been over 400 papers published during the past 15 years dealing with prenatal and early life factors related to CVD mortality and disease risk.

The association between birth weight and disease outcomes is, with few exceptions,[10] consistent with data based upon the older generations born in the early 1920s or 1930s from

Table 27.1 Early fetal origin hypotheses developing studies

Author and title of study	Year of publication	Study population	Main observations and interpretations
Forsdahl. Are poor living conditions in childhood and adolescence an important risk factor for arteriosclerotic heart disease? [2]	1977	20 northern counties in Norway; men and women aged 40–69 who lived their infancy, childhood and youth in 1896 to 1925.	In the counties where infant mortality (INFmo) was high, the same generation had both a high total mortality and ischaemic heart disease (IHD) mortality in middle age. Variations in IHD mortality rate between counties is linked to variations in poverty in childhood and adolescence because INFmo is a reliable index of standard of living. Forsdahl suggested that poverty followed by prosperity is a risk factor for IHD.
Barker et al. Infant mortality, childhood nutrition, and ischaemic heart disease in England and Wales.[3]	1986	England and Wales; county boroughs (CBs, larger towns), London boroughs (LBs), urban areas (metropolitan boroughs and urban districts), rural areas within counties. IHD rates in 1968-78 (35–74 years); INFmo in 1921-25.	On division of the country into 212 local authority areas a strong geographical relation was found between IHD mortality rates at ages 35–74 years and INFmo in 1921-25. IHD mortality rates are highest in the least affluent areas. It was suggested that poor nutrition in early life increases susceptibility to the effects of an affluent diet in later life, and that predisposition to IHD is related to nutrition during prenatal period and early childhood.
Barker et al. Weight in infancy and death from ischaemic heart disease.[4]	1989	Six districts of Hertfordshire, England; 5654 men born in 1911-30.	One of the first articles about hypothesis of an effect of early life factors on IHD. Men with the lowest weights at birth and at 1 year had the highest death rates from IHD. The standardised mortality ratio (SMR) fell from 104 in men whose birth weight was 2.5 kg or less to 62 in those who weighed between 4.0–4.3 kg, but rose slightly in the highest birth weight category. The paper showed the relation for the first time. Though inaccuracies, eg, in birth weight measurements, exist this gives evidence of the importance of fetal life on subsequent diseases. The interpretation was that greater early growth will reduce deaths from IHD. Later in 1990s it was shown that those who where thin at birth but caught up during infancy were particularly prone to IHD risk.
Barker et al. Growth in utero, blood pressure in childhood and adult life, and mortality from cardiovascular disease.[13]	1989	England, Wales, and Scotland. (1) In 1970 one week sample, n=9921 in the analyses. (2) In 1946 one week stratified sample (MRC national survey), n=3259.	In children at 10 years and adults at 36 years systolic blood pressure was inversely related to birth weight (independent of gestational age). Within England and Wales 10 year olds living in areas with high cardiovascular disease (CVD) mortality were shorter and had higher resting pulse rates than those living in other areas. Their mothers were also shorter with higher diastolic blood pressure. This suggested there are persisting geographical differences in the childhood environment that predispose to differences in CVD mortality.
Barker et al. Fetal and placental size and risk of hypertension in adult life.[12]	1990	Preston, Lancashire, UK n(men and women)=449	In both sexes systolic and diastolic blood pressure were strongly related to placental weight and birth weight. The highest blood pressures occurred in the people who had been small babies with large placentas. Discordance between placental and fetal size may lead to circulatory adaptation in the fetus, altered arterial structure in the child, and hypertension in the adult. It was discussed that women's nutrition in childhood may be linked to blood pressure in the next generation.
Hales et al. Fetal and infant growth and impaired glucose tolerance at age 64.[14]	1991	468 men born in 1920-30, (in Hertfordshire, England) aged 64 had a standard 75 g oral glucose tolerance test.	Men who were found to have impaired glucose tolerance or diabetes had had a lower mean birth weight and a lower weight at 1 year. Reduced early growth was also related to a raised plasma concentration of 32-33 split proinsulin. These trends were independent of current body mass. The results may be a consequence of fetal undernutrition and programming of the endocrine pancreas. The researchers favoured environmental explanation for their findings instead of genetic determination, on the one hand because disturbance of insulin production was manifested by growth failure in early life long before the onset of adult glucose intolerance, and on the other hand because maternal nutrition was thought to have a strong influence on fetal and infant growth.
Barker et al. The relation of small head circumference and thinness at birth to death for cardiovascular disease in adult life.[8]	1993	Sheffield, England n(men)= 1586	SMR for cardiovascular disease fell from 119 in men who weighed 5.5 pounds (2495 g) or less at birth to 74 in men who weighed more than 8.5 pounds (3856 g). The fall was significant for premature cardiovascular deaths up to 65 years of age. SMR also fell with increasing head circumference and increasing ponderal index. They were not related to the duration of gestation. The findings showed that reduced fetal growth is followed by increased mortality from CVD. Based on this further evidence for the first time it was proposed that CVD originates through programming of the body's structure by the environment during fetal life.

Theoretical models on the evolution of chronic disease

- Lifestyle model in the 1960s-70s

- Biological programming in fetal and infant life model in 1980s-90s

- Social programming model in the 1990s

- Life course model in 2000, incorporating both biological and social environments, and their interactions

different countries. However, it is not known how these observations apply to younger generations assuming that younger generations must have had better nutritional status in early life. The historical cohorts on which these observations are mainly based are liable to bias owing to selective survival and availability of data records.

Early life factors and intermediate heart disease risk factors/conditions

The associations between markers of fetal growth and intermediate risk factors are less consistent than evidence for morbidity and mortality. These include birth measures in relation to plasma concentrations of cholesterol, apolipoprotein B,[w14] and fibrinogen,[11] blood pressure,[12 13] and liability to impaired glucose tolerance and diabetes.[14–16]

Blood pressure has been suggested as one link between the intrauterine environment and the risk of CVD. Baker and colleagues studied the correlation between birth weight and subsequent blood pressure in three adult populations in Hertfordshire, Preston, and Sheffield in the UK[w15] as well as in children of different ages.[4 17 w16] Other studies replicating Barker's have been made on various child populations.[18 19 w17–19] The key findings include an inverse independent relation between birth weight and subsequent systolic blood pressure, amplified by age,[12 18 19 w17–19] and an association of lower birth weight and thinness at birth with an increased risk of insulin resistance,[16 w20 w21] which is an important risk factor for heart diseases. Observations are not consistent; weak, non-linear or insignificant correlations between birth weight and blood pressure have been reported,[20 w22] particularly among younger populations.

A correlation between possible undernutrition and serum cholesterol has been noted in men and women in some studies,[w14 w21] but there are also studies which show no relation.[w23] The association between body length at birth and cholesterol might reflect abnormal intra-uterine growth, in which retarded trunk and visceral growth is associated with alterations in lipid metabolism. Abdominal circumference at birth, which reflects visceral growth, has been related to serum cholesterol concentration in adults.[5]

Lower birth weight and weight at 1 year of age have been associated with subsequent development of type 2 diabetes mellitus in adult life. In the Hertfordshire study, the men with impaired glucose tolerance and diabetes had lower weight gain prenatally and during infancy than men without.[14] The plasma 32-33 split proinsulin concentration fell with increasing weight at 1 year. All the findings were independent of current body mass index (BMI).[14] In the Preston study, impaired glucose tolerance was also related to lower birth weight and smaller head circumference.[21] Gestational age had no influence on the results. A follow up study of 297 women aged 60–71 years suggests, in accordance with previous studies, that those who had lower birth weight had higher plasma concentrations of glucose and insulin.[w21] Obesity in adult life adds to the disadvantage of low birth weight; the women who were light at birth but are currently obese have the least favourable risk factor profile.[w21] A longitudinal study of diabetes and its complications conducted among the American Indian population in Arizona, however, showed the prevalence of non-insulin dependent diabetes mellitus to be greatest not only in those with the lowest birth weights, but also in those with the highest birth weights.[22] This study is supported by a study on Mexican American families.[23]

Patients with type 2 diabetes and hypertension often have other abnormalities, such as high plasma insulin concentrations, high serum triglyceride concentrations, low serum HDL (high density lipoprotein) concentrations, and high body mass indices and waist-to-hip ratios. This combination of abnormalities has been called syndrome X or "small baby syndrome",[w24] but may be better known as insulin

Table 27.2 Summary of the main associations between birth weight and other growth measures and heart disease

Exposure	Type of association	Outcome
● Birth weight	Inverse linear; in some studies inverse J shaped	CHD mortality and morbidity; in particular among men, weaker in women
	Inverse (linear), J shaped or U shaped	Fasting glucose, insulin, insulin resistance, impaired glucose tolerance, type 2 diabetes, metabolic syndrome
	Inverse linear, but not consistently	Blood pressure
● Birth length	Inverse	CHD particularly in women, LDL cholesterol
	Positive or negative (placental weight acts as effect modifier), effect marginal	Blood pressure
● Head circumference	Inverse	CVD mortality in men, impaired glucose tolerance
● Ponderal index	Inverse, inverse U shaped	CHD (CVD) mortality, impaired glucose tolerance, insulin resistance, type 2 diabetes
● Abdominal circumference	U shaped	CHD morbidity
	Inverse	LDL cholesterol, plasma fibrinogen
● Catch up growth in particular if thin at birth	Positive	CHD mortality, blood pressure
● Weight at 1 year	Inverse	CHD mortality among men; type 2 diabetes mellitus, plasma fibrinogen, factor VII

CHD, coronary heart disease; CVD, cardiovascular disease; LDL, low density lipoprotein.

182

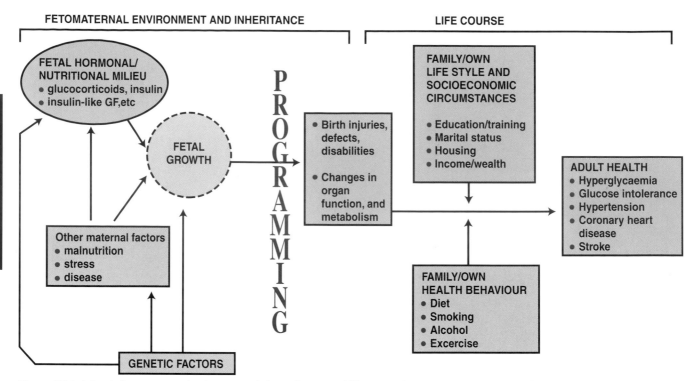

Figure 27.1. Intrauterine programming by prenatal determinants and life course factors in heart diseases (GF, growth factor).

resistance or metabolic syndrome. Metabolic syndrome is characterised by compensatory hyperinsulinaemia[w24] and is associated with increased mortality from CHD.[w25] The association of both type 2 diabetes and hypertension with reduced fetal growth has raised the possibility that these and other components of the syndrome may have a common origin in suboptimal development at a particular stage of intrauterine life.[14 21] In the Preston study,[21] the prevalence of metabolic syndrome in both men and women decreased progressively as their birth weights increased. The association between metabolic syndrome and low birth weight was independent of gestational age and possible confounding variables, including cigarette smoking, alcohol consumption, and social class currently or at birth.

Several reports, however, have been more equivocal about the relation of birth related factors to CVD and its risks, particularly studies in adolescents and young adults, and the authors have questioned the basis and rationale for these associations and the underlying mechanisms.[24 25 w22 w23 w26–30]

The main associations between birth weight and other growth measures and heart disease are summarised in table 27.2.

Suggested biological/environmental mechanisms underlying the evolution of heart disease risk

Nutritional factors during pregnancy

There are numerous factors and mechanisms which affect both fetal growth,[w31–33] and adult CVD outcomes,[w4 w34] which makes the analyses of the associations and their interpretation extremely complex (fig 27.1). Among them, in the light of early programming, are: (1) re-stricted maternal nutrition itself; and (2) maternal or pregnancy induced physiological, metabolic or hormone related conditions which may impair fetal nutrition or otherwise affect growth.

A primary fetal origin hypothesis from the early 1990s stated that adult disease such as CVD is programmed by poor maternal nutrition during pregnancy, leading to fetal growth retardation and a permanent effect on the body's structure, physiology, and metabolism.[5 w8] Based on rodent experiments and human studies it nowadays also covers other mechanisms.

Maternal nutrition
In rodents, dietary changes during gestation induce not only growth retardation but also permanent changes in metabolism[w35] which can be transmitted through several generations.[w36] Though well supported by animal studies,[26] the evidence for similar processes in humans is patchy and complex.[w23 w37] Among indicators of *maternal nutrition* in humans, low pre-pregnancy weight, height, and BMI are associated with lower birth weight,[w31 w38] which in itself is associated with heart disease risk.[w30] However, in men born in the 1920s and '30s, high maternal BMI together with low ponderal index was associated with their offspring's highest standardised mortality ratio for CHD. One explanation for this contradictory finding may be that, as suggested by animal studies,[w39] the mothers themselves may have been smaller at birth and, as a result, accumulated more fat. Maternal height, reflecting long term nutrition, may be an even better indicator of disturbed long term nutrition than weight in relatively well nourished populations. For example, Forsen and colleagues reported that offspring of short, heavy mothers have higher rates of CHD than those of taller women.[27] Small studies in humans, directly examining nutritional

intake, suggested that women who have a high intake of carbohydrates in early pregnancy and a low intake of dairy protein in late pregnancy tend to have infants who are thin at birth.[w40 w41]

Fetal nutrition

Other indicators of possible disturbed fetal nutrition not directly related to maternal nutrition (for example, pregnancy induced hypertension, pre-eclampsia)[w33 w42] have rarely been studied in relation to adult disease risk in humans. Evidence that hypertension during pregnancy in humans affects adult CVD risk is inconsistent,[w43-47] although animal data are supportive.[26] One difficulty, to date, has been separating pregnancy induced hypertension from essential hypertension because few studies record blood pressure measurements during pregnancy, at least not during early pregnancy, or present data on pre-pregnancy hypertension. High maternal blood pressure has, however, been associated with low birth weight of offspring,[w31 w42] which in itself is associated with high blood pressure in adult life, but it is unclear to what extent this reflects maternofetal undernutrition during pregnancy or genetic factors.

Growth patterns

The growth of the fetus is a complex process which is still insufficiently understood. A key concept in the "fetal origin hypothesis" is fetal undernutrition, and its relation with adult diseases. The human evidence, as described above, is based on studies where birth measures have been related to different adult heart disease outcomes in different populations. This is strongly supported by the animal experiments, and stresses the importance of the fetomaternal environment. Barker[5] has differentiated undernutrition during pregnancy by trimesters, and he suggests that the down regulation of growth during the first trimester leads to a proportionately small child who has increased risk of raised blood pressure and may possibly die of haemorrhagic stroke. Undernutrition during the second trimester leads to a disturbed fetoplacental relation, and insulin resistance or deficiency; consequently birth weight is reduced and the baby is thin, and has an increased risk of raised blood pressure, non-insulin dependent diabetes, and death from CHD. Undernourished babies during the last trimester in turn may have growth hormone resistance or deficiency, and consequently they are short but birth weight is within the normal range. These adults may have raised blood pressure, raised LDL (low density lipoprotein) cholesterol concentration, and increased risk of CHD and thrombotic stroke.

Later growth patterns, particularly catch-up growth,[w48] have been reported to relate to heart disease risk. For example, children who are thin at birth but become obese in later life or have high catch-up growth in infancy[w48] appear to be at higher risk. However, it is not known why catch-up growth is detrimental, but one possibility is that fetal growth restriction leads to reduced cell numbers, and subsequent catch-up growth is achieved by overgrowth of a limited cell mass.

Hormonal evidence related to fetal growth and later heart disease risk

Fetal growth is also affected by several hormones, growth factors, and genetic factors (fig 27.1). A recently proposed underlying mechanism, based mainly on animal studies, suggests that increased blood pressure in adult life is caused by increased exposure to corticosteroids during fetal life. This might result from reduced placental 11β-hydroxysteroid dehydrogenase (11β-OHSD) activity or increased corticosteroid release secondary to disturbed nutrition.[w9 w49-51] Increased exposure in turn may lead to permanent tissue damage, and programming of adult disease.[1 w52] There are data supporting similar mechanisms in humans—for example, studies have found that birth weight is correlated with placental 11β-OHSD activity,[w50] and cortisol concentrations in adult life correlate with birth weight[w53] and adult blood pressure.[w54]

Insulin and insulin-like growth factors are likely to have a substantial influence on fetal growth. Insulin stimulates growth through several mechanisms: by increasing uptake and utilisation of nutrients; by direct mitogenic actions; and by increasing the release of other hormones and growth factors.[w55] However, the final role of these factors in the evolution of adult disease risk is largely unknown, although it can be speculated that via the effects on fetal growth the disturbances in the regulation of these factors lead to increased risk of adult chronic diseases.

Genetic evidence

The role of genetic factors is poorly understood even though a familial aggregation of CHD and hypertension is clear. A complementary explanation for the observed associations between fetal growth and adult phenotypes could be provided by genomic variation which alters the function and/or regulation of genes influencing both phenotypes. Recently the first small genetic studies have been published which stress the importance of possible gene–environmental interaction.[w56 w57] Disturbances or variations in genes which regulate either insulin or glucocorticoid action or metabolism may reduce birth weight[w58] and thus possibly increase the risk of insulin resistance in adulthood. In Mexican American families, Stern and colleagues[23] dissected the relation between birth weight and adult insulin resistance into two components: (1) a sporadic, environmental association between *low* birth weight and adult insulin resistance; and (2) a genetic association between *high* birth weight and adult insulin resistance. This is in agreement with the studies suggesting non-linear association between birth weight and impaired glucose tolerance.[22] There is a debate over whether these effects/associations are truly genetic or whether they are caused by the environment—that is, phenotypic. A future challenge is to determine the relative contributions of genes *and* environmental factors to the fetal and adult phenotypes.

184

Other possible models in the evolution of heart diseases and limitations of the studies

In Europe there are more than 20 large longitudinal studies in which the main focus has been or is to study prenatal or early life factors in relation to adult disease risk. Many of them are historical cohort studies, or data collection has started after birth retrospectively at various points of life. The most important historical cohort studies, from the point of view of the fetal origin hypothesis, are the Hertfordshire,[4 14] Preston,[12 21] and Sheffield[8] studies, as well as the Helsinki[27] and Uppsala[28] cohort studies.

The studies to date have had a number of important limitations that complicate interpretation. They have not been able to address the complexities of interactions between environmental and genetic factors in explaining the associations between maternal, fetal, and later life factors in the evolution of adult CVD risk. This is because they have been variously too small; retrospective and therefore subject to survival and selection biases; or prospective, but in children and adolescence and therefore have not been able to examine adult phenotypes. It has also been questioned whether a study with a completely different *a priori* hypothesis should be used at all for other purposes. However, the use of old data for studying early life factors is justified considering the latency between early exposure and adult outcomes. For example, Barker's studies based on early last century cohorts have been extremely valuable hypotheses developing studies, which should now be replicated in younger cohorts reaching adult age.

An important consideration and future challenge to explore from the point of view of the biological programming model is the extent to which associations between the fetal environment and adult health may be confounded by or interact with measures taken later in life.[20 w1 w29] For example, adult weight and height have been reported to be stronger predictors of blood pressure than birth measures,[w47] but observations from different studies are inconsistent. A further question concerns the relative influence of childhood and adult measures of socioeconomic status, and health behaviour. Several studies report a powerful association between markers of social status or wealth in childhood or adulthood, and the risk of adult chronic diseases and mortality.[18 w59] The risk of premature death from CVD appears to be particularly sensitive to socioeconomic influences acting in early life,[w60] but the results from different studies vary.[18 28 w61–63] A recent review of the influence of early-life socioeconomic environment on the risk of adult disease concluded that both early-life and later circumstances are important.[7]

Figure 27.1 shows a simplified framework for the different associations between the various factors in the prenatal period and their effect on adult health. It is evident that no single model is able to explain heart disease risk.

Early life factors and adult heart disease risk: summary

- A number of factors throughout the life course affect adult disease risk, starting in utero

- A number of studies show that fetal growth is related to adult heart disease mortality, morbidity, and risk factors

- Several factors affect fetal growth and subsequently may contribute to adult disease risk

- There are only a few studies in humans with extensive life course data to explore the association between prenatal and infancy exposures and adult disease or risk outcomes

- We do not know the mechanisms by which the observed associations are evoked or mediated in humans, or whether the same relations apply to older and younger cohorts

This is mainly because there is a vast amount of evidence that: (1) socioeconomic and living circumstances have an independent effect on adult health; (2) health behaviour affects disease risk[w3]; (3) genetic factors may have an important role in the programming process and possible gene–environment influences; and (4) the impact of chain effects and clustering of disadvantageous factors on disease risk. The clustering effect differs from programming in that it does not expect necessarily to take into account any critical period. It has been questioned if "critical periods" should be taken into account not only during fetal life but later over the life course.

It is reasonable to assume that early programming is a result of an interaction between fetomaternal environment and individual genotype. The "inborn" predisposition to later disease is in turn modified by factors along the life course. The variate of social and biological programming, the multidisciplinary *life course model* provides an alternative way of exploring the association between early life environment, both social and biological, and adult disease risk. This approach points out that there is a clear need to establish studies by assembling cohorts where measures of pre- and postnatal determinants have been previously recorded in different populations living under different conditions in order to explore pathways and mechanisms in the evolution of heart diseases.

Conclusions

Inconsistencies between and within studies exist, and relations of varying degrees of strength have been described. With the available evidence of the relation between early life factors, intermediate CVD risk factors, disease incidence, and mortality, it remains unclear whether the associations are primarily a manifestation of intrauterine programming of CVD risk due to poor maternal nutrition itself or other influences in utero unrelated to maternal undernutrition, such as defective placentation, and hypertension or other aspects of the genetic, metabolic or circulatory milieu. Studies need to address the extent to which fetal environment and early life experiences act on adult health through independent or intermediary mechanisms, and the extent to which the associations between birth variables and disease risk are independent of later social environment and living habits.

1. **Nyirenda M, Seckl JR.** Intrauterine events and the programming of adulthood disease: the role of fetal glucocorticoid exposure [review]. *Int J Molecular Med* 1998;**2**:607–14.
- *A review of the role of fetal glucocorticoid exposure in the programming of adulthood disease. During fetal development glucocorticoids are involved in control of growth and maturation of fetal organs in preparation for extrauterine life. The experiments have shown that fetal exposure to exogenous glucocorticoids reduces birth weight and causes permanent hyperglycaemia and hypertension in the adult rat offspring. This may provide a new insight into the pathophysiology and control of cardiovascular and metabolic diseases.*

2. **Forsdahl A.** Are poor living conditions in childhood and adolescence an important risk factor for arteriosclerotic heart disease? *Br J Prev Social Med* 1977;**31**:91–5.

3. **Barker DJP, Osmond C.** Infant mortality, childhood nutrition, and ischaemic heart disease in England and Wales. *Lancet* 1986;i:1077–81.

4. **Barker DJP, Winter PD, Osmond C,** et al. Weight in infancy and death from ischaemic heart disease. *Lancet* 1989;ii:577–80.

5. **Barker DJP.** Fetal origins of coronary heart disease. *BMJ* 1995;**311**:171–4.
- *This review article, based on the main hypotheses developing papers, provides a framework of ideas of possible pathways and mechanisms leading from fetal undernutrition to later abnormalities. The consequences of fetal undernutrition are presented separately depending on the trimester of pregnancy.*

6. **Vågerö D, Illsley R.** Explaining health inequalities: beyond Black and Barker. *European Sociology Review* 1995;**11**:1–23.

7. **Davey Smith G.** Socioeconomic differentials. In: Kuh D, Ben-Shlomo Y, eds. *A life course approach to chronic disease epidemiology.* Oxford: Oxford University Press, 1997:242–73.
- *Social class at different stages of life is associated with morbidity and mortality risk in adulthood to a variable degree, depending upon the outcome of interest. For CVD mortality, poor early life social conditions appear to make an important contribution to disease risk in adulthood. An index of life course social position, which combines data regarding social position from different stages of life, is more strongly related to CVD mortality than is any indicator relating to just one point in time. This is an excellent overview and secondary data source analysis of the influence of social position on morbidity and mortality.*

8. **Barker DJP, Osmond C, Simmonds SJ,** et al. The relation of small head circumference and thiness at birth to death from cardiovascular disease. *BMJ* 1993;**306**:422–6.

9. **Osmond C, Barker DJP, Winter PD.** Early growth and death from cardiovascular disease in women. *BMJ* 1993;**307**:1519–24.
- *This study showed that death rates from CVD among women fell progressively between the low and high birth weight groups women (n = 5585, born in 1923–30); earlier the association had been obvious only among men. The results suggested that the association between CVD and birth weight is similar in both sexes. However, in many studies the associations among women are weak or non-significant.*

10. **Vågerö D, Leon D.** Ischemic heart disease and low birth weight: a test of the fetal origins hypothesis from the Swedish Twin Registry. *Lancet* 1994;**343**:260–263.
- *This study tested the fetal origins hypothesis, examining ischaemic heart disease (IHD) mortality among Swedish twins (8174 female and 6612 male twins, born between 1886 and 1925). IHD was not found to be any higher among twins compared to the general population. However, the shorter twin in a twin pair was more likely to die of heart disease than the taller. The study suggested that postnatal influences may well be as important as prenatal influences in producing any effect on IHD mortality, and that the type of growth retardation in utero*

experienced by twins may not constitute a risk for IHD in adulthood. The missing association may also be caused by the fact that in this design socioeconomic confounding is well controlled for, or by the fact that growth retardation experienced by twins is different from that experienced by low birth weight singletons.

11. **Barker DJP, Meade TW, Fall CHD,** et al. Relation of fetal and infant growth to plasma fibrinogen and factor VII concentrations in adult life. *BMJ* 1992;**304**:148–52.
- *This study involved 591 men, born in 1920–30, aged around 64 years, and 148 men born in 1935–43, aged around 50 years. Plasma fibrinogen and factor VII concentrations were inversely related to weight at 1 year and fibrinogen concentration fell progressively as the ratio of placental weight to birth weight decreased, but not for both study populations. Neither plasma fibrinogen nor factor VII concentration was related to birth weight. The results are thought to be caused by impaired liver development during a critical early period, but further studies are needed.*

12. **Barker DJP, Bull AR, Osmond C,** et al. Fetal and placental size and risk of hypertension in adult life. *BMJ* 1990; **301**:259–62.

13. **Barker DJP, Osmond C, Golding J,** et al. Growth in utero, blood pressure in childhood and adult life, and mortality from cardiovascular disease. *BMJ* 1989;**298**:564–7.

14. **Hales CN, Barker DJP, Clark PMS,** et al. Fetal and infant growth and impaired glucose tolerance at age 64. *BMJ* 1991;**303**:1019–22.

15. **Phipps K, Barker DJP, Hales CN,** et al. Fetal growth and impaired glucose tolerance in men and women. *Diabetologia* 1993; **36**:225–8.
- *Standard oral glucose tolerance tests were carried out on 140 men and 126 women born in 1935–43, aged 50. Subjects with impaired glucose tolerance or non-insulin dependent diabetes mellitus had lower birth weight (independent of gestational age), a smaller head circumference, and were thinner at birth (adjusted for body mass index). They also had a higher ratio of placental weight to birth weight. The results may be caused by reduced growth of the endocrine pancreas, which in turn may be a consequence of maternal undernutrition during pregnancy or other failure, such as placental defect, in fetal nutrition.*

16. **Lithell HO, McKeigue PM, Berglund L,** et al. Relation of size at birth to non-insulin dependent diabetes and insulin concentrations in men aged 50–60 years. *BMJ* 1996;**312**:406–10.
- *This study involved 1333 men born in 1920–24 and resident in Uppsala, Sweden, in 1970. There was a weak inverse correlation between ponderal index at birth and 60 minute insulin concentrations in the intravenous glucose tolerance test at age 50 years. This association was stronger in the highest third of the distribution of body mass index than in the other two thirds. Prevalence of diabetes at age 60 years was higher (8%) in men whose birth weight was < 3250 g compared with men with birth weight 3250 g or more (5%). There was a stronger association between diabetes and ponderal index. Correlations were adjusted for body mass index. These results gave fairly strong support to the fetal origin hypothesis.*

17. **Law CM, de Swiet M, Osmond C,** et al. Initiation of hypertension in utero and its amplification throughout life. *BMJ* 1993;**306**:24–7.
- *A study on four different populations aged 0–10 years, 36 years, 46–54 years, and 59–71 years. In all four populations the inverse relation between birth weight and systolic blood pressure was apparent and the relation became larger with increasing age. According to this, the results from older generations would be applicable to younger generations, but this needs replication.*

18. **Whincup PH, Cook DG, Papacosta O.** Do maternal and intrauterine factors influence blood pressure in childhood? *Arch Dis Child* 1992;**67**:1423–9.

19. **Williams S, George I, Silva P.** Intrauterine growth retardation and blood pressure at age seven and eighteen. *J Clin Epidemiol* 1992;**45**:1257–63.
- *This study involved children aged 7 and 18 years, born in 1972–73. At age 7, after adjusting for sex and weight, the differences between normal and intrauterine growth retarded (IUGR) children were 0.9 mm Hg (95% CI –0.1 to 2.2) for systolic and 0 mm Hg (95% CI –1.7 to 2.0) for diastolic blood pressure, respectively. At age 18 the differences were less pronounced. These results give only weak support to the hypothesis of evolution of hypertension already in utero, although the number of IUGR children was comparatively low (at age 7, 70 and at age 18, 68).*

20. **Seidman DS, Laor A, Gale R,** et al. Birth weight, current body weight, and blood pressure in late adolescence. *BMJ* 1991;**302**:1235–7.
- *This study involved 32,580 17 year old subjects (19,734 men and 12,846 women) born in Jerusalem during 1964–71. Diastolic and systolic blood pressures were associated with birth weight, but the correlation coefficients were low. Body mass index was significantly linked with high systolic blood pressure in both men and women. The results can be interpreted that a high body weight rather*

186

than a low birth weight was linked with higher systolic and diastolic pressure in both men and women, which stresses the importance of life course in the evolution of disease risk.

21. **Barker DJP, Hales CN, Fall CHD,** *et al*. Type 2 (non-insulin-dependent) diabetes mellitus, hypertension and hyperlipidaemia (syndrome X): relation to reduced fetal growth. *Diabetologia* 1993;**36**:62–7.

22. **McCance DR, Pettitt D, Hanson RL,** *et al*. Birth weight and non-insulin dependent diabetes: thrifty genotype, thrifty phenotype, or surviving small baby genotype? *BMJ* 1994;**308**:942–5.
• *This study involved 1179 American Indians born in 1940–72 whose glucose tolerance was evaluated at ages 20–39 years. The prevalence of non-insulin dependent diabetes mellitus was greatest in those with the lowest and highest birth weights (a U shaped relation). When age, sex, body mass index, maternal diabetes during pregnancy, and birth year were controlled for, subjects with birth weight < 2500 g had a higher rate than those with weights of 2500–4499 g. The U shaped relation was seen primarily in subjects with a parental history of diabetes. A genetic background seems to have a clear effect on non-insulin dependent diabetes mellitus, but it does not seem to explain the U shaped relation.*

23. **Stern MP, Bartley M, Duggirala R,** *et al*. Birth weight and the metabolic syndrome: thrifty phenotype or thrifty genotype. *Diabetes/Metabolism Research and Reviews* 2000;**16**:88–93.

24. **Whincup PH, Cook DG, Adshead F,** *et al*. Childhood size is more strongly related than size at birth to glucose and insulin levels in 10–11-year-old children. *Diabetologia* 1997;**40**:319–26.
• *This study involved 10–11 year old children. One group (n = 591) was studied fasting, the other (n = 547) was studied 30 minutes after a standard oral glucose load. Neither fasting nor post-load glucose concentrations showed any consistent relation with birth weight or ponderal index at birth. After adjustment for childhood height and ponderal index, both fasting and post-load insulin concentrations fell with increasing birth weight. However, the proportional change in insulin for a 1 SD increase in childhood ponderal index was much greater than that for birth weight. Obesity in children is, evidently, a stronger determinant of insulin concentrations and insulin resistance than size at birth.*

25. **Paneth N, Ahmed F, Stein AD.** Early nutritional origins of hypertension: a hypothesis still lacking support. *J Hypertens* 1996;**14**(suppl 5):121–9.
• *This review focuses on the hypothesis of reduced birth weight and subsequent elevated blood pressure in light of four causal criteria: specificity, consistency, strength, and biological coherence. Aspects of the methodology used in studies of the hypothesis are also examined. According to this study, the evidence thus far provided does not support the hypothesis. Further studies have provided more evidence, but it is still patchy.*

26. **Langley-Evans SC.** Hypertension induced by foetal exposure to a maternal low-protein diet, in the rat, is prevented by pharmacological blockage of maternal glucocorticoid synthesis. *J Hypertens* 1997;**15**:537–44.
• *In this experiment involving rats(14 dams, 136 offspring), the dams were fed a low protein or a control diet after conception. All the pups had a standard diet. At the age of 7 weeks the blood pressures of all the offspring were determined. Blood pressures of rats exposed to maternal low protein diets in utero were raised significantly relative to control rats. These results are consistent with Barker's hypothesis on programming.*

27. **Forsén T, Eriksson JG, Tuomilehto J,** *et al*. Mother's weight in pregnancy and coronary heart disease in a cohort of Finnish men: follow up study. *BMJ* 1997;**315**:837–40.

28. **Leon DA, Koupilova I, Lithell HO,** *et al*. Failure to realise growth potential in utero and adult obesity in relation to blood pressure in 50 year old Swedish men. *BMJ* 1996;**312**:401–6.
• *This study involved 1333 men born during 1920–24 and resident in Uppsala, Sweden, in 1970. There was a small decrease in systolic blood pressure as birth weight increased. Much stronger effects were observed among men who were born at term and were in the top third of body mass index at age 50. Men who were light at birth (< 3250 g) but were of above median adult height had particularly high blood pressure. It is suggested that it is a failure to express one's full growth potential in utero, rather than small size at birth per se, that is related to raised adult blood pressure. This is consistent with already known aetiological factors and still supports the fetal origin hypothesis.*

website
extra

*Additional references
appear on the
Heart website*

www.heartjnl.com

28 Interventional catheterisation. Opening up I: the ventricular outflow tracts and great arteries

John L Gibbs

Interventional catheterisation in the treatment of patients with congenital heart disease has expanded dramatically since Rashkind first introduced balloon atrial septostomy in 1966. In many centres up to half of all cardiac catheterisations in congenital heart disease are therapeutic rather than diagnostic. Developments in plastics and alloy engineering have led to improvements in equipment for balloon or stent treatment and these techniques are playing an increasing role in the management of adults with congenital heart disease. The only existing guidelines, which represent the American consensus of opinion, have been published by the American Council on Cardiovascular Disease in the Young.[1]

Right ventricular outflow obstruction

Pulmonary valve stenosis

Balloon dilatation has proved extraordinarily successful in the treatment of pulmonary stenosis at any age. Improvements in guide wire technology and in balloon design have allowed successful transvenous valvoplasty to be carried out at very low risk even in the premature neonate and, in contrast to treatment of aortic stenosis, ballooning the pulmonary valve is effective even in the presence of cusp calcification in adult life.

There are no absolute indications for intervention in pulmonary stenosis and different centres vary in their threshold for treatment. In general pulmonary stenosis is a well tolerated lesion and the risk of sudden death is much lower than with obstruction to left ventricular outflow. Pulmonary stenosis does not always become more severe with age and may occasionally improve or even resolve spontaneously. Clinical signs and symptoms (usually exercise intolerance if the obstruction is severe), ECG changes, and echocardiographic findings all play a part in timing of intervention. As an approximate generalisation the combination of right ventricular hypertrophy and a peak flow velocity of 4 m/s or greater would encourage most cardiologists in the UK to intervene. Technically pulmonary balloon valvoplasty is usually straightforward,[2] with optimum results being obtained with a balloon diameter between 120–150% of the diameter of the valve. It is rarely necessary to resort to surgery whatever the age of the patient, the exception being severe valve dysplasia when elasticity of the deformed cusps prohibits effective valvotomy (surgical resection of the cusps rather than valvotomy may be required). Pulmonary regurgitation induced by balloon valvoplasty is usually mild, appears to be well tolerated even in the long term, and does not appear to be any more severe than regurgitation after surgical valvotomy.

Some degree of infundibular stenosis often occurs with valvar stenosis. This is frequently related to right ventricular hypertrophy and may gradually resolve spontaneously after valve obstruction is treated; a failure of reduction in right ventricular pressure immediately after ballooning does not necessarily indicate failure of the procedure and patience may be required before making a definitive assessment of the results.[3]

In complex cyanotic heart disease associated with valvar pulmonary stenosis it is sometimes possible to improve pulmonary blood flow by a "limited" valvoplasty, thereby avoiding the need for palliative shunt surgery.[4] The major factor in achieving good results is very careful patient selection and careful judgement of balloon diameter to avoid excessive pulmonary blood flow.

Infundibular stenosis

Infundibular stenosis, because it is usually muscular, is generally treated surgically. However, on rare occasions infundibular stenting can offer effective palliation when surgical "correction" of a complex anomaly is not possible—for example, tetralogy of Fallot with diffuse pulmonary hypoplasia.[5] Young children with hypercyanotic attacks associated with tetralogy of Fallot may benefit from balloon dilatation of the right ventricular outflow tract, even when the obstruction is principally infundibular.[6] The mechanism for this improvement is not clear, but it seems likely that tearing and subsequent scarring of the infundibular muscle is involved.

Balloon dilatation for pulmonary valve stenosis

- Treatment of choice for valvar pulmonary stenosis at any age, even in adults with valve calcification

- Main determinant of success is balloon size
  – A balloon of up to 150% the diameter of the valve may be required, in contrast to dilatation of the aortic valve, when large balloons are dangerous
  – "Limited" balloon valvoplasty may provide good palliation in complex cyanotic heart disease with pulmonary stenosis

- Infundibular stenosis caused by right ventricular hypertrophy associated with valvar stenosis often improves spontaneously within a few weeks of ballooning the valve

- Pulmonary regurgitation after ballooning is probably no worse than after surgical valvotomy

Balloon dilatation for non-valvar right ventricular outflow obstruction

- Ballooning may help in selected patients with tetralogy of Fallot

- Balloon expandable stents occasionally useful for infundibular stenosis in poor candidates for surgery

- Proximal branch pulmonary artery stenoses may respond to balloon angioplasty but are often elastic and may require stenting

- Stenosed right ventricular to pulmonary artery conduits may be dilatable but improvement often short lived; stenting may help but late stent fracture possible

Pulmonary atresia

Surgery remains the treatment of choice for tetralogy with pulmonary atresia. There have been some attempts to establish continuity between the right ventricle and the pulmonary trunk by laser or radiofrequency perforation of the atretic outflow tract, but the risk of perforation of the heart (sometimes fatal) is probably unacceptable in patients with long segment atresia. The rarest form of pulmonary atresia, where the ventricular septum is intact and the pulmonary valve is imperforate, is more amenable to transcatheter treatment. Laser or radiofrequency perforation of the valve followed by balloon dilatation may be very successful in selected cases and may be the only treatment necessary. Duct patency may need to be maintained for several weeks after a successful procedure as pulmonary blood supply remains duct dependent until right ventricular hypertrophy has regressed to some extent. Patience is usually rewarded and aortopulmonary shunt surgery is rarely required.[7] The choice between laser and radiofrequency perforation of the valve is largely one of resources; the laser tends to burn through the valve faster and laser wires tend to be easier to manipulate. The wires' prices are similar but the laser generator is substantially more expensive than the radiofrequency counterpart.

Pulmonary artery stenoses

Pulmonary artery stenosis occurs most frequently in patients with tetralogy of Fallot. It may be present before surgery or may appear early or late after surgical repair (fig 28.1). It may be easily missed, particularly in adults and particularly when it is unilateral. Surgical repair of pulmonary artery stenosis may be technically difficult and narrowing may recur because of patch scarring and shrinkage, so when stenosis of a major branch occurs after surgery most centres would try transcatheter treatment before further surgery. Many pulmonary artery stenoses are elastic and recoil after simple balloon angioplasty,[8] and some operators choose to proceed directly to stent implantation. Stenting may be technically difficult; it carries risks of stent embolisation,

pulmonary artery rupture, and even death. It will not give a good result if the stenosis is too tough to be dilated. It therefore seems wise to try simple ballooning first to ensure that the lesion is dilatable and to be sure that stenting is really required. Experience so far suggests that restenosis caused by intimal proliferation in the stent is uncommon[9] and that when it does occur repeat balloon dilatation is usually helpful. When pulmonary artery stenosis occurs postoperatively there is usually extensive fibrosis around the vessel to offer support after angioplasty. This is not the case for "native" artery stenosis and a less aggressive approach, possibly with serial procedures to enlarge the vessel gradually, is needed if pulmonary artery rupture (potentially fatal) is to be avoided.

Multiple peripheral pulmonary artery stenoses are much more difficult to deal with. Surgery rarely produces obvious benefit. There are rare cases where angioplasty or stenting of a prominent stenosis in a large branch might improve pulmonary perfusion, but the benefits may be offset by induction of segmental pulmonary oedema. There are no conclusive data at present to suggest any improvement in survival or objective improvement in symptoms.

Stenosis localised to the pulmonary trunk rather than its branches may also occur after surgery (most commonly after the arterial switch). This tends to be less responsive to ballooning[10] and proximity to the pulmonary valve

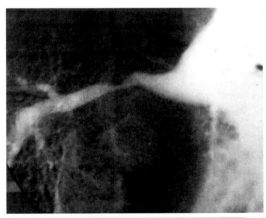

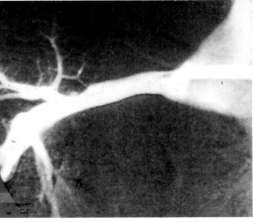

Figure 28.1. Severe stenosis of the right pulmonary artery (top) after surgical repair of tetralogy of Fallot. There was no improvement after balloon dilatation because of elastic recoil, but a balloon expandable stent (bottom) has relieved the stenosis and considerably improved blood flow to the right lung.

or the pulmonary artery bifurcation makes stent implantation difficult. Surgery is usually required.

Conduit obstruction

Conduits between the right ventricle and the pulmonary trunk eventually become obstructed (and calcified) whether they are allografts, homografts, or synthetic. When the conduit itself is stenosed balloon angioplasty or even stent implantation may help and surgical replacement of the conduit may be deferred in some cases by over two years.[11] In some cases obstruction occurs at the proximal or distal anastomosis of the conduit and stenting may be more helpful. There are some concerns over the uneven stresses on stents in such situations (the proximal part of the stent will be within the right ventricular wall) and stent fracture has been reported.[11]

Left ventricular outflow obstruction

Valvar aortic stenosis

There is still divided opinion in the UK over whether surgery or balloon valvoplasty is better treatment for aortic stenosis in children. Logic suggests that surgery allows a careful valvotomy under full vision and that this would be unlikely to be matched by the crude inflation of a balloon, yet clinical data have not shown any clear difference between the two approaches.[12] Severe regurgitation or important residual stenosis may occur after either procedure but no randomised trial to compare the two has been (or is ever likely to be) performed. In neonates early concerns about vascular damage by balloon catheters have proved unfounded, with improved balloon design and with formal arteriotomy using the axillary or carotid arteries in preference to the femoral artery. In contrast to pulmonary valvoplasty it is important to use a balloon no larger (ideally slightly smaller) than the aortic root if cusp avulsion is to be avoided.

Indications to intervene should be similar whether surgery or catheterisation is employed. In neonates the decision is rarely difficult as the circulation is usually duct dependent with severe stenosis. In older children, however, timing is more difficult; the combination of left ventricular hypertrophy, a left ventricular outflow velocity in excess of 4 m/s, and either

ECG repolarisation abnormalities or an abnormal blood pressure response to exercise, would prompt treatment in most centres. The older the patient, the more technically difficult the procedure. This is largely because of difficulty keeping the balloon in a stable position during inflation. Use of a stiff guide wire with a floppy tip curled in the ventricle or injection of adenosine to induce transient ventricular standstill have been advocated. Nonetheless, balloon valvoplasty may produce good palliation in older children,[13] even if the patient has previously undergone balloon valvoplasty or surgical valvotomy.[14] Complications include arterial damage, cardiac perforation, embolic stroke, and induction of severe aortic regurgitation. Bacterial endocarditis related to ballooning appears to be very rare but most operators give prophylactic antibiotics to cover the procedure. Transcatheter treatment is probably best avoided later in life when the valve has become calcified.[15]

Other forms of aortic stenosis

There have been occasional reports of balloon dilatation of discrete, membraneous subaortic stenosis[16] and of supravalvar stenosis, but results are not encouraging and surgery remains the treatment of choice.

Coarctation and recoarctation of the aorta

Native (unoperated) coarctation

In neonates balloon dilatation of coarctation rarely provides more than transient benefit and restenosis occurs as the rule rather than the exception because of constriction of ductal tissue; surgery remains the treatment of choice. In infants, older children, and adults there is divided opinion on the optimum form of treatment.[17–19] Death at surgery for coarctation is very rare now, but it is the associated small risk of spinal cord damage and consequent irreversible paraplegia that has led to balloon angioplasty having some protagonists. Balloon

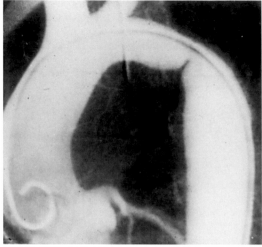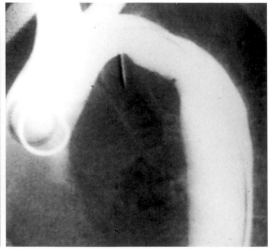

Figure 28.2. Aortography 14 years after subclavian flap repair of coarctation (left). Although often referred to as recoarctation, this appearance is almost certainly caused by residual rather than recurrent stenosis. Discrete, shelf like lesions like this respond well to balloon dilatation (right), with low risk of aortic aneurysm or rupture in patients who have surrounding scar tissue caused by previous surgery.

angioplasty works by tearing the intima and media of the aorta, leaving only the adventitia intact. It is not surprising that balloon dilatation of native coarctation is associated with a risk of false aneurysm formation (up to 20% in some series). Some groups have advocated a graduated approach, using repeated procedures to enlarge the stenosis gradually, but as yet there is no clear evidence that graduated ballooning carries any less risk.

A major factor in aneurysm production is the size of the balloon. Various formulae to aid in the choice of balloon size have been suggested, either related to the diameter of the coarctation itself or to the diameter of the descending aorta at the level of the diaphragm. It is clear that for some partially elastic stenoses it is necessary to employ a balloon larger than the required final vessel diameter. This is probably an important factor in aneurysm formation, but it is not yet clear whether using a stent to overcome elastic recoil[20] (allowing a smaller balloon to be used) will reduce risk of aneurysm. Covered stents, which might be expected to minimise the effects of tearing the aorta, are not yet widely available. An additional factor which should be taken into account when considering balloon angioplasty is that partial relief of coarctation is really not acceptable! If a severe coarctation is partially treated collateral vessels may regress, thereby potentially increasing the risk of spinal cord damage at operation.

Recoarctation

Recoarctation after neonatal surgical repair occurs in up to 10% of cases in most published experience. In contrast to native coarctation, balloon angioplasty is widely favoured for treatment of recoarctation; this is because the aorta is surrounded by supportive fibrous scar tissue and the risk of inducing a false aneurysm is low, particularly if care is taken to avoid oversized balloons (fig 28.2). Aortic rupture and death caused by disruption of the suture line has been reported after dilatation of recoarctation in patients who have had patch repair (as opposed to subclavian flap or end to end anastomosis). Many centres regard patch

repair as an indication for surgical rather than transcatheter treatment.

1. **Allen HD, Beekman RH, Garson A,** *et al.* Pediatric therapeutic cardiac catheterisation. A statement for healthcare professionals from the Council on Cardiovascular Disease in the Young, American Heart Association. *Circulation* 1998;**97**:609–25.
• *An American consensus statement on various aspects of interventional catheterisation in congenital heart disease; who should be doing it, which type of centres should be involved in training, guidelines on skill maintenance, which procedures are widely accepted and which are still controversial, and a brief appraisal of many (but not all) devices in use in the USA at present. A useful, well balanced guide, with only one or two procedures recently pioneered in Europe but not yet employed in the US left uncovered.*

2. **McCrindle BW.** Independent predictors of long term results after balloon pulmonary valvuloplasty. Valvuloplasty and angioplasty of congenital anomalies (VACA) registry. *Circulation* 1994;**89**:1751–9.
• *Multicentre results from 533 patients. Major factor in predicting successful procedure was size of balloon.*

3. **Fawzy ME, Galal O, Dunn B,** *et al.* Regression of infundibular pulmonary stenosis after successful balloon pulmonary valvuloplasty in adults. *Cathet Cardiovasc Diagn* 1990;**21**:77–81.
• *22 adults, all with some degree of infundibular as well as valvar stenosis. In all cases the gradient fell further with follow up, showing that adults behave like children in terms of regression of residual infundibular stenosis after relief of fixed obstruction at valve level.*

4. **Stumper O, Piechaud JF, Bonhoeffer P,** *et al.* Pulmonary balloon valvuloplasty in the palliation of complex cyanotic heart disease. *Heart* 1996;**76**:363-6.

5. **Gibbs JL, Uzun O, Blackburn MEC,** *et al.* Right ventricular outflow stent implantation: an alternative to palliative surgical relief of infundibular pulmonary stenosis. *Heart* 1997;**77**:176–9.

6. **Sluysmans T, Neven B, Rubay J,** *et al.* Early balloon dilatation of the pulmonary valve in infants with tetralogy of Fallot: risks and benefits. *Circulation* 1995;**91**:1506–11.
• *Following on from earlier pioneering studies in the UK, this study describes the effect on cyanosis as well as looking at pulmonary artery growth after balloon dilatation of the outflow tract in tetralogy. It confirmed initial feelings that this is a surprisingly safe procedure and can offer excellent palliation in the minority of patients where surgical repair does not seem immediately appropriate.*

7. **Gibbs JL, Blackburn ME, Uzun O,** *et al.* Laser valvotomy with balloon valvoplasty for pulmonary atresia with intact ventricular septum: five years' experience. *Heart* 1997;**77**:225–8.

8. **Kan JS, Marvin WJ Jr, Bass JL,** *et al.* Balloon angioplasty—branch pulmonary artery stenosis: results from the valvuloplasty and angioplasty of congenital anomalies registry. *Am J Cardiol* 1990;**65**:798–801.
• *182 procedures in 156 patients from 27 centres. Angiographic improvement in appearance of stenosis in most cases but proximal pulmonary artery pressure fell from mean of 69 (25) mm Hg to only 63 (24) mm Hg. On top of that there were complications in 21 cases and five deaths because of pulmonary artery rupture, paradoxical embolism, low cardiac output or cardiac arrest.*

9. O'Laughlin MP, Perry SB, Lock JE, *et al.* Use of endovascular stents in congenital heart disease. *Circulation* 1991;**83**:1923–39.

10. Nakanishi T, Matsumoto Y, Seguchi Mnakazawa M, *et al.* Balloon angioplasty for postoperative pulmonary artery stenosis in transposition of the great arteries. *J Am Coll Cardiol* 1993;**22**:859–66.
- *28 patients. At least 50% fall in gradient achieved in about half the patients, with one non-fatal pulmonary artery rupture and three aneurysmal dilatations of pulmonary artery. Does not make the technique sound very rewarding in this setting.*

11. Powell AJ, Lock JE, Keane JF, *et al.* Prolongation of RV-PA conduit life by percutaneous stent implantation: intermediate term results. *Circulation* 1995;**92**:3282–8.
- *44 patients with obstructed conduits (either homografts or other bioprostheses). Freedom from redo surgery was 65% at 30 months. Nine patients needed repeat dilatation or repeat stenting and stent fracture occurred in seven cases (thought to be related to the uneven stresses on stents in conduits).*

12. Justo RN, McCrindle BW, Benson LN, *et al.* Aortic valve regurgitation after surgical versus percutaneous balloon valvotomy for congenital aortic valve stenosis. *Am J Cardiol* 1996;**77**:1332–8.
- *187 patients who had either surgical or percutaneous valvotomy. Not randomised and not perfectly matched groups of patients either, but no significant difference between the two groups in terms of reduction in gradient or development or progression of aortic regurgitation.*

13. Moore P, Egito E, Mowrey H, *et al.* Midterm results of balloon dilatation of congenital aortic stenosis: predictors of success. *J Am Coll Cardiol* 1996;**27**:1257–63.
- *148 children aged older than 1 month, with 95% eight year survival, 75% free from reintervention at four years and 50% at eight years. Results tend to look more favourable when neonates are excluded, as in this study.*

14. Sreeram N, Kitchiner D, Williams D, *et al.* Balloon dilatation of the aortic valve after previous surgical valvotomy: immediate and follow up results. *Br Heart J* 1994;**71**:558–60.
- *22 cases, results appeared just as rewarding as in patients who had not undergone previous treatment.*

15. Anon. Percutaneous balloon aortic valvuloplasty: acute and 30 day follow up results in 674 patients from the NHLBI balloon valvuloplasty registry. *Circulation* 1991;**84**:2383–97.
- *A multicentre report. Adults only (the majority were over 70 years old); 86% survival at 30 days with appreciable morbidity (stroke, vascular damage) but 75% of survivors appeared to benefit to some extent with regard to exercise tolerance.*

16. Lababidi Z, Weinhaus L, Stoeckle H, *et al.* Transluminal balloon dilatation for discrete subaortic stenosis. *Am J Cardiol* 1987;**59**:423–5.

17. Rao PS. Should balloon angioplasty be used instead of surgery for native aortic coarctation? *Br Heart J* 1995;**74**:578–9.
- *An editorial presenting one American view of ballooning native coarctation from neonates to adults. From a well known protagonist of the technique, suggests that balloon angioplasty has similar results to surgery in terms of relieving stenosis and producing aneurysms. Should be read in conjunction with the following reference from the correspondence columns which argues that published data are by no means conclusive and could be interpreted quite differently.*

18. Qureshi SA, Rosenthal E. Should balloon angioplasty be used instead of surgery for native aortic coarctation? *Heart* 1997;**77**:86.
- *See comment above.*

19. Fawzy ME, Sivanandam V, Galal O, *et al.* One to ten year follow up of balloon angioplasty of native coarctation of the aorta in adolescents and adults. *J Am Coll Cardiol* 1997;**30**:1542–6.
- *43 patients over the age of 15; 7% had suboptimal relief of coarctation (but responded to repeat angioplasty) and 7% developed small aortic aneurysms, although the aneurysms did not seem to increase in size over the study period. The patients all had discrete coarctation rather than tubular stenoses. The conclusion was that it is a safe and effective alternative to surgery for this particular type of coarctation. A pity there is such a paucity of reports of surgical treatment from the current generation of surgeons who appear to produce superlative results at very low risk.*

20. Ebeid MR, Prieto LR, Latson LA. Use of balloon expandable stents for coarctation of the aorta: initial results and intermediate follow up. *J Am Coll Cardiol* 1997;**30**:1847–52.
- *Small study of a new technique, the idea being that using a stent avoids the need to use an oversized balloon and therefore might reduce the risk of aneurysm formation. No aneurysms, good results in terms of relief of obstruction, but only nine patients, so early days yet.*

29 Interventional catheterisation. Opening up II: venous return, the atrial septum, the arterial duct, aortopulmonary shunts, and aortopulmonary collaterals

John L Gibbs

Obstruction to flow in the superior caval vein rarely occurs de novo. It is usually a consequence of scarring related to surgery, to the presence of venous catheters or pacemaker electrodes, or external compression by tumour. When obstruction occurs insidiously there may be no symptoms and no indication to intervene, but with rapid onset obstruction, when collateral veins have not had time to develop and enlarge, venous hypertension in the head and neck will prompt treatment (fig 29.1). Although these stenoses can be dilated using a balloon, stent implantation is usually required to prevent recoil.[1] Self expanding as well as balloon expandable stents have been used with good effect. In the presence of complete obstruction "reconstruction" is sometimes possible by passing a long needle and then a guide wire through the obstruction, followed by ballooning and stenting. Because the vein is usually surrounded by scar tissue accidental perforation is unlikely to cause any more harm than localised haematoma.

Intra-atrial obstruction to systemic venous return may occur after venous inflow redirection surgery for transposition of the great arteries. This is relatively common after Mustard's operation, when patches of material are sewn inside the atria to redirect the systemic veins to the left atrium and the pulmonary veins to the right atrium (fig 29.2). Obstruction is much less likely after Senning's operation, in which redirection is achieved using infoldings of the atrial wall. Obstruction may become evident many years after surgery (during teenage or adult life) and often presents with oedema, ascites or even protein losing enteropathy. Such symptoms are clearly an indication to intervene and rarely occur unless there is obstruction to both superior and inferior venous channels. Total obstruction of the superior channel may occur without being clinically obvious when collateral veins (often azygos or hemiazygos) are well established. Stenoses in the intracardiac venous channels often respond well to balloon dilatation alone, although some degree of elastic recoil is common. Self expanding or balloon expandable stents produce excellent results in such cases[2 3] and stenting appears surprisingly safe. It is easy to imagine that stenting the systemic venous pathways might produce compression of the adjacent pulmonary venous pathways but in practice that does not appear to occur. The precise indications for intervention in asymptomatic patients remains controversial.

Pulmonary venous obstruction

Pulmonary venous obstruction as an isolated anomaly is exceedingly rare; the vast majority of cases occur in association with anomalous pulmonary venous return and it may be seen both before and after surgical repair of anomalous venous connections. Obstruction to an anomalous common pulmonary venous channel is most often associated with infracardiac or supracardiac total anomalous pulmonary venous drainage (TAPVD) and in such circumstances the treatment of choice is almost invariably surgical redirection of the pulmonary veins. When associated with very complex cardiac abnormalities (usually with right atrial isomerism) in the neonate it may be venous obstruction that is the immediate haemodynamic problem, rather than the abnormal site of venous drainage, and there have been occasional reports of balloon dilatation or even stenting of obstructed anomalous pulmonary venous channels. Such procedures may produce some temporary relief of pulmonary

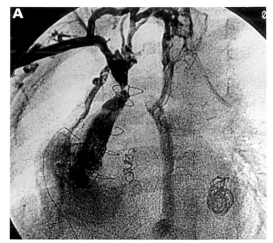

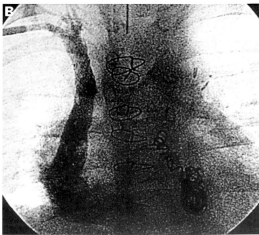

Figure 29.1. (A) Severe, symptomatic obstruction of the superior caval vein, with multiple small collateral channels, in a child who had undergone cardiac transplantation following numerous palliative operations for complex congenital heart disease. There was little improvement after simple balloon dilatation (using axillary venotomy), but stent implantation (B) produced complete relief of obstruction.

oedema but there can be no doubt that surgical redirection of the pulmonary veins offers a much more secure and longer lasting answer.

When pulmonary venous obstruction occurs after surgical repair of TAPVD it is rarely simply a problem of inadequate venous anastomosis, but usually affects the pulmonary veins (often all four) in their distal portions close to the left atrium. Surgical patching of the pulmonary veins, balloon dilatation and stent implantation (both transcatheter and surgically placed) all produce disappointing results, often with only short term improvement.[4][5] The mechanism behind this so called pulmonary veno-occlusive disease, responsible for the relentless recurrence of stenosis, is poorly understood; necropsy studies of the walls of the pulmonary veins show intimal and medial thickening.

Creation of an atrial septal defect

The majority of patients who undergo atrial septostomy are neonates with transposition of the great arteries, but there are other situations where creation of an atrial septal defect may be helpful, even in adolescents or adults. In babies the traditional Rashkind balloon is still favoured, the balloon being pulled back to the right atrium after it has been passed across the foramen into the left atrium and inflated. For older patients, when the atrial septum may be too tough to allow an adequate hole to be torn with the Rashkind balloon, progressive dilatation (as opposed to forced balloon withdrawal) using a balloon introduced over a guide wire may be effective. This is probably safer than the alternative of blade septostomy when a folding blade at the tip of a catheter is withdrawn across the septum, the procedure being repeated with varying orientation of the blade to make a series of cuts. Not surprisingly, complications such as atrial perforation may occur. The defect created by the blade may be enlarged by balloon. In older patients who have an intact atrial septum it may be necessary first to perforate the septum using a transseptal needle or a radiofrequency or laser wire. The risk of septostomy varies considerably, depend-

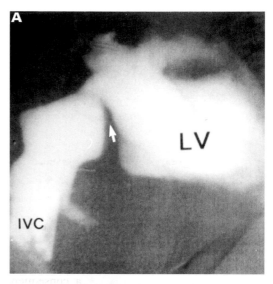

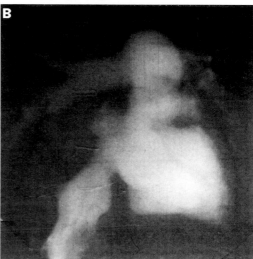

Figure 29.2. (A) Obstruction in the systemic venous pathway in a 14 year old after Mustard's operation for transposition. The patch sewn inside the atria to redirect systemic venous return to the mitral valve and left ventricle has become distorted, causing a shelf like obstruction (arrowed). Balloon dilatation has resulted in sufficient widening of the pathway (B) to relieve completely symptoms of venous hypertension (protein losing enteropathy in this case). IVC, inferior vena cava; LV, left ventricle.

ing on the anatomical abnormality as well as the method employed.

Simple and complex transposition

In simple transposition poor mixing between the pulmonary and systemic circulations may cause severe hypoxaemia and death even if the arterial duct is patent, so it is customary to perform immediate balloon septostomy. In most centres this is done under echocardiographic control.[6] It may be carried out anywhere, without the need for a catheterisation laboratory, is safe, and usually takes only a few minutes. Access to the heart is achieved through the umbilical or femoral vein; the former has the advantage of preserving the femoral vein for later use, although the ductus venosus may be awkward to cross in some cases.

Mitral, pulmonary, and tricuspid atresia

With mitral atresia the left atrium can empty only across the foramen to the right atrium. It

---

Venous obstruction

Systemic circulation

- In the superior caval vein
  - Usually iatrogenic or caused by external compression
  - Ballooning rarely sufficient, stent usually required
- Within the atrium
  - Relatively common after Mustard's operation for transposition
  - Ballooning alone often sufficient to relieve symptoms

Pulmonary circulation

- Rare, often associated with anomalous pulmonary venous return
  - Ballooning, stenting and surgery all very rarely rewarding

is wise to decompress the left atrium even when the foramen does not appear to be obviously restrictive in the early neonatal period. Septostomy can be technically difficult because the left atrium is small. Immediate haemodynamic benefit (a fall in left atrial pressure) may occur but in some cases the sudden decompression of the left atrium produces a dramatic increase in pulmonary blood flow, resulting in acute deterioration or even death. When neonatal septostomy has not been carried out the atrial septum often becomes restrictive with time, giving signs and symptoms of pulmonary venous and arterial hypertension later in life. Decompression of the left atrium is difficult and hazardous in older patients (dilatation by balloon[7] or the Park blade[8] may help) and surgical septectomy may be required.

In patients with pulmonary atresia with an intact ventricular septum or with tricuspid atresia, the only route by which the right atrium can empty is across the foramen to the left atrium. There is divided opinion on the desirability of neonatal septostomy in such cases. In some countries it is routine but in practice it is rare for the foramen to be restrictive in infancy, and it is the author's opinion that septostomy is very rarely required.

The failing Fontan circulation and end stage pulmonary hypertension in older patients

When the chronically elevated systemic venous pressure associated with the Fontan operation (direct anastomosis of the right atrium to the pulmonary trunk) is poorly tolerated, creation of a small atrial septal defect may relieve the symptoms of high systemic venous pressure (albeit at the price of some degree of desaturation caused by right to left atrial shunting). Similarly, creation of a small atrial septal defect may reduce right atrial pressure and increase cardiac output in advanced pulmonary hypertension in adults. Because the atrial septum is intact (necessitating septal puncture), and it is difficult to judge as well as to create the appropriate size of defect, this approach has not been widely adopted. Nonetheless, it may be worth consideration if symptoms are severe.[9]

Arterial duct

Atrial septostomy

- Beneficial in:
  - All neonates with simple transposition or mitral atresia
  - Most neonates with complex transposition
  - Occasional neonates with tricuspid atresia or hypoplasia of the right heart
  - Children or young adults with "failing" Fontan circulation
  - Selected adults with end stage pulmonary hypertension

- Techniques:
  - "Pullback" balloon (Rashkind)
  - Balloon dilatation
  - Park blade catheter

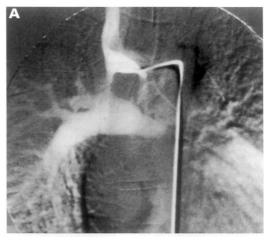

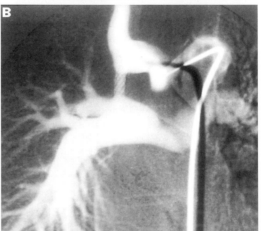

Figure 29.3. (A) Severe obstruction of a classical Blalock–Taussig shunt in a teenager with complex pulmonary atresia. There was almost complete recoil after simple balloon dilatation but stent implantation notably improved blood flow to the right lung (B).

Medical treatment with prostaglandin E allows short term maintenance of duct patency in neonates with duct dependent circulation. Attempts to keep the duct open in the longer term have included simple balloon angioplasty (unreliable),[10] "hot" balloon angioplasty (better but still unreliable),[11] and stent implantation. Stenting seems to keep the duct open effectively when the systemic circulation is dependent—that is, variants of the hypoplastic left heart syndrome.[12] It may be useful as a bridge to transplantation in some cases,[13] but unfortunately it does not prevent heart failure developing and recent results of palliative surgery (the Norwood operation and its modifications) are superior. When the pulmonary circulation is dependent the duct tends to be tortuous and while stenting is possible, it is technically very demanding and sudden death may occur during or after the procedure.[14] Neointimal proliferation producing stenosis within the stent is common, necessitating repeated balloon dilatations to cope with growth of the child. There are only rare circumstances (for instance bilateral pulmonary artery disconnection with bilateral ducts) where it may be a reasonable alternative to a surgical aortopulmonary shunt.

Aortopulmonary shunts

The classical Blalock–Taussig shunt, where the subclavian artery is joined, end to side, to the ipsilateral pulmonary artery, may provide excellent palliation for complex cyanotic heart disease, but stenosis eventually occurs. This may be in the form of discrete stenosis (often at the distal anastomosis), may be diffuse along the length of the shunt, or a combination of these. Balloon angioplasty alone may improve the stenosis in many cases,[15] but elasticity is common and stent implantation may be the only means of improving the shunt diameter (fig 29.3).[16] Dramatic improvement in pulmonary blood flow, cyanosis, and symptoms may occur but the procedure is only indicated in complex disease unsuitable for surgical repair. A modified Blalock shunt, usually fashioned from Goretex tubing, has a limited life because of lack of growth and increasing thickness of the layer of tissue (a mixture of endothelial cells, fibrous tissue, and sometimes laminated thrombus, collectively known as "peel") lining the synthetic tube. Although balloon angioplasty may result in enlargement of the shunt lumen this is often short lived, and there is some risk of inducing abrupt shunt occlusion (usually fatal) if the "peel" is dissected off the wall of the shunt.

Aortopulmonary collaterals

When the pulmonary arteries have failed to develop the lungs are supplied by collateral vessels from the aorta. These vessels are prone to stenoses developing with associated progressive reduction in pulmonary blood flow, with worsening cyanosis and exercise tolerance.[17] The vessels are often extremely thick walled and elasticity is common, although in some cases they cannot be dilated even with high pressure balloons. It is wise to ensure the stenosis is dilatable by simple ballooning before proceeding to stenting, which may be required to maintain an effective increase in blood flow.[18]

1. **Wisselink W, Money SR, Becker O,** *et al.* Comparison of operative and percutaneous balloon dilatation for central venous obstruction. *Am J Surg* 1993;**166**:200–4.

2. **Bu'Lock FA, Tometzki AJ, Kitchener DJ,** *et al.* Balloon expandable stents for systemic venous pathway stenosis late after Mustard's operation. *Heart* 1998;**79**:225–9.
 • *Good results in terms of angiographic improvement after stent implantation, and the risks appear to be low. In some patients the stenosis was detected only on routine late angiography and there is controversy over the place of stent implantation in asymptomatic patients (see below).*

3. **Rosenthal E, Qureshi SA.** Stenting of systemic venous pathways after atrial repair for complete transposition. *Heart* 1998;**79**:211–12.
 • *A useful overview of the subject, highlighting that indications to intervene are not clear cut.*

4. **Driscoll DJ, Hesslein PS, Mullins CE.** Congenital stenosis of individual pulmonary veins: clinical spectrum and unsuccessful treatment by transvenous balloon dilatation. *Am J Cardiol* 1982;**49**:1767–72.

5. **Cullen S, Ho SY, Shore D,** *et al.* Congenital stenosis of pulmonary veins: failure to modify natural history by intraoperative placements of stents. *Cardiology in the Young* 1994;**4**:395–8.

6. **Beitzke A, Stein JL, Suppan C.** Balloon atrial septostomy under two dimensional echocardiographic control. *Int J Cardiol* 1991;**30**:33–42.
 • *44 newborns all had successful septostomies under echo control. This, and other reports like it, led to most centres abandoning the catheter laboratory for neonatal septostomy.*

7. **Thanopoulos BD, Georgakopoulos D, Tsaousis GS,** *et al.* Percutaneous balloon dilatation of the atrial septum: immediate and midterm results. *Heart* 1996;**76**:502–6.

8. **Park SC, Neches WH, Mullins CE,** *et al.* Blade atrial septostomy: collaborative study. *Circulation* 1982;**66**:258–66.

9. **Kerstein D, Lew PS, Hsu DT,** *et al.* Blade balloon atrial septostomy in patients with severe primary pulmonary hypertension. *Circulation* 1995;**91**:2028–35.
 • *15 children and adults with advanced primary pulmonary hypertension, with either syncopal attacks or right heart failure. After blade septostomy cardiac output increased and there appeared to be a benefit in survival too, when compared with approximately matched patients who had conventional treatment. There were two procedural deaths, one before the septostomy was performed and one because of massive desaturation after a single pass of the blade, not surprising for such a sick group of patients.*

10. **Walsh KP, Sreeram N, Franks R,** *et al.* Balloon dilatation of the arterial duct in congenital heart disease. *Lancet* 1992;**339**:331–2.

11. **Abrams SE, Walsh KP, Diamond MJ,** *et al.* Radiofrequency thermal angioplasty maintains arterial duct patency: an experimental study. *Circulation* 1994;**90**:442–8.

12. **Gibbs JL, Wren C, Watterson KG,** *et al.* Stenting of the arterial duct combined with banding of the pulmonary arteries and atrial septectomy or septostomy: a new approach to palliation for the hypoplastic left heart syndrome. *Br Heart J* 1993;**69**:551–5.

13. **Ruiz CE, Gamra H, Zhang HP,** *et al.* Brief report: stenting of the ductus arteriosus as a bridge to cardiac transplantation in infants with the hypoplastic left heart syndrome. *N Engl J Med* 1993;**328**:1605–8.

14. **Gibbs JL, Rothman MT, Rees M,** *et al.* Stenting of the arterial duct: a new approach to palliation for pulmonary atresia. *Br Heart J* 1991;**67**:240–5.

15. **Marx GR, Allen HD, Ovitt TW,** *et al.* Balloon dilatation angioplasty of Blalock-Taussig shunts. *Am J Cardiol* 1988;**62**:824–7.

16. **McLeod K, Blackburn MEC, Gibbs JL.** Enlargement of a classical Blalock Taussig shunt by implantation of a stent after failed balloon angioplasty. *Cardiology in the Young* 1994;**4**:411–12.

17. **Brown SC, Eyskens B, Mertens L,** *et al.* Percutaneous treatment of stenosed major aortopulmonary collaterals with balloon dilatation and stenting: what can be achieved? *Heart* 1998;**79**:24–8.
 • *12 patients with 25 stenosed collaterals. Encouraging increase in oxygen saturation in the majority. Notable that some stenoses improved with ballooning alone, some were undilatable even with very high pressure balloons, and one patient developed an aneurysm.*

18. **Redington AN, Somerville J.** Stenting of aortopulmonary collaterals in complex pulmonary atresia. *Circulation* 1996;**94**:2479–84.
 • *12 severely cyanosed patients, in whom stent implantation was possible in 11. Saturations as well as exercise duration increased. It is not clear how long the improvement will last, but anything that can help these very difficult patients is good news.*

195

SECTION VII: IMAGING TECHNIQUES

30 Myocardial perfusion imaging

Raymond J Gibbons

Non-invasive images of the myocardium that reflect myocardial perfusion can be obtained either by using conventional nuclear medicine radiopharmaceuticals and cameras or by positron emission tomography (PET). This review will focus on myocardial perfusion imaging using conventional approaches; a subsequent article in this series will focus on PET.

Imaging fundamentals

Comprehensive reviews of imaging fundamentals and procedures are available.[1][2] The two most commonly used isotopes for myocardial perfusion imaging are thallium-201 and technetium-99m. Thallium-201 is generated by a cyclotron. It is then transported as a finished product to the location where it is used, which is feasible because it has a half life of 73 hours. The isotope decays by a reasonably complex scheme, but most of the photons have an energy of about 80 keV, which is a low energy. Technetium-99m is bound to other compounds for the purposes of myocardial perfusion imaging. It is formed on site by elution from a molybdenum-99 generator. Technetium-99m is a meta-stable compound which is constantly formed from molybdenum-99 within the generator. Technetium-99m has a half life of about six hours, and emits photons with a 140 keV energy. This energy is much higher than the emissions of thallium, but much lower than the 511 keV emissions of PET radiopharmaceuticals. The differences in physical properties between thallium-201 and technetium-99m are relevant to the choice of radiopharmaceutical, which will be discussed later.

Both thallium-201 and technetium-99m radiopharmaceuticals are most commonly imaged using single photon emission computed tomography (SPECT). This technique employs many of the same back projection techniques that have been applied to conventional radiographs for CT scanning. Although multiple view planar images were first employed for myocardial perfusion imaging, they have been largely replaced by SPECT, which is superior from the standpoint of localisation, quantification, and image quality. Regardless of the radiopharmaceutical used, SPECT imaging is performed at rest and during stress to produce images of myocardial regional uptake that reflect relative regional myocardial blood flow. During maximal exercise or vasodilator stress, myocardial blood flow is typically increased three- to fivefold compared to rest. In the presence of a significant coronary stenosis, myocardial perfusion will not increase appropriately in the territory supplied by the artery with the stenosis, creating heterogeneous uptake. In patients who are unable to exercise, either one of the two coronary vasodilators, adenosine or dipyridamole, may be used to increase blood flow. Asthma, or chronic lung disease with a significant bronchospastic component, is a contraindication to the use of either one of these two agents. In such circumstances, dobutamine is used as an alternative, although it does not increase blood flow to the same degree.

Thallium-201 is a potassium analogue that is taken up by viable myocardial cells in direct proportion to coronary blood flow. The initial thallium injection is performed at peak stress, when hypoperfused myocardium will have less uptake than myocardium with normal perfusion. Over the next few hours "redistribution" of thallium occurs as a result of a fairly complex process. Thallium will wash out of the myocardium at a rate dependent on local myocardial perfusion. At the same time, thallium will be redelivered to the myocardium from a large reservoir in the blood pool. The final result of this process is that a region of ischaemic but viable myocardium which initially has less than normal uptake will become equal to normal regions over time. This "redistribution" is then detected on subsequent imaging. In contrast, areas of infarction or fibrosis will have reduced uptake initially that does not change over time. Reinjection of a small additional amount of thallium before acquisition of delayed images or repeat images after a longer delay of 24 hours may be used to enhance the detection of ischaemic but viable myocardium.

Several technetium-99m labelled agents have been developed, including teboroxime, tetrofosmin, and sestamibi. Teboroxime has a very short myocardial retention time which requires very rapid imaging. This practical limitation has limited its use. Sestamibi is the most studied of these agents, and is currently the most widely used. Tetrofosmin was developed after sestamibi and has been the subject of far fewer studies. Either tetrofosmin or sestamibi distribute to the myocardium in relation to blood flow. Their uptake requires a viable myocardial cell and an intact cell membrane. Both of these agents have far less redistribution than thallium, as they are bound within the myocardial cell in a nearly irreversible fashion. As a result, they must be injected twice, once at rest, and once during stress. Uptake on the resting injection will reflect relative resting blood flow to areas of viable myocardium.

A variety of different imaging protocols have been employed with thallium-201 and technetium-99m agents in order to optimise the detection of ischaemia and infarction. These are discussed below.

Clinical applications

Although myocardial perfusion imaging can be used in a wide variety of clinical settings, this review will focus on its primary application in adults with coronary artery disease. SPECT perfusion imaging may be used in patients with known or suspected stable angina for the purposes of both diagnosis and risk stratification. It may be employed in patients with acute ischaemic syndromes (unstable angina/ myocardial infarction) for acute triage as well as risk stratification.

Diagnosis of stable angina
Patients with known or suspected stable angina have been the subject of clinical practice guidelines issued by the British Cardiac Society[3] and jointly by the American College of Cardiology and the American Heart Association.[4] The interested reader is referred to these documents for a more comprehensive description of the evaluation and treatment of this clinical problem. SPECT myocardial perfusion imaging is often useful for the diagnosis of coronary artery disease in such patients. It should be used selectively as part of a careful strategy that begins with a clinical estimation of the likelihood of significant coronary artery disease on the basis of the patient's history of chest pain, risk factor assessment, and physical examination.

The proper choice of non-invasive tests should carefully consider the patient's ability to exercise and the resting ECG. In patients who are able to exercise, the exercise ECG is the preferred initial diagnostic test in most patients. However, there are important patient subsets in whom SPECT myocardial perfusion imaging is preferred. Exercise SPECT myocardial perfusion imaging is preferred in patients with > 1 mm ST depression or pre-excitation syndrome on their resting ECG, because of the reduced specificity of additional ST depression in these circumstances. Exercise SPECT myocardial perfusion imaging is also preferred in patients who have undergone percutaneous transluminal coronary angioplasty (PTCA) or coronary artery bypass grafting (CABG), be-

---

Stress SPECT perfusion imaging as the initial test for the diagnosis of coronary artery disease

- $\geq$ 1 mm ST depression at rest

- Pre-excitation (Wolff-Parkinson-White) syndrome

- Prior revascularisation (PTCA/CABG)

- Left bundle branch block

- Ventricular pacing

- Unable to exercise

- (Possibly) left ventricular hypertrophy or digoxin use with < 1 mm ST depression at rest

---

cause of its superior ability to localise ischaemia, and its increased sensitivity in patients with one vessel coronary artery disease. Patients with < 1 mm ST depression on their resting ECG, but with digoxin use or resting left ventricular hypertrophy, should also be considered for SPECT myocardial perfusion imaging, although the advantage of SPECT perfusion imaging in such patients is less well established. Patients with ventricular pacing or left bundle branch block should be assessed with SPECT perfusion imaging, as their exercise ECGs are uninterpretable. However, since these electrocardiographic abnormalities may cause perfusion defects during exercise stress in the absence of coronary artery disease, adenosine or dipyridamole SPECT perfusion imaging is preferred.[5] Adenosine or dipyridamole SPECT perfusion imaging is preferred in patients who are unable to exercise.

Multiple studies have examined the sensitivity and specificity for SPECT perfusion imaging for the detection of coronary artery disease. The reported sensitivity has generally ranged from 70–90%, and the reported specificity from 60–90%. These reports should be interpreted cautiously, as they do not reflect the effects of a type of bias called work up verification, or post-test referral, bias.[6] Such bias occurs whenever the results of a non-invasive test are used to decide which patients should have the diagnosis of coronary artery disease verified or ruled out by coronary angiography. Thus, patients with positive results on non-invasive tests are referred for coronary angiography, and patients with negative results are not. This selection process reduces the number of true negative results. The effect of this bias is to raise the measured sensitivity and lower the measured specificity in relation to their true values.

Risk stratification

SPECT perfusion imaging is also useful for the purpose of non-invasive risk stratification to identify patients who have the greatest risk for subsequent death and myocardial infarction.

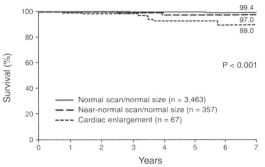

Figure 30.2. Cardiac survival in patients with intermediate risk exercise ECGs, subgrouped on the basis of their findings on perfusion imaging. The three subgroups shown—patients with normal perfusion scans and normal heart size; patients with near normal scans and normal heart size; and patients with cardiac enlargement—were significantly different from one another (p < 0.001). Both of the subgroups with normal heart size had a low risk of subsequent cardiac death, with an annual cardiac mortality of less than 0.5%. Reproduced from Gibbons *et al*[12] with permission of the American Heart Association.

High risk (> 3% annual mortality) features on stress SPECT perfusion imaging

- Post-stress ejection fraction < 35% (technetium-99m)

- Stress induced large perfusion defect

- Stress induced multiple perfusion defects of moderate size

- Large, fixed perfusion defect with left ventricular dilatation or increased lung uptake (thallium-201)

- Stress induced moderate perfusion defect with left ventricular dilatation or increased lung uptake (thallium-201)

Modified from ACC/AHA/ACP-ASIM guidelines for the management of patients with stable angina[3]

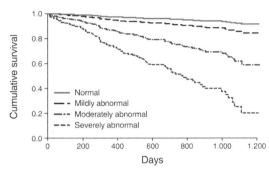

Figure 30.1. Cumulative survival in 5183 consecutive patients who underwent dual isotope (rest thallium-stress sestamibi) SPECT perfusion imaging as a function of the scan results. The rate of death increased significantly with worsening scan abnormalities. Reproduced from Hachamovitch *et al*. Incremental prognostic value of myocardial perfusion single photon emission computed tomography for the prediction of cardiac death. *Circulation* 1998;**97**:535, with permission of the American Heart Association.

As for diagnosis, perfusion imaging should be employed as part of a strategy which includes careful clinical assessment as well as a resting ECG. Normal stress SPECT myocardial perfusion images are highly predictive of a benign prognosis. Multiple studies involving thousands of patients followed for several years have found that a normal stress perfusion study is associated with a subsequent rate of cardiac death and myocardial infarction of less than 1% per year, which is nearly as low as that of the general population.[7] Although the published data are limited, the only exceptions would appear to be patients with normal perfusion images in the presence of either a high risk treadmill ECG score or severe resting left ventricular dysfunction.

In contrast, several different abnormal findings on stress SPECT perfusion imaging have been associated with severe coronary artery disease, and subsequent cardiac events. Large stress induced perfusion defects,[8] as well as defects in multiple coronary artery territories, are adverse prognostic signs (fig 30.1). Transient post-stress ischaemic left ventricular dilatation is also associated with an adverse prognosis.[9] In patients studied with thallium-201, increased lung uptake on postexercise or pharmacologic stress images is an indicator of stress induced global dysfunction, and it provides independent and incremental prognostic information compared to clinical, elec-

trocardiographic, and catheterisation data.[10] The results of SPECT perfusion imaging can be used to identify a "high risk" patient subset. These patients, who have a greater than 3% annual mortality rate, should be considered for early coronary angiography, as their prognosis may be improved by revascularisation.[11]

SPECT perfusion imaging is also of proven utility in selected situations following treadmill exercise testing. Patients with an intermediate risk treadmill score comprise between a third and two thirds of all patients undergoing exercise ECG testing. Approximately 50% of such patients will have normal or near normal images on exercise SPECT perfusion imaging. The subsequent cardiac event rate in these patients is extremely low, and coronary angiography is not warranted[12] (fig 30.2).

Acute ischaemic syndromes

Triage of acute chest pain

The emergency department evaluation of patients with chest pain but without electrocardiographic ST elevation is challenging. Although serum markers and transient ST depression may help to identify a subset of patients who clearly merit hospital admission, many patients with an intermediate risk of short term cardiac events will lack these findings. Hospital admission rates for such patients, who consume a large amount of health care resources, vary widely. A variety of different chest pain unit triage systems have been developed. Myocardial perfusion imaging is an integral part of many of these. One of the largest reported series performed resting SPECT sestamibi imaging as part of a comprehensive strategy that relied on initial clinical assessment and ECG findings to categorise the patients into one of five levels of risk.[13] Gated rest sestamibi imaging was performed on all patients assigned to two of these five levels. More than 75% of these patients had normal SPECT perfusion images and were discharged home without adverse events. The quarter of patients with abnormal images were admitted to the hospital, and had a significant rate of death and myocardial infarction in the ensuing year. A large, multicentre trial (ERASE chest pain), which utilises a similar strategy, is currently underway with results expected shortly.

Although the early results from these studies are certainly promising, it must be recognised that emergency department imaging is not universally available and is often associated with potential patient delays. A strategy using SPECT perfusion imaging is less useful in patients with prior myocardial infarction, and more costly than strategies based on treadmill exercise testing, which have also yielded positive results.[14] Most importantly, these strategies should use SPECT perfusion imaging selectively on the basis of clinical and electrocardiographic findings, rather than in an indiscriminate fashion for all patients.

Risk stratification as part of a clinical management strategy

Several randomised trials have examined the utility of SPECT perfusion imaging as part of a non-invasive or conservative strategy to risk stratify patients in order to decide which are candidates for coronary angiography and invasive treatment. The TIMI IIIb trial randomised 1473 patients with non-Q wave myocardial infarction or unstable angina to an early invasive strategy, using coronary angiography or an early conservative strategy which reserved coronary angiography for patients with recurrent ischaemia or an abnormal stress thallium test.[15] The combined end point of death, myocardial infarction, or ischaemia on a treadmill performed six weeks later showed no difference between the two strategies.

Subsequently, the VANQWISH trial randomised 920 patients with non-Q wave myocardial infarction to an early invasive strategy using coronary angiography and an early conservative strategy that utilised stress thallium imaging to select patients for coronary angiography.[16] There was again no significant difference in outcome between the two strategies, and all cause mortality was actually slightly lower in patients in the conservative strategy group (fig 30.3). On the basis of both of these randomised trials, stress SPECT perfusion imaging would appear to have great utility for the non-invasive assessment of patients with unstable angina and non-Q wave myocardial infarction. The advantages of such a conservative strategy are further reinforced by data from the OASIS registry,[17] which found that early coronary angiography was more prevalent in institutions and countries where catheterisation laboratories were available. This increased rate of catheterisation did not reduce the rate of subsequent death or myocardial infarction, but did lead to an increased incidence of stroke.

Myocardial viability

SPECT perfusion imaging is often used to evaluate the possible contribution of ischaemia

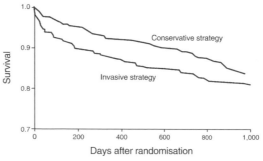

Figure 30.3. Survival of patients in the VANQWISH trial, as a function of randomisation to the invasive strategy (early coronary angiography) or the conservative strategy (selective coronary angiography using perfusion imaging). There was no significant difference in outcome comparing the two strategies. (Reproduced from Boden *et al*[6] with the permission of the Massachusetts Medical Society.)

to ventricular dysfunction. The detection of viable myocardium—either stunned or hibernating—in such cases implies that revascularisation will lead to improved regional and global function.

The presence of stress induced ischaemia has long been recognised as a highly specific indicator of viable myocardium. However, because its sensitivity was clearly less than 100%, the criteria to detect viable myocardium were eventually expanded to include "fixed" defects—that is, those without evidence of stress induced ischaemia, on resting (technetium-99m) or redistribution (thallium-201) images that were only mild to moderate in severity.[18] Despite these expanded definitions, and a wide variety of imaging protocols (see below), SPECT imaging has a slightly lower sensitivity than PET for the detection of stunned or hibernating myocardium. Although some recent studies have suggested that the specificity (and positive predictive value) of SPECT perfusion imaging is as low as 50%, these estimates are probably erroneously low because of the effect of post-test referral bias. Although the redistribution of thallium-201 can potentially detect ischaemia at rest, which technetium-99m cannot, the prevalence of this finding, and its overall clinical significance, are not well established. In most patients, resting thallium-201 and technetium-99m images provide similar information (fig 30.4).

Controversies

Stress echocardiography or stress SPECT

Both stress echocardiography and stress myocardial perfusion imaging are feasible and effective alternatives to treadmill exercise testing in suitable patients. As indicated previously, imaging studies should be used selectively in patients who will benefit most from the technology, which is associated with considerable additional expense. Both stress echocardiography and stress SPECT imaging studies have advantages and disadvantages. The choice between the two tests depends on many factors, including these relative advantages and disadvantages, the individual patient, local expertise, and the anticipated impact of an

Figure 30.4.
Comparison of segmental activity on a resting technetium-99m sestamibi scan with segmental activity on the redistribution image from a resting thallium-201 scan in segments with abnormal contractile function. There was a significant correlation ($r = 0.78$) between segmental activity on the two scans, although there was some variability. More importantly, activity in those segments with dysfunction which improved after revascularisation generally exceeded 60% of peak counts on both scans. In contrast, dysfunctional segments that did not improve following revascularisation, presumably because they were fibrotic, generally had activity at less than 60% of peak counts on both scans. Reproduced from Udelson *et al*. Predicting recovery of severe regional ventricular dysfunction. Comparison of resting scintigraphy with thallium-201 and technetium-99m sestamibi. *Circulation* 1994;**89**:2552, with permission of the American Heart Association.

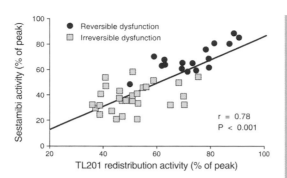

Relative advantages of thallium-201 and technetium-99m

- Thallium
  - lower cost
  - greater evidence base
  - assessment of lung uptake
  - less bowel/liver uptake
  - detection of ischaemia at rest

- Sestamibi
  - better images
  - assessment of left ventricular ejection fraction/regional function
  - better quantification
  - faster imaging protocols

Relative advantages of stress echocardiography and SPECT perfusion imaging

- Echocardiography
  - higher specificity
  - availability/convenience
  - structural/valvar evaluation
  - lower cost

- SPECT
  - higher sensitivity
  - higher success rate
  - better evaluation of ischaemia in presence of regional dysfunction
  - greater evidence base

Modified from ACC/AHA/ACP-ASIM guidelines for the management of patients with stable angina[3]

imaging study on clinical decision making. Ongoing technical developments related to both techniques should lead to improved diagnostic accuracy.

Choice of radiopharmaceutical

Both thallium-201 and technetium-99m based perfusion agents are widely available. Although some laboratories have chosen to use one or the other exclusively, the clinician is often faced with a choice between the two. Most of the advantages of technetium-99m perfusion agents have been better established for sestamibi, although they should also theoretically apply equally well to tetrofosmin. In general, the better image quality and ventricular function assessment that is achieved with technetium-99m perfusion agents are the most important considerations, and account for the increasing use of these agents in most nuclear cardiology laboratories.

Choice of imaging protocol

Laboratories which employ thallium-201 generally use one of three protocols. The traditional protocol involves stress imaging, redistribution imaging three or four hours later, and, when necessary, delayed imaging approximately 24 hours later to evaluate fixed defects. The most common modification of this protocol involves performance of the optional delayed images on the same day following a reinjection of a small amount of thallium in patients with fixed defects. The third thallium protocol is commonly used by large volume laboratories. The three to four hour redistribution images are only performed after reinjec-

tion of a small amount of thallium. Delayed imaging at 24 hours is still performed when necessary. Thus, all of these three protocols involve stress and delayed images with a third set of images in a subset of patients.

Laboratories which employ sestamibi generally use one of four different protocols. The original protocol developed for technetium-99m perfusion agents involve two injections of radiopharmaceutical—one at rest and one during stress—on different days. For patient convenience, this was subsequently modified to perform both studies on the same day by using a low dose for the first study and a high dose for the second study. The sequence of images may be either rest-stress, which is the most common, or stress-rest. The fourth protocol is the so called "dual isotope" protocol, in which thallium imaging is first performed following resting injection. The technetium-99m based perfusion agent is then injected during stress testing, which follows immediately thereafter, and subsequently imaged. Each of these protocols has its proponents, who usually emphasise the practical logistical consequences, as the available scientific evidence has not established the clear superiority of any one of these protocols.

Any one of these protocols may be used to detect stress induced ischaemia (and therefore myocardial viability), which is usually sufficient for clinical decision making. In an occasional patient with known severe coronary artery disease and significant left ventricular dysfunction, only resting imaging may be required in order to demonstrate normal or near normal uptake of either radiopharmaceutical (and therefore viability) in dysfunctional regions that are presumed to be ischaemic.

Technical developments

There are a number of newer technical developments that are already available or proposed for SPECT imaging. Gating of SPECT images is now widely available, and software for processing the images is available on most camera systems.[19] The increased cost and logistical difficulty of gating are generally felt to be justified by the ability to measure ejection fraction and to assess regional wall motion. The assessment of regional wall motion is primarily helpful in the case of mild fixed defects to make certain that they represent diaphragmatic or breast attenuation. A careful review of the literature suggests that the actual percentage of cases whose interpretation is modified is small.[20]

Attenuation of the diaphragm, breast, or other soft tissue is a major limitation of SPECT imaging with either thallium-201 or technetium-99m, although it is more pronounced with the former, because of its lower energy emission. Although systems for attenuation correction are now available on several commercial camera systems, they have not yet proven to be of clear benefit. Further developments in this regard are anticipated.

Differences in image reconstruction involving iterative processes have been proposed to replace back projection. They may help to address the problem of extracardiac activity which sometimes reduces the quality of technetium-99m images. Partial volume effects and "balanced ischaemia" (a near uniform reduction in flow that is not detected by a relative flow technique) are occasionally significant limitations of SPECT perfusion images with no definitive solution on the horizon.

I thank Professor Paolo Camici for his review and critique of this article.

1. **Maddahi J.** Myocardial perfusion imaging for the detection and evaluation of coronary artery disease. In: Marcus ML, Schelbert HR, Skorton DJ, *et al*, eds. Cardiac imaging—principles and practice, 2nd ed. Philadelphia: WB Saunders, 1996.
   • *An excellent, comprehensive book chapter detailing the usefulness of myocardial perfusion imaging.*

2. **O'Connor MK, Miller TD, Christian TF,** *et al.* Cardiovascular system. In: O'Connor MK, ed. *The Mayo Clinic manual of nuclear medicine.* New York: Churchill Livingstone, 1996.
   • *This book chapter, based on the Mayo Clinic laboratory procedure manual, provides a step by step practical guide to the performance of radionuclide angiography and perfusion imaging.*

3. **Gibbons RJ, Chatterjee K, Daley J,** *et al.* ACC/AHA/ACP-ASIM guidelines for the management of patients with chronic stable angina: a report of the American College of Cardiology/American Heart Association task force on practice guidelines (committee on the management of patients with chronic stable angina). *J Am Coll Cardiol* 1999;**33**:2092–197.
   • *A detailed, lengthy, evidence based set of practice guidelines which represent a joint effort of the two major American cardiology organisations and the largest American internal medicine organisation. This is the first set of national guidelines on this topic issued in the United States.*

4. **de Bono D.** Investigation and management of stable angina: revised guidelines 1998. Joint working party of the British Cardiac Society and Royal College of Physicians of London. *Heart* 1999;**81**:546–55.
   • *A succinct set of guidelines for the evaluation and management of patients with stable angina.*

5. **O'Keefe JH Jr, Bateman TM, Barnhart CS.** Adenosine thallium-201 is superior to exercise thallium-201 for detecting coronary artery disease in patients with left bundle branch block. *J Am Coll Cardiol* 1993;**21**:1332–8.

6. **Roger VL, Pellikka PA, Bell MR,** *et al.* Sex and test verification bias: impact on the diagnostic value of exercise echocardiography. *Circulation* 1997;**95**:405–10.
   • *A landmark study from the Mayo Clinic echocardiography laboratory demonstrating the impact of post-test referral bias on the measurement of sensitivity and specificity. The authors used two different methods to correct for referral bias, which both demonstrate that the true sensitivity of exercise echocardiography is less than 50%.*

7. **Brown KA.** Prognostic value of thallium-201 myocardial perfusion imaging: a diagnostic tool comes of age. *Circulation* 1991;**83**:363–81.
   • *A classic review article detailing the published literature on the prognostic value of thallium-201 perfusion imaging in patients with known or suspected coronary artery disease, after myocardial infarction, or for preoperative risk stratification.*

8. **Hachamovitch R, Berman DS, Kiat H,** *et al.* Exercise myocardial perfusion SPECT in patients without known coronary artery disease. Incremental prognostic value and use in risk stratification. *Circulation* 1996;**93**:905–14.

9. **Krawczynska EG, Weintraub WS, Garcia EV,** *et al.* Left ventricular dilatation and multivessel coronary artery disease on thallium-201 SPECT are important prognostic indicators in patients with large defects in the left anterior descending distribution. *Am J Cardiol* 1994;**74**:1233–9.

10. **Pollock SG, Abbott RD, Boucher CA,** *et al.* Independent and incremental prognostic value of tests performed in hierarchical order to evaluate patients with suspected coronary artery disease: validation of models based on these tests. *Circulation* 1992;**85**:237–40.
    • *A rigorous analysis of the incremental value of stress induced ischaemia and increased lung:heart ratio on thallium-201 myocardial perfusion imaging. The authors demonstrate that lung:heart ratio contributes significantly to prognostic models even after adjustment for all known clinical, exercise, and catheterisation information.*

11. **Yusuf S, Zucker D, Peduzzi P,** *et al.* Effect of coronary artery bypass graft surgery on survival: overview of 10-year results from randomised trials by the coronary artery bypass graft surgery trialists collaboration [published erratum appears in *Lancet* 1994;**344**:1446]. *Lancet* 1994;**344**:563–70.
    • *A rigorous meta-analysis of all the randomised trials comparing coronary artery bypass graft surgery with medical treatment. This analysis demonstrates that the patients for whom surgery reduces mortality are those in whom the annual mortality with medical treatment is highest. In contrast, "low risk" patients on medical treatment (< 1% annual mortality) do not derive any mortality benefit from coronary artery bypass grafting.*

12. **Gibbons RJ, Hodge DO, Berman DS,** *et al.* Long-term outcome of patients with intermediate-risk exercise electrocardiograms who do not have myocardial perfusion defects on radionuclide imaging. *Circulation* 1999;**100**:2140–5.

13. **Tatum JL, Jesse RL, Kontos MC,** *et al.* Comprehensive strategy for the evaluation and triage of the chest pain patient. *Ann Emerg Med* 1997;**29**:116–25.

14. **Farkouh ME, Smars PA, Reeder GS,** *et al.* A clinical trial of a chest-pain observation unit for patients with unstable angina. Chest pain evaluation in the emergency room (CHEER) investigators. *N Engl J Med* 1998;**339**:1882–8.
    • *A randomised trial of a chest pain observation unit in 424 patients with intermediate-risk unstable angina. Patients randomised to the chest pain unit were observed carefully for six hours prior to stress testing. The chest pain unit resulted in fewer hospitalisations, less resource use, and no increase in the rate of subsequent cardiac events.*

15. **TIMI IIIB Investigators.** Effects of tissue plasminogen activator and a comparison of early invasive and conservative strategies in unstable angina and non-Q wave myocardial infarction. Results of the TIMI IIIB trial. *Circulation* 1994;**89**:1545–56.

16. **Boden WE, O'Rourke RA, Crawford MH,** *et al.* Outcomes in patients with acute non-Q-wave myocardial infarction randomly assigned to an invasive as compared with a conservative management strategy. Veterans Affairs non-Q-wave infarction strategies in hospital (VANQWISH) trial investigators [published erratum appears in *N Engl J Med* 1998;**339**:1091]. *N Engl J Med* 1998;**338**:1785–92.

17. **Yusuf S, Flather M, Pogue J,** *et al.* Variations between countries in invasive cardiac procedures and outcomes in patients with suspected unstable angina or myocardial infarction without initial ST elevation. OASIS (organization to assess strategies for ischaemic syndromes) registry investigators. *Lancet* 1998;**352**:507–14.

18. **Bonow RO, Dilsizian V, Cuocolo A,** *et al.* Identification of viable myocardium in patients with chronic coronary artery disease and left ventricular dysfunction. Comparison of thallium scintigraphy with reinjection and PET imaging with 18F-fluorodeoxyglucose. *Circulation* 1991;**83**:26–37.
    • *Landmark article comparing thallium perfusion imaging and positron emission tomography (PET) in the identification of viable myocardium. Thallium defects that were irreversible on exercise-redistribution imaging were almost always viable by PET if the reduction in thallium activity was only mild or moderate. Thallium reinjection identified viability in approximately half of the irreversible defects with a severe reduction in thallium activity; the results were concordant with PET in 88% of these segments.*

19. **Chua T, Kiat H, Germano G,** *et al.* Gated technetium-99m sestamibi for simultaneous assessment of stress myocardial perfusion, post-exercise regional ventricular function and myocardial viability. Correlation with echocardiography and rest thallium-201 scintigraphy. *J Am Coll Cardiol* 1994;**23**:1107–14.

20. **DePuey EG, Rozanski A.** Using gated technetium-99m-sestamibi SPECT to characterize fixed myocardial defects as infarct or artifact. *J Nucl Med* 1995;**36**:952–5.
    • *Systematic evaluation of the impact of gating on the interpretation of sestamibi SPECT images in 551 consecutive patients. The authors emphasised the reclassification of fixed defects on the basis of the results of gated SPECT. Careful tabulation of the data shows that a total of 22 patients, or 4%, had their perfusion images interpreted differently on the basis of the results of gating.*

website extra

Additional references appear on the Heart website

www.heartjnl.com

31 Positron emission tomography and myocardial imaging

Paolo G Camici

Imaging with positron emission tomography (PET) offers unrivalled sensitivity and specificity for research into biochemical pathways and pharmacological mechanisms in vivo. Cardiac and neurological research with PET has flourished over the past 20 years, but it is only more recently that cardiology has begun to benefit from the advantages provided by PET. From the physical point of view, scanning of the heart presents a challenge because of greater complications in correcting for photon attenuation and scattered radiation, and because of movement of the heart and lungs.

Methodological background

The success of PET is based on the properties of the isotopes used (table 31.1). Their short physical half lives make it possible to administer a tracer dose high enough to obtain useful data, but such that the radiation burden to the patient is acceptably low. Positron emitters do not exist in nature and they must be produced artificially by means of a particle accelerator (generally a cyclotron).[1] Production of isotopes with the shortest half lives has to be carried out in the vicinity of the scanner and necessitates the installation of cyclotron and radiochemistry facilities. However, ^{18}F compounds can be delivered from a relatively remote site of production. The commercial success of PET has been driven by ^{18}F labelled fluorodeoxyglucose (FDG) which is used to measure glucose metabolism in tissues. Because of the longer half life of ^{18}F (table 31.1), many centres rely on production from a centralised cyclotron, thus avoiding the expense of individual facilities. However, research centres aiming to derive most from the power of PET require on site production of a range of tracers.

Positron emission and detection

Positrons are emitted with a continuous range of energies up to a maximum, which is characteristic of each particular isotope (table 31.1). The positron is successively slowed down by Coulomb interaction with atomic electrons and "annihilates" with an electron when its energy has been reduced close to zero, resulting in a pair of photons flying off in opposite directions with an energy of 511 keV. Positrons emitted from a tracer injected into the body are not measured directly, but indirectly from the photons emitted when the positron annihilates with an electron (fig 31.1). Detectors placed on either side of the active volume are connected in a so called coincidence circuit so that if both detectors record an event within a very short interval (about 10^{-8} seconds), it is assumed that a positron annihilation has taken place.

Attenuation correction: a main feature of PET

The distance between the emitting atom and the point of annihilation depends on positron energy (table 31.1). This distance, together with the photon angular spread, "blur" the true tracer distribution slightly and, depending on the type of PET detector and the radioisotope used, can lower the resolution by 1–3 mm. This small loss of resolution, however, is relatively minor compared to the consequences of photon scattering. Photons of 511 keV travelling through a composite medium such as the thorax will be scattered by interaction with atomic electrons and undergo change of direction and loss of energy. If a photon is scattered it is "lost" to the original line of response (the

Unique features of PET

- Positron annihilation/coincidence detection
- Short physical half life/lower radiation dose to patients
- Attenuation correction
- Correction for partial volume effect
- Capability of making absolute measurements of tracer concentration
- Multiple physiological tracers

Table 31.1 Properties of isotopes used in PET imaging

| Isotope | Half life (min) | Positron energy (MeV) | | Mean range in tissue (mm) | Examples of labelled compounds |
		Mean	Maximum		
^{15}O	2.03	0.74	1.74	2.97	H$_2$^{15}O— blood flow ^{15}O$_2$—oxygen consumption C^{15}O—blood volume
^{13}N	10.0	0.49	1.20	1.73	^{13}NH$_3$—blood flow
^{11}C	20.4	0.39	0.97	1.23	^{11}C-HED—presynaptic catecholamine reuptake (uptake 1) ^{11}C-CGP 12177—β adrenoceptors ^{11}C-MQNB—muscarinic receptors ^{11}C-acetate—oxygen consumption
^{18}F	109.8	0.25	0.64	0.61	^{18}F-FDG—glucose metabolism ^{18}F-FDopa—dopamine storage

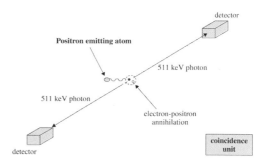

Figure 31.1. Physics of positron emission, annihilation, and coincidence detection. Adapted from Camici *et al.*[2]

line joining the two detectors depicted in fig 31.1), and the apparent radioactivity measured along that line of response will be reduced. This effect is known as "attenuation". Scatter and attenuation are problems common to all sorts of radionuclide imaging techniques and are responsible for most of the artifacts associated with single photon emission computed tomography (SPECT), particularly when low energy isotopes (for example, thallium-201) are used. In contrast to SPECT, correction for attenuation is relatively straightforward in PET because of the mechanism of coincidence detection. A radioactive source is placed in the detector field of view and measurements are taken with and without the inactive patient in position. The ratio of counts recorded for the two situations gives the total attenuation factor.[2]

Partial volume effect

The partial volume effect occurs whenever the dimensions of the object to be imaged are comparable to the resolution of the camera. Although the detector will accurately record the total activity in the object, it will distribute it over an area larger than the actual size of the object. Hence, the detected concentration of activity per unit volume will be less than the actual value. In PET (or SPECT) imaging, quantification of radionuclide concentration is complicated by partial volume effects caused by the small thickness of the ventricular wall relative to the spatial resolution of the cameras and the motion of the heart. In addition, because of the changes in wall thickness throughout the cardiac cycle, the recovery coefficient (the radioactivity concentration recorded relative to the actual concentration) will vary. The partial volume effect is therefore particularly important in patients with coronary artery disease who have regional motion abnormalities and thinning of the left ventricular walls.[3] A number of strategies have been developed to correct for it.

Tomographs and data acquisition

The earliest tomographs consisted of a single ring of detectors with thick lead shielding on either side to stop photons arising from outside the plane of the ring (which can only yield random or scattered coincidences). Most PET scanners consist of bismuth germanate detectors. The 511 keV photons have a high probability of being stopped by this high density material and then giving up their energy. This energy is transformed into visible light (scintillation) which is amplified by a photomultiplier tube, just as in a conventional nuclear medicine gamma camera. Data acquisition in such systems is organised as a series of planes or slices through the patient. A detector can also be in coincidence with detectors in other rings of a multi-ring scanner. Conventionally, the raw data are formatted into matrices known as sinograms, each element of which contains the number of events ("counts") recorded in each line of response. Each row of the sinogram represents a one dimensional view (or projection) of the patient at a given

angle and the sinogram encompasses all angles around the patient. The standard process of image reconstruction extrapolates or back-projects the projection data into the "image space" (field of view) of the tomograph, as well as applying a spatial frequency filter to remove blurring.[1 2]

Most PET scanners operate in frame mode where a number of (usually) contiguous time frames are defined before acquisition commences. Frame lengths are chosen to try to accommodate the varying kinetic components at different times after injection. However, especially with rapidly decaying tracers (such as ^{15}O and ^{11}C), it is more efficient to store each event separately in list mode. List mode acquisition offers data of the highest possible temporal resolution which can be: (1) subsequently rebinned into different frame sequences, as desired, for image reconstruction; and (2) partitioned into different gates on the basis of cardiac and respiratory signals to reduce motion artifacts caused by cardiac and respiratory movement.

Positron labelled tracers

A tracer is a measurable substance used to mimic, follow or trace a chemical compound or process without disturbing the process under study. In the case of PET this is made possible by: (1) the high sensitivity of PET imaging which enables the measurement of radio-labelled tracers administered in picomolar concentrations which are sufficiently low so as not to disturb the processes under study; and (2) the ability of current cameras to perform rapid dynamic imaging—that is, to provide good temporal resolution. Positron emitting radionuclides are incorporated into tracers by rapid radiochemical procedures. These can be administered to subjects either by intravenous injection or by inhalation. The tracer substitutes for the natural or endogenous substrate and gives information on the cellular pathway that would have been followed by that substrate.

From counts to physiological parameters

After administration of a known amount of the tracer, its myocardial and arterial concentrations can be measured as a function of time using the PET camera. Measurement of the radiotracer concentration in arterial blood can be made from regions of interest positioned in either the left atrium or ventricle and provide information on the supply of tracer to the myocardium over the time course of the PET study. This measurement is termed the "arterial input function". The myocardial uptake of the tracer over time is termed the "tissue response" and can also be determined from analysis of the PET images. The tissue response to an arterial input function can be quantified using a tracer kinetic model, which describes the dynamic biological behaviour of the tracer in tissue in mathematical terms. These kinetic models are based upon careful validation in animal studies utilising both in vitro and in vivo models. The application of these models to the raw data allows transformation of the initial radioactivity

Cardiac applications of PET

- Myocardial blood flow

- Free fatty acid, glucose, and oxygen metabolism

- Identification of hibernating myocardium

- Cardiac autonomic function:
  –postsynaptic β adrenoceptors
  –presynaptic nerve terminals
  –cholinergic receptors

measurements (counts) into absolute units (for example, myocardial blood flow in ml/minute per gram of tissue). This ability to provide accurate measurements per unit mass of tissue is a major advantage of PET imaging.

Applications of PET to cardiology

There has been much discussion about the dual roles of "research" and "clinical" PET. A number of centres have installed PET systems purely for clinical diagnosis, mainly in the determination of myocardial viability, but also for applications in oncology and neurology. Diagnostic testing of this kind is clearly derived from original work carried out at research establishments. The terms "research" and "clinical" should, therefore, be regarded as complementary. In the author's institution the balance between research and diagnosis is approximately 80% versus 20%.

Myocardial blood flow

Oxygen-15 labelled water ($H_2^{15}O$) and nitrogen-13 labelled ammonia ($^{13}NH_3$) are the tracers most widely used for the quantification of regional myocardial blood flow with PET. Tracer kinetic models have been successfully validated in animals against the radiolabelled microsphere method over a wide flow range for both $H_2^{15}O$ and $^{13}NH_3$.[4] Assessments of myocardial blood flow in normal volunteers using either tracer at rest or during pharmacologically induced coronary vasodilatation are similar (table 31.2).[5] $H_2^{15}O$ is theoretically superior to $^{13}NH_3$ in that water is a metabolically inert and freely diffusible tracer which has a virtually

complete myocardial extraction independent of both flow rate and myocardial metabolic state.[4] On the other hand, the quality of myocardial $^{13}NH_3$ images is superior to that of $H_2^{15}O$. Both tracers have short physical half lives (table 31.1) which allow repeat measurements of myocardial blood flow in the same session.

Before the advent of PET technology, investigations of regional coronary blood flow in man were restricted to measurements in the epicardial coronary arteries. However, it is well established that the major regulatory site of tissue perfusion is at the level of the microcirculation which is not amenable to catheterisation.[4] With the development of quantitative myocardial blood flow measurement using PET, it is possible to challenge the function of the coronary microvasculature by measuring the coronary vasodilator reserve (CVR), calculated as the ratio of near maximal flow during pharmacologically induced coronary vasodilatation to baseline flow. PET studies in healthy human volunteers have established that CVR in response to intravenous dipyridamole or adenosine is 3.5–4.0 (fig 31.2A) (table 31.2).[5] These data are similar to those reported using the Doppler catheter technique for measuring epicardial coronary flow velocity.[4]

Use of PET in normal volunteers has highlighted the effects of age, sex, and alteration in sympathetic tone on myocardial blood flow and CVR. Thus, it has been shown that myocardial blood flow at baseline and at hyperaemia remains relatively constant up to 60 years of age. Above this age, there is a significant increase in basal flow associated with an increase in systolic blood pressure and a significant reduction in hyperaemic myocardial blood flow and CVR.[6]

The measurement of CVR is useful for the assessment of the functional significance of coronary stenoses in patients with coronary artery disease (fig 31.3).[7] In addition, PET is particularly helpful in those circumstances where the CVR is diffusely (and not regionally) blunted, for example, hypertrophic cardiomyopathy or hypertensive heart disease caused by a widespread abnormality of the coronary microcirculation (fig 31.2B, C).[8] It may aid in the differentiation of pathological from physiological left ventricular hypertrophy and in the exclusion of myocardial ischaemia in patients with chest pain and angiographically normal

Table 31.2 PET measurements of myocardial blood flow in normal subjects

Author	Tracer	Agent	Number subjects	Age	MBF$_{bas}$	MBF$_{hyp}$	MBF$_{hyp/bas}$
Bergmann et al	$H_2^{15}O$	Dip	11	25	0.9 (0.2)	3.6 (1.2)	4.1 (1.2)
Geltman et al	$H_2^{15}O$	Dip	16	25 (4)	1.2 (0.3)	4.6 (1.6)	3.8 (1.1)
Camici et al	$^{13}NH_3$	Dip	12	51 (8)	1.0 (0.2)	2.7 (0.9)	2.9 (1.0)
Sambuceti et al	$^{13}NH_3$	Dip	14	49 (7)	1.1 (0.3	3.7 (0.8	3.6 (0.9
Chan et al	$^{13}NH_3$	Ado	20	35 (16)	1.1 (0.2)	4.4 (0.9)	4.4 (1.5)
Chan et al	$^{13}NH_3$	Dip	20	35 (16)	1.1 (0.2)	4.3 (1.3)	4.3 (1.9)
Araujo et al	$C^{15}O_2$	Dip	11	26 to 42	0.8 (0.1)	3.5 (1.1)	4.2 (1.2)
Merlet et al	$H_2^{15}O$	Dip	6	51 (5)	0.9 (0.1)	3.5 (0.8)	4.0 (0.7)
Muzik et al	$^{13}NH_3$	Ado	6	26 (3)	0.8 (0.2)	3.6 (1.0)	
Uren et al	$H_2^{15}O$	Dip/Ado	43	47 (20)	1.0 (0.2)	3.2 (1.3)	3.4 (1.3)
Radvan et al	$C^{15}O_2$	Dip	8	27 (5)	0.8 (0.2)	3.1 (08)	3.8 (0.8)
Czernin et al	$^{13}NH_3$	Dip	18	31 (9)	0.8 (0.2)	3.0 (0.8)	4.1 (0.9)
Czernin et al	$^{13}NH_3$	Dip	22	64 (9)	0.9 (0.3)	2.7 (0.6)	3.0 (0.7)

Ado, adenosine; Dip, dipyridamole; MBF$_{bas}$, baseline myocardial blood flow; MBF$_{hyp}$, hyperaemic myocardial blood flow; MBF$_{hyp/bas}$, coronary flow reserve. Data are mean (SD). Adapted from Camici et al.[5]

A

Normals

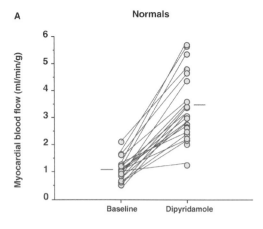

B

Hypertrophic cardiomyopathy

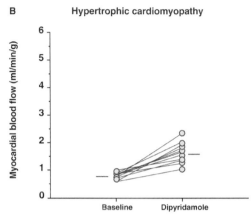

C

Left ventricular hypertrophy

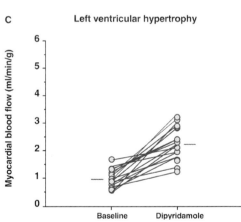

Figure 31.2. Myocardial blood flow under baseline conditions and during hyperaemia induced by intravenous dipyridamole in normal subjects (A), in patients with hypertrophic cardiomyopathy (B), and patients with left ventricular hypertrophy secondary to arterial hypertension or aortic stenosis (C). The diffuse blunting of flow reserve in these patients with angiographically normal coronary arteries is suggestive of widespread microvascular dysfunction. Adapted from Choudhury *et al.*[8]

$Y = 6.73 - 0.13x + 7.8x^2$ $r = 0.77$ (n = 35)

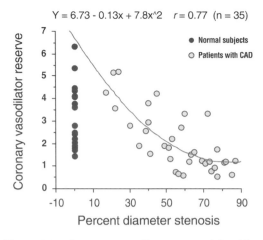

Figure 31.3. Coronary vasodilator reserve falls with increasing percent diameter stenosis and is exhausted for stenoses > 80%. Normal control values of coronary vasodilator reserve are shown at zero percent diameter stenosis on the left. CAD, coronary artery disease. Adapted from Uren *et al.*[7]

coronary arteries.[4][5] Finally, the improved spatial resolution of the latest generation of PET cameras means that there is now a realistic prospect of quantification of transmural distribution of myocardial blood flow.

Myocardial metabolism

The utilisation of exogenous glucose by the myocardium can be assessed using PET with the glucose analogue FDG.[1] FDG is transported into the myocyte by the same trans-sarcolemmal carrier as glucose and is then phosphorylated to FDG-6-phosphate by the enzyme hexokinase. This is essentially a unidirectional reaction and results in FDG-6-phosphate accumulation within the myocardium, as no glucose-6-phosphatase (the enzyme that hydrolyses FDG-6-phosphate back to free FDG and free phosphate) has yet been identified in cardiac muscle. Thus, measurement of the myocardial uptake of FDG is proportional to the overall rate of trans-sarcolemmal transport and hexokinase phosphorylation of exogenous (circulating) glucose by heart muscle.

A number of kinetic modelling approaches have been used for the quantitation of glucose utilisation rates using FDG.[1] The major limitation of these approaches is that quantification of glucose metabolism requires the knowledge of the lumped constant, a factor which relates the kinetic behaviour of FDG to naturally occurring glucose in terms of the relative affinity of each molecule for the trans-sarcolemmal transporter and for hexokinase. Unfortunately, the value of the lumped constant in humans under different physiological and pathophysiological conditions is not known, thus making precise in vivo quantification of myocardial metabolic rates of glucose practically impossible. Current measurements of the uptake of FDG (particularly if obtained under standardised conditions) allow comparison of absolute values from different individuals and may help to establish the absolute rates of glucose utilisation (in FDG units) in normal and pathologic myocardium.[9]

PET for the identification of hibernating myocardium

In the current era of coronary revascularisation and thrombolysis, it has become increasingly apparent that restoration of blood flow to asynergic myocardial segments may result in improved regional and global left ventricular function.[9-11] The greatest clinical benefit is seen in those patients with the most severe forms of dysfunction. Initial studies indicated that myocardial ischaemia and infarction could be distinguished by analysis of PET images of the perfusion tracer $^{13}NH_3$ and the glucose analogue FDG acquired after an oral glucose load. Regions which showed a concordant reduction in both myocardial blood flow and FDG uptake ("flow-metabolism match") were labelled as predominantly infarcted, whereas regions in which FDG uptake was relatively preserved or increased despite having a perfusion defect ("flow-metabolism mismatch") were considered to represent jeopardised viable myocardium.[12] The uptake of FDG by the myocardium, however, depends on many factors such as dietary state, cardiac workload, response of the tissue to insulin, sympathetic drive, and the presence and severity of ischaemia. These factors contribute to variability in FDG imaging in the fasted or glucose loaded state, confusing data interpretation

With the recent suggestion that semiquantitative and quantitative analyses of FDG uptake may enhance detection of viable myocardium, there was an urgent need to standardise the study conditions rigorously. Furthermore, many patients with coronary artery disease are insulin resistant—that is, the amount of endogenous insulin released after feeding will not induce maximal stimulation owing to partial resistance to the action of the hormone. This may result in poor FDG image quality after an oral glucose load. To circumvent the problem of insulin resistance, an alternative protocol has been recently applied to PET viability studies. The protocol is based on the use of the hyperinsulinaemic euglycacmic clamp—essentially the simultaneous infusion of insulin and glucose acting on the tissue as a "metabolic challenge" and stimulating maximal FDG uptake.[9] This leads to optimisation of image quality and cnables PET studies to be performed under standardised metabolic conditions, which allows comparison of the absolute values of the metabolic rate of glucose (μmol/g/min) among different subjects and centres (fig 31.4).

By comparing FDG images obtained under these conditions with regional wall motion information (derived from echocardiography or conventional radionuclide ventriculography), the need for a simultaneous flow scan is obviated. It is also possible to reduce the period of image acquisition to approximately 30 minutes, giving a total scan time of about an hour.

When to use PET for the identification of hibernation
Basically, three techniques are used to assess myocardial hibernation: dobutamine echocardiography, SPECT with thallium-201, and PET with FDG. These methods probe different aspects of myocyte viability, namely the presence of inotropic contractile reserve, sarcolemmal integrity, and preserved uptake of exogenous glucose, respectively. In patients with normal or moderate impairment of left ventricular function, their predictive value for the identification of hibernating myocardium appears to be similar (positive predictive value 69–83%, negative predictive value 81–90%).[11] Dobutamine stress echocardiography is the least expensive and most widely available technique for the detection of hibernating myocardium. Although it has good predictive accuracy in patients with mild to moderate left ventricular dysfunction, there is evidence that in patients with pronounced left ventricular dysfunction it has a higher false negative rate than nuclear techniques. In particular, PET is regarded as the method with the greatest predictive value in patients with heart failure and very poor ejection fraction.[13] Using PET with FDG during hyperinsulinaemic euglycaemic clamp, we have shown that a threshold value for the metabolic rate of glucose of 0.25 μmol/g/min allowed the best prediction of improvement in functional class of at least one grade after revascularisation.[14]

PET for the investigation of the autonomic nervous system
Several β blocker drugs have been labelled with carbon-11 to act as radioligands for imaging by PET.[1] The most promising of these is CGP 12177. This is a non-selective β adrenoceptor antagonist which is particularly suited for PET studies because of its high affinity and low lipophilicity, thus enabling the functional receptor pool on the cell surface to be studied. A graphical method for quantification of β

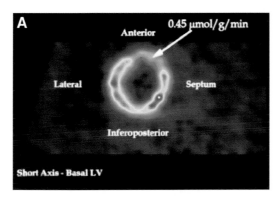 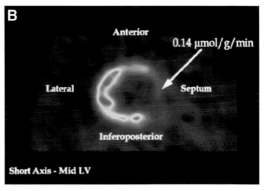

Figure 31.4. Myocardial viability in two patients with coronary artery disease and severe chronic left ventricular dysfunction assessed by PET with ^{18}F labelled FDG during hyperinsulinaemic euglycaemic clamp. Both patients had previous myocardial infarctions. The scan in panel A shows that FDG uptake in the previously infarcted anteroseptal segment is 0.45 μmol/g/min, suggesting the presence of viable myocardium. In the scan in panel B the uptake of FDG in the anterior wall and the interventricular septum is significantly reduced (0.14 μmol/g/min), suggesting absence of viability in this large area. A cut off point of 0.25 μmol/g/min is routinely used in our laboratory to differentiate between viable and non-viable myocardium.[13]

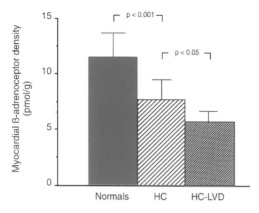

Figure 31.5. Mean left ventricular β adrenoceptor density in normal subjects and in patients with hypertrophic cardiomyopathy with preserved systolic function (HC) or with left ventricular dysfunction (HC-LVD). Adapted from Choudhury *et al.*[16]

adrenoceptor density (B_{max}, pmol/g) from the PET data has been developed. This approach requires two injections of [11]C-(S)-CGP 12177, one at a high specific activity followed by a second at a lower specific activity.[15] Studies in our institution in a group of healthy subjects over a broad range of ages have yielded mean (SD) B_{max} values of 8.4 (2.0) pmol/g, a figure which is comparable with the values measured using in vitro binding.[15] In addition, studies in patients have demonstrated diffuse down regulation of myocardial β adrenoceptors in hypertrophic cardiomyopathy and in congestive cardiac failure, two disorders in which there is a broad range of evidence for chronically raised levels of sympathetic nervous system activation. It has further been hypothesised that abnormal sympathetic activation may actually precede the development of systolic dysfunction in patients with hypertrophic cardiomyopathy. The relation between left ventricular function and myocardial β adrenoceptor density has been investigated and a significant correlation between left ventricular fractional shortening (echocardiography) and β adrenoceptor density (PET) was shown (fig 31.5).[16]

PET has also been used to investigate the integrity of pre-synaptic sympathetic innervation of the heart. Three tracers have been used for this purpose: [18]F labelled fluorometaraminol, ^{18}F labelled fluorodopamine and ^{11}C labelled hydroxyephedrine (^{11}C-HED). These tracers compete with endogenous noradrenaline for the transport into the presynaptic nerve terminal via the neuronal uptake-1 transport system. Once within the neuron these compounds are metabolised and trapped, and hence serve as markers of sympathetic innervation. Recent studies have demonstrated decreased retention of ^{11}C-HED in patients after cardiac transplant which is consistent with the heart being denervated. However, with time, some sympathetic re-innervation occurred particularly in the anteroseptal regions of the heart.[17] This has recently been correlated with recovery of the sensation of angina pectoris in these patients. Both pre- and postsynaptic myocardial autonomic function can be assessed non-invasively by combining different

tracers—for example, ^{11}C-HED and [11]C-(S)-CGP 12177.[18]

PET studies using ^{11}C labelled MQNB have been used to quantify the density of myocardial muscarinic cholinergic receptors in both experimental animals and in man.[1] It would be desirable for these studies to be extended to patient groups given the possible pathophysiological role of muscarinic receptors in arrhythmogenesis and control of sympathetic nerve function.

1. **Schelbert HR.** Principles of positron emission tomography. In: Marcus ML, Schelbert HR, Skorton DJ, Wolf GL, eds. *Cardiac imaging.* Philadelphia: WB Saunders Company, 1991:1140–270.
• *A very comprehensive chapter on the various aspects of PET scanning in this companion to Braunwald's "Heart disease".*

2. **Camici PG, Rosen SD, Spinks TJ.** Positron emission tomography. In: Murray IPC, Ell PJ, eds. *Nuclear medicine in clinical diagnosis and treatment,* 2nd ed. London: Churchill-Livingstone, 1998:1353–67.

3. **Parodi O, Schelbert HR, Schwaiger M,** *et al.* Cardiac emission computed tomography: underestimation of regional tracer concentration due to wall motion abnormalities. *J Comput Assist Tomogr* 1984;**8**:1083–92.

4. **De Silva R, Camici PG.** The role of positron emission tomography in the investigation of coronary circulatory function in man. *Cardiovasc Res* 1994;**28**:1595–612.

5. **Camici PG, Gropler RJ, Jones T,** *et al.* The impact of myocardial blood flow quantitation with PET on the understanding of cardiac diseases. *Eur Heart J* 1996;**17**:25–34.

6. **Uren NG, Camici PG, Melin JA,** *et al.* The effect of ageing on the coronary vasodilator reserve in man. *J Nucl Med* 1995;**36**:2032–6.

7. **Uren NG, Melin JA, De Bruyne B,** *et al.* Relation between myocardial blood flow and the severity of coronary artery stenosis. *N Engl J Med* 1994;**330**:1782–8.
• *Describes the relation between stenosis severity measured by quantitative coronary angiography and coronary flow reserve measured non-invasively by PET, in patients with coronary artery disease.*

8. **Choudhury L, Rosen SD, Patel DP,** *et al.* Coronary flow reserve in primary and secondary left ventricular hypertrophy: a study with positron emission tomography. *Eur Heart J* 1997;**18**:108–16.

9. **Marinho NVS, Keogh BE, Costa DC,** *et al.* Pathophysiology of chronic left ventricular dysfunction: new insights from the measurement of absolute myocardial blood flow and glucose utilization. *Circulation* 1996;**93**:737–44.
• *Shows the ability of PET to provide quantitative estimates of regional myocardial glucose utilisation that can be used to assess viability even in the absence of a flow scan. In addition, it demonstrates that baseline myocardial blood flow in patients with hibernating myocardium and previous infarction is, in most cases, within normal limits.*

10. **Camici PG, Wijns W, Borgers M,** *et al.* Pathophysiological mechanisms of chronic reversible left ventricular dysfunction due to coronary artery disease (hibernating myocardium). *Circulation* 1997;**96**:3205–14.
• *A detailed review on the pathophysiology of hibernating myocardium.*

11. **Wijns W, Vatner SF, Camici PG.** Hibernating myocardium. *N Engl J Med* 1998;**339**:173–81.
• *This is a more clinically oriented review on the subject of myocardial hibernation.*

12. **Tillisch J, Brunken R, Marshall R,** *et al.* Reversibility of cardiac wall-motion abnormalities predicted by positron tomography. *N Engl J Med* 1986;**314**:884–8.

13. **Fath-Ordoubadi F, Pagano D, Marinho NVS,** *et al.* Coronary revascularisation in the treatment of moderate and severe post-ischaemic left ventricular dysfunction. *Am J Cardiol* 1998;**82**:26–31.

14. **Fath-Ordoubadi F, Beatt KJ, Spyrou N,** *et al.* Efficacy of coronary angioplasty for the treatment of hibernating myocardium. *Heart* 1999;**82**:210–16.

15. **Choudhury L, Rosen SD, Lefroy D,** *et al.* Myocardial beta adrenoceptor density in primary and secondary left ventricular hypertrophy. *Eur Heart J* 1996;**17**:1703–9.

16. **Choudhury L, Guzzetti S, Lefroy D,** *et al.* Myocardial beta-adrenoceptor and left ventricular function in hypertrophic cardiomyopathy. *Heart* 1996;**75**:50–4.

17. **Schwaiger M, Hutchins GD, Kalff V,** *et al.* Evidence for regional catecholamine uptake and storage sites in the transplanted human heart by positron emission tomography. *J Clin Invest* 1991;**87**:1681–90.

18. **Schafers M, Dutka D, Rhodes CG,** *et al.* Myocardial pre- and postsynaptic autonomic dysfunction in hypertrophic cardiomyopathy. *Circ Res* 1998;**82**:57–62.

website
extra

Additional references appear on the Heart website

www.heartjnl.com

32 Non-invasive coronary artery imaging with electron beam computed tomography and magnetic resonance imaging

P J de Feyter, K Nieman, P van Ooijen, M Oudkerk

Recent developments in hardware and software have increased the diagnostic capabilities of magnetic resonance imaging (MRI) and electron beam computed tomography (EBT) to visualise the cardiac anatomy, including the coronary arteries. Visualisation of the heart puts any diagnostic technique to the test, because the continuous cardiac motion distorts the image and high temporal resolution is required to "freeze" the heart to produce a sharp image.

In particular, non-invasive visualisation of the coronary arteries is difficult because of the small size of the coronary arteries (2–5 mm in diameter), the complex, tortuous course making it often impossible to "catch" the coronary artery in one slice (tomogram), and the cardiac and respiratory motion causing loss of sharpness or motion artefacts.

In this article image acquisition and processing techniques of MRI and EBT will be presented. The clinical role of both techniques in cardiac imaging will be discussed, together with a brief introduction of the technical aspects.

Magnetic resonance imaging: physics and technique

MRI has excellent temporal and spatial resolution and is capable of visualising the cardiac anatomy. The advantages of MRI are its ability to acquire images non-invasively, in the absence of ionising radiation, and in any tomographic plane without interference from surrounding bone or soft tissues. The basic concepts and clinical role of MRI can be found in excellent recent review articles.[1-5] In this paper we limit ourselves to a brief summary of MRI concepts.

MRI scanner
The MRI scanner consists of a magnet, gradient coils, and a body coil. The large magnet produces a strong homogeneous magnetic field, is cylindrical, and for imaging the patient is placed within the bore of the magnet. Gradient coils vary the strength of the magnetic field from one point to another and they determine the spatial information of the emitted MR signal necessary for the construction of the image. The bodycoil acts as an antenna, and transmits and receives radiofrequency (RF) waves.

Basic principles of MRI
Nuclei with an odd number of protons (such as hydrogen) posses a property called spin angular momentum—that is, the nucleus spins around its axis. Since the odd nuclei are positively charged, the spinning motion causes a magnetic momentum around it and acts as a small magnet. The strength of this magnetic moment is a property of the type of nucleus. Hydrogen nuclei possess a large magnetic moment, and are very abundant in the human body thereby making hydrogen the nucleus of choice for MRI. In the absence of an externally applied magnetic field (B_O) these individual magnetic moments have no preferred orientation, but when placed in strong external magnetic field these magnetic moments align with the orientation of the external field. However, the spins do not exactly align but are at an angle to the external magnetic field (fig 32.1). This causes the spin to precess around the axis of the external magnetic field with a unique (resonant) frequency.

The unique frequency of this precession is governed by the Larmor frequency equation $f = g \times M$, where f = frequency, g = gyromagnetic ratio (unique for each nucleus), and M = strength of magnetic field. The spins precess at random and give rise to a rather small secondary magnetic field (net tissue magnetisation, M) which at equilibrium is aligned longitudinally, along the axis of the main magnetic field (B_O) which is much larger, so that tissue magnetisation is "overruled" by the main magnetic field B_O, making tissue magnetisation undetectable in the longitudinal axis. To "detect" this tissue magnetisation to produce an MR image it is necessary to disturb this equilibrium. An RF pulse emitted from the RF transmitter coil with a resonant frequency equal to the unique frequency of the precessing spins rotates the net longitudinal tissue magnetisation into the transverse plane (X-Y plane) and synchronises the precession (fig 32.2). This allows the transverse magnetisation to be detected and measured. Termination of the RF

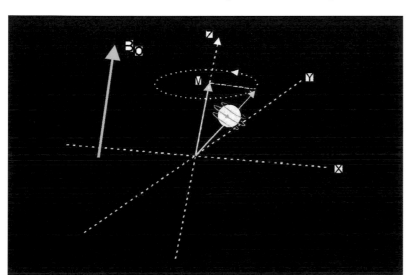

Figure 32.1. Spin angular moment causing a magnetic dipole. B_O, external magnetic field which causes spin to precess at an angle to B_O. M, net tissue magnetisation aligned along Z axis.

pulse causes the perturbed nuclei to return (relax) to the original longitudinal alignment in the magnetic field and incoherent precession. As they relax a signal is emitted which is detected by the RF receiver. This is the MR signal from which the image is reconstructed.

Different tissues relax at different rates, thus providing contrast between tissues. This signal needs to be processed to allow three dimensional location of the source (tissue protons) of the signal. A supplemental magnetic field gradient is applied (by the gradient coils) which causes a predictable variation of the magnetic field and thus a predictable resonant frequency of protons along an axis. This allows exact location of protons enabling precise image reconstruction.

Cardiac MRI

MR coronary imaging: technique

Cardiac and respiratory motion are formidable problems making robust MR coronary angiography very difficult. Today conventional diagnostic coronary angiography is the undisputed standard of reference because a selective injection of contrast media reproduces in real time (no motion artefacts) the entire coronary artery (including collaterals), with an in-plane resolution of 0.15×0.15 mm.

Coronary imaging with an image acquisition of 25–50 images per second (that is, 20–40 ms per acquisition), such as can be achieved with conventional diagnostic coronary angiography, would result in a nearly motion free image, but unfortunately such ultrafast MR acquisition techniques are not yet available. To circumvent these motion problems several other approaches must be used. To reduce cardiac motion disturbances one chooses a "quiet" window in the cardiac cycle during which the heart does not contract. This window is usually in mid and late diastole and lasts for about 100 ms to 150 ms. This window can be selected by triggering to the ECG signal so that the acquisition is performed in that predetermined window. This requires a stable heart rhythm and precludes patients with arrhythmias.

Respiratory motion artefacts can be reduced by using two acquisition approaches: (a) breathholding, and (b) respiratory gating. Breathholding for 20 seconds is possible in the majority of patients.

Respiratory gating techniques make use of a navigator technique, which monitors the movement of the diaphragm during respiration so that images are acquired only at the same predetermined diaphragm level. Potential navigator techniques allow longer acquisition times, during normal breathing, but irregularities in breathing pattern during long acquisition periods "shift" the diaphragm level, which may be (partly) overcome by adaptive windowing (to correct for diaphragm shift).

Another problem is the presence of epicardial fat, which produces a bright MR signal, which may interfere with the signal of blood within the coronary arteries. Fat saturation—that is, a strong RF pulse that selectively satu-

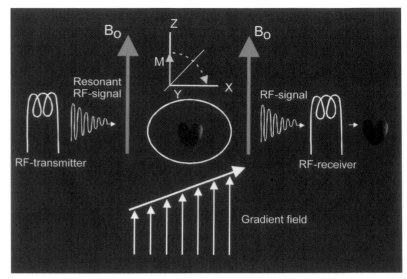

Figure 32.2. The patient (heart) is placed within a strong external magnetic field (B_O). The RF transmitter rotates the net tissue magnetisation in the transverse plane, and after termination, relaxation occurs which emits a signal detected by the RF receiver. The gradient coils produce a supplemental magnetic field gradient to allow precise location of the excited protons. The received signals have certain signal intensity (brightness) and location, both of which are processed to form the desired image.

rates the magnetisation of fat bound hydrogen atoms, but not waterbound hydrogen atoms—effectively suppresses this fat signal and is often used in MR coronary imaging.

MR coronary imaging to detect a coronary stenosis

The detection of haemodynamically significant lesions with different MR techniques appears to be the "Holy Grail" of MR imaging (fig 32.3). So far, the results of detecting stenoses have been disappointing with sensitivities ranging from as low as 33% to as high as 90%.[1 2 6] Overall the MR techniques are not robust enough to allow clinically reliable identification of a coronary lesion. The inability to reliably detect coronary stenosis is caused by: (1) the unacceptable quality of the images (mainly caused by problems of cardiac and respiratory motion) which makes interpretation unreliable or sometimes even impossible; (2) partial voluming of tortuous vessels; (3) intravoxel phase dispersion caused by complex or turbulent flow at coronary stenosis; (4) overlapping of adjacent anatomic structures, in particular the circumflex artery which is obscured by overlapping of the coronary sinus; (5) an inability to distinguish normal antegrade coronary flow from collateral filling of a vessel occurring beyond a severe stenosis or total occlusion; and (6) MR signal of the vessel wall or coronary plaque mimicking the blood signal of the vessel lumen.

Future of MR coronary imaging

There are three factors that must always be considered in MR coronary imaging: acquisition time, signal to noise ratio, and resolution. Improvement of one of the three is at the expense of one or both of the other two, and therefore MR imaging is about trying to find the optimal compromise.

Ultrafast new MR scanners will allow: (a) shorter acquisition windows (less than 100 ms)

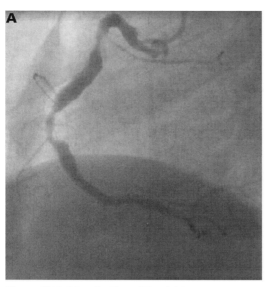
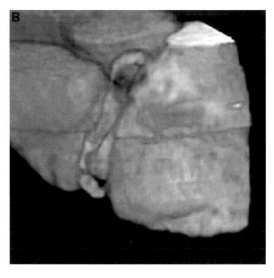

Figure 32.3. Visualisation of the right coronary artery with (A) a fast sequence MR coronary angiography technique, and (B) three dimensional reconstruction. Two significant stenoses are clearly visible.

which may dramatically reduce motion artefacts; and (b) three dimensional acquisition which offers the advantage of higher signal to noise ratio, and more isotropic pixel resolution. Small volume scan acquisition oriented along the coronaries, obtained during one breath hold, is feasible and appears promising.[7] The low contrast to noise ratio is expected to be improved by blood pool contrast media, so that the vessel lumen becomes more visible and protruding lesions can be distinguished. High

gradient scanners are expected to improve the current spatial resolution of typical sequence of $1.5 \times 1.5 \times 3$ mm to an in-plane resolution of less than 1 mm. However, it may take several years before MR coronary angiography will evolve into a reliable clinical tool.

MR imaging to establish proximal course of coronary arteries

MR imaging is a reliable, patient friendly technique to assess the anomalous origin or

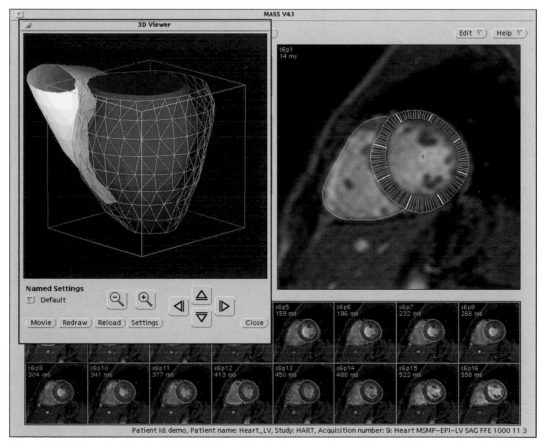

Figure 32.4. Computer display of the MASS analytical software package. The small images along the bottom represent the individual frames over a cardiac cycle at a certain anatomical level. The left ventricular endocardial and epicardial contours were generated using semiautomatic contour detection. From the contours in all the frames and slices, a three dimensional model can be reconstructed that can also be used as a functional display representing regional wall thickening/thinning. Reproduced from van der Geest et al. *J Comput Assist Tomogr* 1997;21:756-65, with permission of the publishers.

Clinical role of MRI in cardiac disease

- Established role—evaluation of atria, ventricles, and pericardium:
    - congenital heart diseases
    - cardiac tumours (masses)
    - pericardial disease
    - left ventricular volume, mass
    - left ventricular function: wall thickness/systolic thickening
    - right ventricular function

- Emerging role:
    - visualisation of coronary arteries
    - visualisation of bypass grafts
    - dobutamine stress MRI for coronary ischaemia to detect wall motion, abnormalities or myocardial contractile reserve

- Potential role:
    - epicardial coronary flow velocity (rest/stress)
    - myocardial perfusion (rest/stress)
    - specific contrasts for myocardial necrosis or viable tissue

---

proximal abnormal course of the right and left coronary arteries accurately.[8]

MR imaging of saphenous vein grafts

MR imaging of vein grafts is relatively easy because the grafts have a large diameter (4–8 mm) and are minimally affected by cardiac and respiratory motion. The patency of grafts can be established by MR with a sensitivity of 85–90% and a specificity of 60–100%.[1 2] However, these examinations only provide information on graft patency and no information about non-occluding stenoses or graft patency of a sequential graft distal to a first coronary anastomosis, thus limiting the application in clinical practice.

MR imaging of right and left ventricle

Newer MR techniques (gradient echo imaging or echo planar imaging) allow acquisition of short axis (or long axis) slices within 50 ms with adequate image quality to assess quantitative evaluation of left ventricular function.[4]

The use of end diastolic and end systolic measurements allows calculation of stroke volume, ejection fraction, and ventricular mass. Wall motion abnormalities can be evaluated quantitatively by cine MR imaging (fig 32.4).[9] Myocardial tagging allows for detection of very subtle wall motion abnormalities. MRI permits accurate delineation of epicardial and endocardial borders so that wall motion and systolic wall thickening can be analysed quantitatively. Stress MRI (using dobutamine) is emerging as a technique to detect coronary artery disease,[10 11] and evaluation of myocardial contractile reserve by stress MRI appears useful for evaluating myocardial viability.[12 13] Myocardial perfusion imaging is emerging as a valuable tool to assess distribution of myocardial perfusion with high resolution.[14 15] The anatomy and function of the right ventricle in particular is notoriously difficult to assess

adequately. However, MR imaging allows evaluation of the right ventricle, which may prove to be useful to monitor congenital heart disease (fig 32.4).

MR imaging of the cardiac anatomy

The presence of tumours or other masses involving the cardiac chambers, the pericardium, and extra cardiac structures can be reliably assessed with MRI.[16]

Limitations of MR imaging

Devices and metallic objects within the body may present a potential hazard for the patient. These objects may cause image artefacts, induce electric currents, cause excessive heating, or may move within the tissues. Patients with pacemakers and implantable defibrillators should not undergo MR imaging. Claustrophobia occurs in 2% of the patients, but the "open" configuration of new scanners will reduce this problem.

Electron beam tomography: physics and technique

EBT is a tomographic *x* ray technique whereby only the structures in a selected slice (tomogram) of the patient are imaged sharply. The *x* ray photons passing through the body are differentially absorbed by the tissue, thus creating object contrast from which an image is reconstructed.

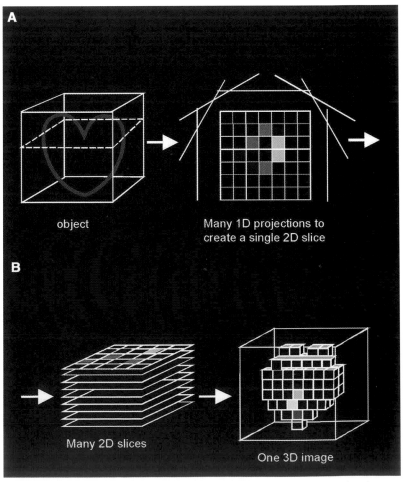

Figure 32.5. Schematic of EBT scanning to reconstruct a three dimensional image. ID, one dimensional; 2D, two dimensional; 3D, 3 dimensional.

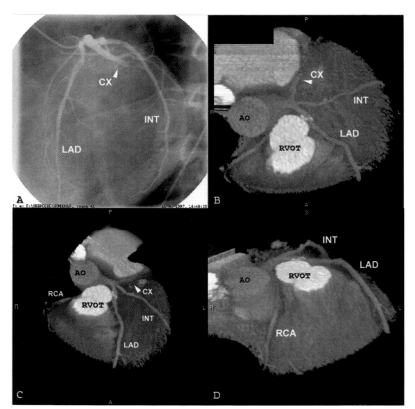

Figure 32.6. EBT of coronary arteries with view from top (B), from a more anterior angle (C), and from a lateral angle (D). The left circumflex (CX) artery is totally occluded. A: corresponding coronary angiography. AO, aorta; INT, intermediate coronary branch; LAD, left anterior descending coronary artery; RCA, right coronary artery, RVOT, right ventricular outflow tract.

The EBT scanner is a dedicated ultrafast cardiac scanner, which is able to acquire tomograms within 100 ms.[17] This fast acquisition is achieved because, unlike "conventional" computed tomographic (CT) scanners, there is no need to rotate the x ray source around the patient (which is energy and time consuming); rather the patient is positioned within a fixed source detector combination where x rays are produced with an electronically steered electron beam. The acquisition is obtained at a predetermined relative motion free diastolic acquisition period, which is determined by high resolution ECG with triggering usually set at 80% of the RR interval. Breathholding is necessary during acquisition of the tomograms to avoid respiratory motion artefacts. The tomogram thickness is set at 1.5 or 3 mm. Scanning is performed with the patient in supine position on the table. After each tomogram the table increment is set at 1.5 or 2 mm, resulting in contiguous non-overlapping slices or slices with 1 mm overlap. One tomogram is made during each RR interval. To completely cover the heart 40 to 60 transaxial tomograms are made during one breath hold. The data are obtained after injection of 150 ml contrast medium at 4 ml/s through an antecubital vein.

The high contrast in-plane resolution is approximately 0.8×0.8 mm (6 line pairs/cm). The radiation exposure is estimated to be one third of that of a diagnostic coronary angiogram.

The image is constructed from many one dimensional projections, which are used to reconstruct a single slice of data (fig 32.5). A three dimensional data set is obtained by stacking many two dimensional tomograms from which three dimensional reconstructions are made usually using a surface shaded rendering or a volume rendering technique.

EBT to assess coronary arteries

During contrast injection the mean CT density within the coronary arteries is about 165–200 Hounsfield units (HU) while the mean density of the myocardium (85–100 HU) and connective tissue (100 HU) is much lower, thus allowing visualisation of the contrast filled coronary lumen.

So far the results of healthy volunteers and approximately 300 patients have been published. In 75–80% of the cases the image quality is sufficient to allow reliable interpretation of the coronary arteries (fig 32.6).[17-19]

The sensitivity to detect significant coronary stenosis ranges from 75–90% and the specificity from 80–94%.

The diagnostic accuracy of EBT coronary angiography is highest in the left main artery and proximal and mid parts of the left anterior descending coronary artery, and moderate in proximal and mid parts of the right (RCA) and left circumflex (LCX) arteries. The distal coronary segments cannot be visualised.

Misdiagnosis is caused by cardiac motion artefacts (in particular of the RCA and LCX), inadvertent respiratory motion, overlapping anatomical structures, triggering problems due to irregular heart rhythm, and lumen interpretation problems in cases of severe overlying calcifications. Total coverage of the heart requires a rather long breath hold (for example, with a heart rate of 60 bpm and slice thickness of 3 mm, a 20 second breath hold covers 6 cm from base to apex) which is not always possible in patients.

EBT to assess bypass graft patency

Initially EBT was able to establish only the patency of coronary venous and arterial bypass graft patency by assessment of the individual transaxial angiograms. The diagnostic accuracy was high with a sensitivity of 95% and a specificity of 86–97%.[17] The recently introduced three dimensional rendering techniques were able to reconstruct the graft completely and thus allow assessment of non-occluding obstructions (fig 32.7). The diagnostic accuracy to detect significant graft obstructions was high, with sensitivity ranging from 92–100% and specificity from 91–100%.

EBT for quantification of coronary calcification

To detect coronary calcium usually 20–30 contiguous, 3 mm EBT slices acquired at 100 ms are obtained. The tomograms, which are acquired during one breath hold, are triggered from an ECG at 80% of the RR interval to minimise cardiac motion. Coronary calcium in the wall has a high density relative to blood and thus is easily detected (fig 32.8). The EBT scanner software allows the quantification of calcium area and density. CT attenuation of tissue is about ± 50 HU and arbitrarily a

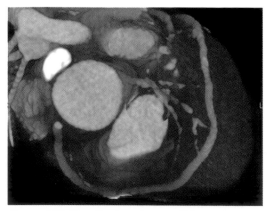

Figure 32.7. Visualisation of sequential venous bypass graft without significant stenoses.

density of 130 HU and more are assumed to be calcium. The calcium scoring algorithm from Agatson is frequently used to calculate the amount of calcium.[20] Calcium densities of 130–200 HU are assigned a score of 1, between 201–300 HU a score of 2, between 301–400 HU a score of 3, and > 401 HU a score of 4. These peak calcium density values are multiplied by the actual area (mm[2]) of calcification per coronary tomographic segment to obtain the score. The score can be given per specific coronary artery or for the entire coronary system (the sum of the individual scores).

EBT is extremely sensitive in defining coronary vascular calcification, and the presence of coronary calcium is always indicative of coronary atherosclerosis.[21] The presence of calcification does not equate with the presence of a significant coronary stenosis, however, and the absence of calcification does not exclude a coronary lesion, including a vulnerable plaque, but the likelihood of the latter is low. There is a direct relation between the magnitude of the calcium score and the extent of the underlying coronary plaque burden and the presence of a severe coronary stenosis. However, site and extent of calcification do not equate with site specific stenosis, and a calcific plaque does not mean a stable plaque.

There appears to be a relation between the presence of coronary calcification and the occurrence of adverse coronary events in asymptomatic individuals.[21 22] The place and role of EBT as a screening tool to predict coronary events, independent of the conventional risk factors such as hypertension, smoking, hypercholesterolaemia, diabetes, and family history, is controversial and requires more data before EBT can be recommended in low risk asymptomatic patients.

Future EBT coronary imaging

Although EBT has a high temporal (100 ms) and high in-plane spatial resolution (0.8 mm × 0.8 mm), with image acquisition triggered to the ECG, its performance is not yet sufficiently robust for reliable coronary visualisation. Technical improvements may be expected, such as doubling the number of detector elements, so that the in-plane resolution may improve from 6 line pairs/cm to 10 line pairs/cm or reducing the tomogram acquisition time from 100 ms to 50 ms.

Clinical role of EBT in cardiac disease

- Established role:
  - detection and quantification of coronary calcium

- Emerging role:
  - visualisation of coronary arteries
  - visualisation of bypass grafts

- Under investigation:
  - quantification of calcium in symptomatic patients and asymptomatic individuals

- Potential role:
  - left ventricle anatomy and function
  - right ventricle anatomy and function
  - myocardial perfusion

Coronary imaging with EBT is promising because calcium quantification provides information on the plaque burden of the coronary arteries, and contrast enhanced CT may reliably determine the severity of obstructive disease.

Conclusion

A major question, given the cost constraints for a potential interested party, is which technique—MRI or EBT—should one purchase?

This largely depends on the purpose for which the technique will be used. If one is interested in visualising coronary arteries or venous bypass grafts EBT seems more robust than MRI.

Visualisation of the heart chambers and cardiac masses can be achieved equally effectively by both techniques. MRI is superior for studying left ventricular function and perfusion, and obviously flow can only be determined by MRI (although it is still in its early phase of development).

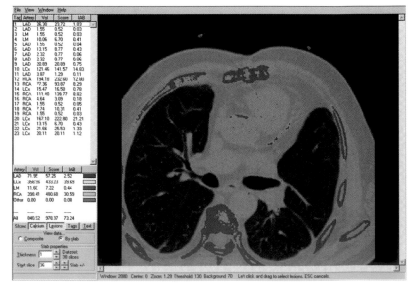

Figure 32.8. Example of coronary calcification score. Blue dots in the left anterior descending artery represent calcification.

1. **van Geuns RJ, Wielopolski PA, de Bruin HG,** *et al.* Basic principles of magnetic resonance imaging. *Prog Cardiovasc Dis* 1999;**42**:149–56.
   - *The basic principles of MRI are presented in a simplified schematic approach.*

2. **van Geuns RJ, Wielopolski PA, de Bruin HG,** *et al.* Magnetic resonance imaging of the coronary arteries: techniques and results. *Prog Cardiovasc Dis* 1999;**42**:157–66.
   - *The basic concepts, clinical results, possibilities, and limitations of MR coronary angiography are reviewed.*

3. **Brown MA, Semelka RC.** MR imaging abbreviations, definitions, and descriptions: a review. *Radiology* 1999;**213**:647–62.

4. **European Society of Cardiology/Association of European Paediatric Cardiologists.** The clinical role of magnetic resonance in cardiovascular disease. Task Force of the European Society of Cardiology, in collaboration with the Association of European Paediatric Cardiologists. *Eur Heart J* 1998;**19**:19–39.
   - *The clinical role of MRI in cardiovascular disease is highlighted and general recommendations are given about the explicit role of MRI in the diagnosis of cardiovascular disease, taking into account other existing diagnostic tools. This article is highly recommended.*

5. **Wielopolski PA, van Geuns RJM, de Feyter PJ,** *et al.* Review article: coronary arteries. *Eur Radiology* 2000;**10**:12–35.
   - *This article presents the current state of art of MRI for diagnosis of cardiovascular disease.*

6. **Manning WJ, Li W, Edelman RR.** A preliminary report comparing magnetic resonance coronary angiography with conventional angiography. *N Engl J Med* 1993;**328**:828–32.
   - *This is the first report showing a rather high sensitivity and specificity of MR coronary angiography in patients.*

7. **Wielopolski PA, van Geuns RJ, de Feyter PJ,** *et al.* Breath-hold coronary MR angiography with volume-targeted imaging. *Radiology* 1998;**209**:209–19.

8. **Post JC, van Rossum AC, Bronzwaer JG,** *et al.* Magnetic resonance angiography of anomalous coronary arteries. A new gold standard for delineating the proximal course? *Circulation* 1995;**92**:3163–71.

9. **van der Geest RJ, Reiber JH.** Quantification in cardiac MRI. *J Magn Reson Imaging* 1999;**10**:602–8.

10. **van Rugge FP, van der Wall EE, Spanjersberg SJ,** *et al.* Magnetic resonance imaging during dobutamine stress for detection and localization of coronary artery disease. Quantitative wall motion analysis using a modification of the centerline method. *Circulation* 1994;**90**:127–38.

11. **Hundley WG, Hamilton CA, Thomas MS,** *et al.* Utility of fast cine magnetic resonance imaging and display for the detection of myocardial ischemia in patients not well suited for second harmonic stress echocardiography *Circulation* 1999;**100**:1697–702.

12. **Baer FM, Theissen P, Schneider CA,** *et al.* Dobutamine magnetic resonance imaging predicts contractile recovery of chronically dysfunctional myocardium after successful revascularization. *J Am Coll Cardiol* 1998;**31**:1040–8.

13. **Geskin G, Kramer CM, Rogers WJ,** *et al.* Quantitative assessment of myocardial viability after infarction by dobutamine magnetic resonance tagging. *Circulation* 1998;**98**:217–23.

14. **Saeed M, Wendland MF, Yu KK,** *et al.* Identification of myocardial reperfusion with echo planar magnetic resonance imaging. Discrimination between occlusive and reperfused infarctions. *Circulation* 1994;**90**:1492–501.

15. **Wu KC, Zerhouni EA, Judd RM,** *et al.* Prognostic significance of microvascular obstruction by magnetic resonance imaging in patients with acute myocardial infarction. *Circulation* 1998;**97**:765–72.

16. **Hoffmann U, Globits S, Frank H.** Cardiac and paracardiac masses. Current opinion on diagnostic evaluation by magnetic resonance imaging. *Eur Heart J* 1998;**19**:553–63.

17. **Rensing BJ, Bongaerts AH, van Geuns RJ,** *et al.* Intravenous coronary angiography using electron beam computed tomography. *Prog Cardiovasc Dis* 1999;**42**:139–48.
   - *This excellent review describes the technique and summarises the studies with EBT regarding both the visualisation of venous bypass grafts and coronary arteries and the diagnostic value in detecting significant obstructions.*

18. **Rensing BJ, Bongaerts A, van Geuns RJ,** *et al.* Intravenous coronary angiography by electron beam computed tomography: a clinical evaluation. *Circulation* 1998;**98**:2509–12.

19. **Moshage WE, Achenbach S, Seese B,** *et al.* Coronary artery stenoses: three-dimensional imaging with electrocardiographically triggered, contrast agent-enhanced, electron-beam CT. *Radiology* 1995;**196**:707–14.
   - *This is the first report about the clinical results of visualising the coronary arteries with contrast enhanced electron beam tomography.*

20. **Agatston AS, Janowitz WR, Hildner FJ,** *et al.* Quantification of coronary artery calcium using ultrafast computed tomography. *J Am Coll Cardiol* 1990;**15**:827–32.

21. **Wexler L, Brundage B, Crouse J,** *et al.* Coronary artery calcification: pathophysiology, epidemiology, imaging methods, and clinical implications. A statement for health professionals from the American Heart Association writing group. *Circulation* 1996;**94**:1175–92.
   - *This is a thorough review of a committee of the American Heart Association about the pathophysiology of coronary calcium, the role and place of EBT to detect and quantify calcium, its relation to extent and severity of coronary atherosclerosis, and its prognostic value.*

22. **Rumberger JA, Brundage BH, Rader DJ,** *et al.* Electron beam computed tomographic coronary calcium scanning: a review and guidelines for use in asymptomatic persons. *Mayo Clin Proc* 1999;**74**:243–52.
   - *A critical review regarding EBT coronary calcium scanning from a clinical perspective: calcium as a measure of atherosclerosis, or as a prognostic indicator of cardiac events. Interpretation guidelines are offered to help guide initiation of a clinically active programme in high risk individuals.*

SECTION VIII: GENERAL CARDIOLOGY

33 Myocarditis, pericarditis and other pericardial diseases

Celia M Oakley

This article discusses the diagnosis and management of myocarditis and pericarditis (both acute and recurrent), as well as other pericardial diseases.

Myocarditis

Myocarditis is the term used to indicate acute infective, toxic or autoimmune inflammation of the heart. Reversible toxic myocarditis occurs in diphtheria and sometimes in infective endocarditis when autoimmune mechanisms may also contribute. Persistent viral infection of the myocardium was first demonstrated a decade ago.[1] Slow growing organisms such as chlamydia and trypanosomal infection in Chagas' disease are causes of chronic myocarditis. Noninfective causes in sarcoidosis and the collagen vascular diseases need to be sought.

Acute myocarditis and acute pericarditis are not always associated (likewise meningitis and encephalitis do not always occur together) and the clinical emphasis is usually on one or the other.

Myocarditis can be caused by many different viruses and the microbial pathogenesis may be complex. Most cases of myocarditis with onset in otherwise healthy people probably have an infectious origin, although the pathogenesis is not yet fully understood (such as the finding of a link between chlamydia and heart disease through antigenic mimicry). In western countries enteroviruses, especially coxsackie B 1–6 serotypes, are the most frequent, and the recent identification of a common coxsackie virus B and adenovirus receptor has explained why these very different virus types both cause myocarditis.[2–4]

Prevalence and clinical features

The prevalence of acute myocarditis is unknown because most cases are not recognised on account of non-specific or no symptoms (but sudden death may occur). Myocarditis may develop as a complication of an upper respiratory or gastrointestinal infection with general constitutional symptoms, particularly fever and skeletal myalgia, malaise, and anorexia. This systemic acute phase response increases energy production but compromises performance. Since myocarditis may not develop for several days or weeks after the symptoms and after a return to normal work and leisure activity, there is a risk of overexertion, which may be dangerous.

Diagnosis is easiest during epidemics of coxsackie infections but difficult in isolated cases. These are not seen by cardiologists unless they develop arrhythmia, collapse or suffer chest pain, the majority being dealt with in the primary care system.

Acute onset of chest pain is usual and may mimic myocardial infarction or be associated with pericarditis. Arrhythmias or conduction disturbances may be life threatening despite only mild focal injury, whereas more widespread inflammation is necessary before cardiac dysfunction is sufficient to cause symptoms.

Investigations

The ECG may show sinus tachycardia, focal or generalised abnormality, ST segment elevation, fascicular blocks or atrioventricular conduction disturbances. Although the ECG abnormalities are non-specific, the ECG has the virtue of drawing attention to the heart and leading to echocardiographic and other investigations. Echocardiography may reveal segmental or generalised wall motion abnormalities or a pericardial effusion. Echocardiography allows other causes of heart failure to be excluded but pronounced focal changes in wall motion may lead to confusion with myocardial infarction, especially if the ECG changes also suggest this.[5]

The chest x ray may be normal, show cardiac enlargement, pulmonary venous congestion or pleural effusions.

Evidence of myocyte necrosis may be found with an increase in creatine kinase or appearance of troponin, indicating myocytolysis. The highest enzyme concentrations occur early and will probably have returned to normal by about a week after onset.[6] Cardiac autoantibodies can be demonstrated only later in the disease process.

A viral origin of myocarditis can only be proved if the virus is detected within an altered myocardium. This has become possible through molecular analyses of necropsy, transplant, and endomyocardial biopsy specimens using new techniques of viral gene amplification, which have shown persistence of viral mRNA.[1] The histological diagnosis of myocarditis (fig 33.1) was clarified by the Dallas criteria,[7] but these unfortunately did not include immunohistochemistry to demonstrate a T cell mediated immune response.

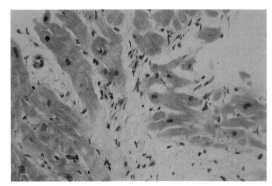

Figure 33.1. Acute myocarditis showing sheets of pale staining myocytes. Lymphocytes are seen which were identified as CD4 and CD8 cells on immunohistology.

Myocardial failure in myocarditis

Contributory causes of myocardial dysfunction include:

(1) a direct cytotoxic effect of the agent, be it viral, bacterial, etc;

(2) a secondary immune response, which can be triggered by any one of many different agents including non-infective ones;

(3) cytokine expression in the myocardium, which plays a crucial role—for example, tumour necrosis factor α (TNF α) and nitric oxide synthase.[4]

(4) aberrant induction of apoptosis, which may also play a part, particularly in individuals who go on to develop a chronic cardiomyopathy.[4] The proportion of patients who do this is completely unknown, but a genetic predisposition to ongoing inflammation, and possibly also to viral persistence, would explain the recognition of a 25–30% familial incidence of dilated cardiomyopathy.[8]

Detection of a causal agent is uncommon during the early phase (or even later). Demonstration of a viral origin is dependent upon gaining serial antibody titres against specific viruses and on showing a gradual fall in titre during convalescence. Even if endomyocardial biopsy is carried out, persisting viral mRNA will be found in only 25–50% of patients with biopsy proven acute myocarditis.[9]

Management

The treatment of acute myocarditis is largely supportive. Effective antiviral agents are unavailable and usually inappropriate, but they need to be more extensively investigated for clinical use. Immunosuppressive agents would be inappropriate if the myocarditis were caused by the direct effect of persisting virus but potentially useful to suppress an ongoing autoimmune inflammatory response. Discouraging results were obtained in a randomised controlled trial of the use of immunosuppressive agents in the treatment of biopsy proven acute myocarditis.[10] The trial was weakened by failure to include immunohistochemical techniques in the biopsy criteria and by frequent protocol violations. The use of steroids in an acutely ill patient therefore remains a discretionary clinical option in addition to the use of diuretics, angiotensin converting enzyme (ACE) inhibitors, β adrenergic blocking agents, and spironolactone.

It is recommended that whenever myocarditis is suspected exercise should be avoided.[11] Interestingly, in a large Finnish epidemiological study of myocarditis, which included nearly 700 000 healthy young men, there were 10 sudden unexpected deaths of which only one was associated with acute myocarditis (and there were no cases of hypertrophic cardiomyopathy or arrhythmogenic right ventricular cardiomyopathy).[5]

The future development of effective treatment will depend on ability to make an early diagnosis before establishment of a myopathic process and on knowledge of whether the cause is infective or autoimmune.[12]

Endocardial fibroelastosis in infancy and childhood, which was associated with persistent mumps virus infection, has been almost eradicated by vaccination and the development of vaccines against the other common viruses may help reduce the incidence of myocarditis in childhood.

Prognosis

Recovery from acute myocarditis often surprises and delights after life threatening illness. Some recover seemingly normal ventricular function, but some cardiovascular reserve must have been lost because biopsies during the acute phase show myocytolysis. It is also uncertain how many will progress to dilated cardiomyopathy.[13]

In a recent study 147 cases of myocarditis were followed up for an average of 5.6 years. Out of 15 cases classed as fulminant, 93% were alive without transplant 11 years after biopsy compared with 45% of 132 less severe cases. Left ventricular dilatation was not as great in the fulminant cases, who were more likely to recover, as in the clinically milder cases who had bigger ventricles.[14]

Other causes of acute myocarditis

Lyme disease caused by *Borrelia burgdorferi*, a tick borne organism carried by deer, may cause an acute myocarditis, typically with a long PR interval as occurs with acute rheumatic fever. Left ventricular dysfunction is usually transient but the organism has been cultured from endomyocardial biopsy material in a patient with a dilated cardiomyopathy.

Chagas' disease, common in rural parts of Central and South America, results from infection by *Trypanosoma cruzi*. Although best known as a cause of heart block and cardiomyopathy in the chronic phase, it can also cause a severe acute myocarditis and sudden death. During this phase, but not the chronic one, trypanosomes can be shown lying within the myocytes.

Kawasaki disease (Japanese mucocutaneous lymph node syndrome) can cause a diffuse myocarditis in its first or second stages. Occlusion of proximal coronary artery aneurysms is the usual cause of death. Treatment with immunoglobulins during the early phases may help to prevent aneurysms from forming. The cause is still unknown but is probably infective.

Peripartum cardiomyopathy (PPCM) is a rare life threatening condition of unknown origin which occurs in women without known pre-existing heart disease. It is defined as the development of cardiac failure in the last month of pregnancy or within five months of delivery, in the absence of an identifiable origin or recognisable heart disease before the last month of pregnancy. The condition is rare and personal series are small.

Recent work has shown evidence of acute myocarditis in a majority of patients when endomyocardial biopsy is carried out early in the illness.[15] The onset is most often

Clinical pericardial syndromes are:

- Acute pericarditis

- Relapsing pericarditis

- Cardiac tamponade

- Chronic pericardial effusion without compression

- Effusive constrictive pericarditis

- Constrictive pericarditis

Some important causes of pericarditis

- Idiopathic

- Infectious
  - viral
  - bacterial
  - fungal
  - parasitic

- Immunological
  - relapsing pericarditis
  - post-infarction (Dressler's syndrome)
  - post-cardiotomy syndrome associated with the connective tissue disorders
  - rheumatic fever
  - Still's disease
  - rheumatoid arthritis
  - systemic lupus erythematosus (SLE)
  - mixed connective tissue disease
  - polyarteritis and the Churg-Strauss variant

- Neoplastic

- Post-irradiation

- Traumatic

- Uraemic

- Drug induced

postpartum and the origin probably immunological without an infective precipitant. This can be related to fetal–maternal incompatibility following the period of maternal immunosuppression during the pregnancy. A mortality of up to 50% has been reported but PPCM may not be as rare as is commonly thought, since subclinical cases may never be diagnosed. The use of immunosuppressive agents, in addition to full treatment for the often fulminating heart failure, is appropriate. Although transplantation has been carried out, a large measure of recovery is common in survivors as in acute myocarditis outside pregnancy. The use of ventricular assist devices as a bridge to recovery rather than transplantation is indicated for the most seriously affected patients.

A genetic predisposition may exist in these patients and occasionally patients give a history of relatives with dilated cardiomyopathy. Clinical recovery may be slow and delayed even up to a year or more after the birth. Even when it appears to be complete, a measure of cardiovascular reserve has been lost, as is indicated by the myocytolysis found on biopsy. Recurrence in future pregnancies is not invariable but there are few data. Pregnancy should therefore be discouraged in any patient with residual myocardial dysfunction and, if possible, delayed for some years.

Summary

Acute myocarditis has many different clinical presentations but, most commonly by far, mimics the onset of acute myocardial infarction. It may present with acute heart failure but only rarely as dilated cardiomyopathy of recent onset. Subclinical myocarditis is common and strenuous exercise should be avoided during acute infections.

Pericardial diseases

Pericarditis is very much a part of general medicine, developing as an acute illness or complicating rheumatic renal and malignant disease or treatment with certain drugs. Echocardiography has done much to reveal pericardial (and myocardial) involvement in "non-cardiac" conditions and to demonstrate the physiology of tamponade and constriction.

Acute pericarditis

The features of acute pericarditis are pericardial pain, pericardial friction, and concordant ST segment elevation on the ECG.

As in acute myocarditis, there are numerous causes but frequently none is found. Acute idiopathic pericarditis is usually benign but may rapidly constrict or pursue a relapsing course before burning out. Rarely it may be associated with a clinically occult diffuse myocarditis (rather than the more usual epicarditis which is responsible for the typical ECG changes). Pericardiocentesis in such cases may be followed by collapse and cardiogenic shock and is ill-advised. Echo should prevent mistakes by checking ventricular contractile function as well as the features of tamponade.

The patient is usually febrile and the pain may be mild or severe. It is typically exacerbated by inspiration and relieved by leaning forward. A friction rub may come and go. Signs of tamponade are unusual.

The chest radiograph may be normal or the heart shadow may be slightly enlarged. There may be pleural effusions but pulmonary congestion, if present, indicates associated myocarditis.

The ECG shows generalised ST segment elevation. This is a current of injury from the superficial layers of the myocardium. The changes are usually generalised. The QRS is normal unless there is a large pericardial effusion. With resolution the ST segment becomes isoelectric and there may be T wave inversion which sometimes persists. Arrhythmias may develop.

> ### The ECG in acute pericarditis is mimicked by:
>
> - early repolarisation
>
> - acute early anterior myocardial infarction
>
> - acute myocarditis

The ECG changes of acute pericarditis may be mimicked by early repolarisation seen most often in young males. Elevated concave upward ST segments are located in the precordial leads with reciprocal depression in AVR; T waves are peaked and slightly asymmetrical with a notch and a slur on the R wave. The axis is usually vertical with counter clockwise rotation, a short and depressed PR interval, prominent U waves, and sinus bradycardia. The ST segment becomes isoelectric with exercise or administration of isoprenaline. Early repolarisation is a benign condition.

Both changes of early repolarisation and of acute pericarditis mimic those of early acute anterior myocardial infarction. Echocardiography provides the most rapid and certain means of differentiation in most cases but not in all. Acute myocarditis also commonly mimics acute myocardial infarction. Enzyme release is usual in those who show ST segment elevation on ECG[16] and echo may show regional akinesia. Coronary angiography differentiates, and endomyocardial biopsy can be performed at the same time.

Other investigations include exclusion of known causes of acute pericarditis, particularly tuberculosis which may require pericardial aspiration. In that case, the pericardium should be aspirated to dryness and all the fluid sent to the laboratory so that it can be spun down and the sediment stained for microbacteria. A tuberculin test may be negative in acute tuberculous pericarditis, which is now being seen more commonly in immigrants and HIV positive patients and is increasingly found to be caused by variant and resistant forms of mycobacteria.

Relapsing pericarditis

Relapsing or recurrent pericarditis causes episodes of chest pain with or without a friction rub, sometimes with pericardial and even pleural effusions. Each episode may last several days and be accompanied by fever. Pericarditis of any cause may be followed by this disabling condition, which is frequently not diagnosed especially if an initiating bout of acute pericarditis has not been documented. It may complicate recovery from acute myocardial infarction (Dressler's syndrome) or cardiac surgery (the postcardiotomy syndrome). Each may be followed by one or several recurrences but the most recalcitrant cases tend to be idiopathic.

The condition is benign and does not lead to constriction. It can sometimes recur for several years before burning out and is then very debilitating, with a major impact on general well being, family life, and work.

Management

Mild cases of relapsing pericarditis respond to aspirin or other non-steroidal anti-inflammatory drugs. Steroids are dramatically effective but should be reserved for severe cases and used only to treat acute attacks, as maintenance steroids do not prevent relapses and create a tendency to ever increasing dosage.

Colchicine is the treatment of choice and can also provide effective prophylaxis. It was introduced because of its efficacy in familial Mediterranean fever (polyserositis). Patients who have been treated with steroids can be weaned off them and on to colchicine. The dose for acute attacks is 1 mg followed by 0.5 mg two or three hourly to a maximum of 10 mg.[17] The maintenance dose is 0.5 mg twice daily. If necessary, colchicine can be combined with indomethacin.

Pericardiectomy has been tried but fails to prevent relapses of pain. This is to be expected as the inflammation may be a reaction to epicardial (or viral) material recognised as foreign, so there is no reason why removal of the fibrous pericardium should make a difference.

Cardiac tamponade

Tamponade may occur in pericarditis of any cause but is uncommon in idiopathic and post-infarction pericarditis. It is usual in acute pyogenic, tuberculous, and malignant pericarditis. Acute haemopericardium may cause tamponade following cardiac rupture after myocardial infarction, in dissection of the aortic root or after cardiac surgery. Metastatic carcinoma, as well as primary tumours, may present with tamponade.

Patients with tamponade may complain of shortness of breath, weakness, heaviness in the chest, or present with hypotension or even cardiogenic shock.

Examination reveals pulsus paradoxus, a high venous pressure in the neck, and a quiet heart with faint heart sounds. It is readily diagnosed in patients known to be at risk but often missed in a previously fit individual or, for example, in a patient with septic shock where the shock is actually caused by pericardial tamponade rather than by septicaemia.[18]

Echocardiography is diagnostic, and has shown that inspiratory increase of blood flow into the heart is accommodated in the right atrium and admitted to the right ventricle at the expense of left ventricular volume as the ventricular septum moves sharply towards the left ventricle, reducing left ventricular stroke volume. Diastolic collapse of the right atrium and right ventricular walls are seen when pericardial pressure rises to exceed the intracardiac pressure, terminating further flow into the heart and thereby reducing or removing the Y descent of the venous pulse, which shows very small volume excursion and may therefore be difficult to see.

Pericardiocentesis should be performed in the cardiac catheterisation laboratory under ultrasound guidance, in addition to fluoroscopy and ECG, and preferably with simultaneous cardiac pressure monitoring. The subxiphoid approach is the safest. Pericardioscopy

225

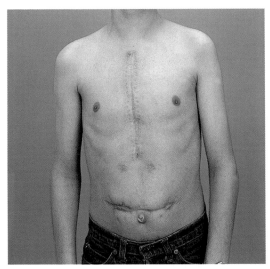

Figure 33.2. Constrictive pericarditis caused by infection presented 10 years after operation to relieve ileal atresia as a neonate. The patient had developed septicaemia as an infant but purulent pericarditis had not been recognised.

Differential diagnosis of constrictive pericarditis

- Primary restrictive cardiomyopathy
  - pulmonary congestion
  - pulmonary hypertension and tricuspid regurgitation with large right (and left) atrium

- Amyloid heart disease
  - absent third sound (until very advanced)
  - low ECG voltage
  - thickening of myocardium on echo

has been used to facilitate diagnostic pericardial biopsy. Triamcinolone can prevent recurrence of immunologically based effusions and cisplatin can deter re-accumulation of malignant effusions.[19]

Chronic pericardial effusion without compression

Large lax effusions occasionally occur, may cause few symptoms, and are found accidentally. It is unusual to find a cause. A very few may be associated with myxoedema.

Effusive constrictive pericarditis

When pericardial effusion is associated with thickening of the visceral pericardium the patient may have persistent cardiac compression, even after pericardiocentesis. It may be seen in tuberculous pericarditis, rheumatoid patients or after mediastinal irradiation.

Constrictive pericarditis

When thickening and scarring of the parietal and/or visceral pericardium compresses the heart and restricts cardiac filling, stroke volume becomes limited despite a considerable rise in filling pressure. Constriction is usually generalised but rarely may be localised, owing to constricting bands usually in the left or right atrioventricular grooves or round the entry of the superior or inferior vena cava.

A tuberculous origin is uncommon now in the west and most cases are idiopathic. A few are associated with rheumatoid arthritis, collagen vascular disease or uraemia, or rarely follow cardiac surgery or irradiation.

The heart is small and pulmonary venous congestion rare. The diastolic pressures in the four cardiac chambers will be similar and the left atrial pressure is rarely high enough to cause pulmonary congestion.

The signs are predominantly right sided and congestive, a high jugular venous pressure with prominent X and Y descents, hepatomegaly, and peripheral oedema. There may be ascites.

The heart is small and quiet with a sharp early third heart sound, which may be confused with pulmonary closure (fig 33.2).

Differentiation from a restrictive cardiomyopathy is not usually difficult as in cardiomyopathy the left sided diastolic pressures are usually much higher than those on the right, unless there is considerable tricuspid regurgitation. The latter is rare in constrictive pericarditis.

In amyloid heart disease a left ventricular third sound is not heard because slow ventricular filling continues through diastole, except in very advanced cases who develop a restrictive physiology. Echocardiography quickly differentiates.

Pericarditis is common in the connective tissue diseases. Acute pericarditis is occasionally the presenting manifestation in Still's disease, when the presence and persistence of severe constitutional symptoms and development of arthritis make the diagnosis clear. Acute pericarditis is common in systemic lupus, particularly during acute flares, and in the Churg-Strauss variant of polyarteritis, but is usually painless in rheumatoid arthritis. Constriction may occur in any of these disorders but is most often seen in association with rheumatoid arthritis because of its greater prevalence.

A number of drugs can induce a lupus syndrome with pericarditis. The best known example is with hydralazine, but it may also be caused by procainamide, methyldopa, and minoxidil. It is reversible on stopping the drug.

1. **Kawai C.** From myocarditis to cardiomyopathy: mechanisms of inflammation and cell death in learning from the past for the future. *Circulation* 1999;**99**:1091–100.
   - *The molecular analysis of necropsy and endomyocardial biopsy specimens has clarified the causal link between myocarditis and dilated cardiomyopathy.*

2. **Huber SA, Gauntt CJ, Sakkinen P.** Enteroviruses and myocarditis. Viral pathogenesis through replication, cytokine induction and immunopathogenicity. *Adv Virus Res* 1998;**51**:35–80.

3. **Bachmaier K, Neu N, de la Masa LM,** *et al.* Chlamydia infections and heart disease linked through antigenic mimicry. *Science* 1999;**283**:1335 9.

4. **Bowles NE, Towbin JA.** Molecular aspects of myocarditis. *Current Opinion in Cardiology* 1998;**13**:179–84.
   - *The pathogenesis of myocarditis remains elusive. The crucial roles of cytokine expression and of aberrant induction of apoptosis are being defined.*

5. **Karjalainen J, Heikkila J.** Incidence of three presentations of acute myocarditis in young men in military service: a 20 year experience. *Eur Heart J* 1999;**20**:1120–5.
   - *The usual presentation mimics myocardial infarction (98 cases); only one presented with sudden death and nine as dilated cardiomyopathy of recent origin.*

6. **Smith SC, Ladenson JH, Mason JW,** *et al.* Elevations of cardiac troponin I associated with myocarditis. Experimental and clinical correlations. *Circulation* 1997;**95**:163–8.
 • *Many patients have elevated troponin or creatine kinase MB if studied during the first week of the disease. When found in a patient with chest pain and ECG ST segment elevation on presentation, the clinical similarity with myocardial infarction caused by coronary thrombosis may be complete.*

7. **Aretz HT, Billingham ME, Edwards WD.** Myocarditis: a histopathological definition and classification. *Am J Cardiovasc Pathol* 1987;**1**:3–14.

8. **Mason JW.** Myocarditis. *Adv Intern Med* 1999;**44**:293–310.

9. **Brodison A, Swann JW.** Myocarditis: a review. *J Infection* 1998;**37**:99–103.
 • *Means of early identification are needed to prevent progression to chronic heart failure by more satisfactory therapies.*

10. **Mason JW, O'Connell JB, Herskowitz A,** *et al.* A clinical trial of immunosuppressive therapy of myocarditis. The myocarditis treatment trial investigators. *N Engl J Med* 1995;**333**:269–75.

11. **Friman G, Ilback NG.** Acute infection: metabolic responses, effects on performance, interaction with exercise and myocarditis. *Int J Sports Med* 1998;**19**(suppl 35):172–82.

12. **Anandasabathy S, Frishman WH.** Innovative drug treatments for viral and auto-immune myocarditis. *J Clin Pharmacol* 1998;**38**:295–308.
 • *Better means of distinguishing between viral and autoimmune causes are needed so that treatment can be appropriate. A useful review of treatments.*

13. **Lieberman EB, Hutchins GM, Herskowitz A,** *et al.* Clinico-pathological description of myocarditis. *Am J Cardiol* 1991;**18**:1617–26.

14. **McCarthy RE, Boeehmer P, Hruban RH,** *et al.* Long term outlook of fulminant myocarditis as compared with acute (non-fulminant) myocarditis. *N Engl J Med* 2000;**342**:690–5.

15. **Midei MG, De Ment SH, Feldman AM,** *et al.* Peripartum myocarditis and cardiomyopathy. *Circulation* 1990;**81**:922–8.
 • *Changes of acute myocarditis are found in a high proportion of cases if biopsies are obtained within a month of onset.*

16. **Karjalainen J, Heikkila J.** "Acute pericarditis" myocardial enzyme release as evidence for myocarditis. *Am Heart J* 1986;**111**:546–52.
 • *Myocardial enzyme release is uncommon without simultaneous ST-segment elevation in suspected acute myocarditis.*

17. **Adler Y, Finkelstein Y, Guindo J,** *et al.* Colchicine treatment for recurrent pericarditis. A decade of experience. *Circulation* 1998;**97**:2183–5.
 • *Colchicine is probably the treatment of first choice for recurrent pericarditis, especially when the origin is idiopathic.*

18. **Arsura EL, Kilgore WB, Strategos E.** Purulent pericarditis misdiagnosed as septic shock. *Southern Med J* 1992;**92**:285–8.
 • *Failure to recognise purulent pericarditis and tamponade may be fatal in bacteraemic patients. In contrast to patients with septic shock, patients with tamponade have high systemic vascular resistance and low cardiac output.*

19. **Maisch B, Pankuneit S, Brilla C,** *et al.* Intrapericardial treatment of inflammatory and neoplastic pericarditis guided by pericardioscopy and epicardial biopsy results from a pilot study. *Clin Cardiol* 1999;**22**(supp 1):117–22.

34 Heart disease in the elderly

Michael Lye, Christina Donnellan

We are an aging population. It is estimated that 20% of people in Europe will be over 65 years of age in the year 2000. The proportion of the population over 80 years, the so-called "old old", is increasing most rapidly. Life expectancy at all ages is also increasing. At 65 years life expectancy ranges from 14.9 to 18.9 years and at 80 years from 6.9 to 9.1 years for men and women, respectively. Cardiovascular disease is the most frequent single cause of death in persons over 65 years of age[1], and most importantly it is responsible for considerable morbidity and a large burden of disability, particularly in the community.

Cardiovascular pathologies such as hypertension and cerebrovascular disease, and heart diseases such as coronary artery disease, arrhythmias, and heart failure, increase in incidence with increasing age.[w1] The aging process itself also effects the cardiovascular system. It is difficult to differentiate "normal" aging, which is inevitable, from age related pathology, which is potentially preventable or treatable.[w2] Age related changes are most likely to be seen in the "old old" who have escaped cardiovascular pathology earlier in life. This group demonstrates the dual processes, often interacting, of biological aging of the cardiovascular system and age related pathology. This combination modifies the pathophysiology of disease such that knowledge of that condition and treatment thereof, derived from studies in "young old" (65–75 years) are not readily applicable to the "old old". Older patients differ from "trial" patients of any age by virtue of their other comorbidities and multiple drug usage, which are invariably exclusion criteria for entering treatment studies.

Age related structural changes

Cardiac
- Increased left ventricular wall thickness, independent of any increase in blood pressure.[2] This is attributed to hypertrophy of individual myocytes with a progressive loss of myocyte numbers. There is also an accumulation of interstitial connective tissue and, in the "old old", accumulation of amyloid deposits.[w3]
- Increased fibrosis and calcification of the valves, particularly the mitral annulus and the aortic valve.[w3] [w4] Recently it has been shown that aortic sclerosis without outflow obstruction is not the benign condition once thought and is associated with significantly increased cardiovascular and total mortality.[w5]

- Loss of cells in the sinoatrial node. By 75 years of age, only 10% of the cells that were present at 20 years remain. There is loss of muscle cells and mild increases in fibrous tissue in the internodal tracts. The remainder of the conducting system is also affected but to a lesser extent.[w4] These changes occur in the absence of coronary artery disease.

Vascular
- Increased stiffness of peripheral and central arteries, caused by proliferation of collagen cross links, smooth muscle hypertrophy, calcification, and loss of elastic fibres.[w6]
- Increase in number of sites for lipid deposition cause endothelial changes that reduce laminar blood flow. These changes are independent of atherosclerosis.[w6]
- More diffuse coronary artery changes. The earliest changes usually appear in the left coronary artery during youth or adulthood, whereas the right and posterior coronary arteries do not usually become involved until after the age of 60 years.

Age related functional changes

Left ventricular systolic function
- In patients carefully screened to exclude coronary artery disease and hypertension, there is little change in left ventricular systolic function with increasing age, although cardiac output may decrease in parallel with a reduction in lean body mass.[1] [w7] The determinants of cardiac output which may be influenced by age include heart rate, preload and afterload, muscle performance, and neurohormonal regulation.
- Increases in heart rate in response to exercise or stress caused by non-cardiovascular illnesses, particularly infections, are attenuated with increasing age.[3] [w8] Stroke volume increases only by "moving up" the Frank Starling curve.[w9] [w10] Thus end diastolic volume increases. These age related changes in cardiac response to exercise are mimicked by β adrenergic blockade,[w11] but β adrenergic agonists do not reverse this aging process.[w12] The decline in exercise performance with age may additionally relate to peripheral factors, blood flow, and muscle mass rather than being solely the consequence of cardiac performance changes.

Diastolic function
- The rate and volume of early diastolic filling decrease with age.[1] [w13] The structural changes described above account for some of

Features of a normal aging process[w2]
- Universal within the species
- Intrinsic to the individual
- Deleterious to survival
- Progressive and irreversible

this decline, but recent findings of partial reversibility with calcium channel blockers[4] or exogenous angiotensin II receptor antagonists[w14] illustrate the dynamic and therefore potentially reversible nature of the process.

- The aged heart requires atrial contraction to maintain adequate diastolic filling, so atrial fibrillation, so common in older people, has a disproportionate effect on cardiac function.[w7]

- Reduced ventricular compliance results in higher left ventricular diastolic pressures at rest and during exercise.[w8] [w13] As a result, pulmonary and systemic venous congestion may occur in the presence of normal systolic function.[w15] With increased afterload on the left ventricle, left ventricular hypertrophy occurs, even in the absence of hypertension or aortic stenosis.[w16 w17] Diastolic dysfunction, at least in the early stages, may be a feature of normal aging. Later, however, it is a pathological process leading to significant left ventricular hypertrophy. At this stage coronary heart disease, hypertension or other pathology is probably involved.

- Age related decreases in capillary density and coronary reserve may cause myocardial ischaemia and thus further diastolic abnormalities in the absence of coronary atherosclerotic disease.[2] [w18] Age associated decreases in the rate of maximal capacity of calcium sequestration by the sarcoplasmic reticulum and/or an age associated increase in net trans-sarcolemmal calcium influx may also contribute to diastolic ventricular abnormalities.[w19 w20]

Heart failure

Chronic heart failure is a disease of "old old" people, and unlike coronary artery disease, the incidence continues to rise with increasing age. Only 17% of people with heart failure are less than 65 years of age,[5] yet most of the interventional studies of the treatment of chronic heart failure have focused on this minority group and extrapolated the results to the older majority.[w21 w22] "Diastolic" heart failure is probably the primary haemodynamic dysfunction in the elderly. Among patients over 80 years of age with clinically defined heart failure, up to 70% have preserved systolic function,[w21] whereas probably less than 10% of patients below 60 years of age have preserved systolic function.[6] It is important to be aware of this high prevalence of diastolic dysfunction as it has implications for treatment. Over 75% of elderly patients with heart failure have hypertension and/or coronary artery disease, and patients with diastolic dysfunction may present with decompensated heart failure caused by uncontrolled blood pressure or progression of ischaemic heart disease.[w23]

Clinical presentation

The symptoms and signs of heart failure are similar in young and elderly people, but non-specific presentation is more common in the elderly.[1] [w24] Community based studies have indicated that perhaps up to half of "old old" patients with activity limiting heart failure are undiagnosed and therefore untreated.[7] There is an expectation by old people themselves, by their relatives, and unfortunately by some of their doctors that many of the features of heart failure in older people are a result of normal aging—"what do you expect at his age?" Patients may present with confusion, depression, fatigue, weight loss, immobility or "social crisis".[w25] Patients with chronic heart failure caused by systolic dysfunction tend to present with gradual worsening of daytime symptoms and paroxysmal nocturnal dyspnoea, whereas those with diastolic dysfunction may present with a more abrupt onset of symptoms.

It is difficult to distinguish between systolic and diastolic heart failure clinically. Some patients may have a combination of both, especially in later stages of the disease. As in younger patients, a normal 12 lead ECG virtually excludes significant heart failure. All older patients should have access to echocardiography to aid diagnosis. This will allow diagnosis of causal factors such as valvar lesions, and provide an assessment of haemodynamic (systolic versus diastolic) function. Normal or preserved systolic function in heart failure has been assumed to imply diastolic dysfunction, but this is no longer adequate as we now have guidelines from the European Society of Cardiology giving clear echocardiographic criteria for diastolic heart failure—at least applicable to the "young old" patient.[8]

Management

Diuretics

The management of systolic heart failure in elderly patients, as in younger patients, involves the use of diuretics, vasodilators, and oxygen supplementation (table 34.1). Most elderly patients will require a loop diuretic because of the age related and heart failure mediated reduction in glomerular filtration rate. Thiazide diuretics are ineffective when the glomerular filtration rate is less than 30–40 ml/min. There is an age related decrease in total body potassium content, as predicted by a proportional reduction in lean body mass, but not in plasma potassium concentrations.[w26] Potassium retention is more of a problem than hypokalaemia in older patients, particularly with the combined use of angiotensin converting enzyme (ACE) inhibitors and potassium sparing diuretics or supplements. Additionally potassium sparing diuretics should be avoided in the elderly because of the increased risks of

Table 34.1 Evidence of benefit for symptoms and mortality for drugs used in heart failure in patients more than 75 years of age

| Drugs | Benefit | | |
	Yes	No	Unknown
Diuretics	Symptoms	–	Mortality
Digoxin	Symptoms	Mortality	–
ACE inhibitors	Symptoms/Mortality	–	–
AIIAs	–	Mortality	Symptoms
β Blockers	–	–	Symptoms/mortality
Spironolactone	–	–	Symptoms/mortality

ACE, angiotensin converting enzyme; AIIAs, angiotensin II receptor antagonists.

Adverse effects of diuretics in older people
● Incontinence
● Urinary retention
● Hyponatraemia
● Hyperkalaemia

hyponatraemia and uraemia as well as hyperkalaemia. While metabolic adverse effects of diuretics should be appreciated the physical effects are invariably more important to the older patient. Thus for the patient whose mobility is impaired by arthritis, Parkinson's or even heart failure itself, being rendered incontinent by high dose loop diuretics does not aid compliance. Similarly acute retention in both men and women does not create a good doctor–patient relationship. It is best therefore to start with a low dose and titrate upwards gradually on the basis of effect on body weight, for example.

ACE inhibitors

ACE inhibitors have demonstrated haemodynamic, functional, and mortality benefits in heart failure patients.[w27] [w28] Unfortunately they are often under prescribed to older patients or, if given, are administered at suboptimal doses.[5] First dose hypotension is not a particular problem in older patients since low dose initiation of ACE inhibitors, preferably with short acting captopril, has become standard practice. Renal function should be monitored closely following their introduction.[w29] Cough, which may be poorly described and confused with early paroxysmal nocturnal dyspnoea, is a frequently seen problem in elderly patients. In old age generalised atherosclerosis may increase the risk of renal artery stenosis, thus increasing the risk of renal failure precipitated by ACE inhibitors. The place of angiotensin II receptor antagonists in routine management of heart failure patients of any age remains problematic. The beneficial effect of losartan seen in ELITE I was borne out in ELITE II, but losartan was shown to be no better than captopril in this larger study. Both trials, however, demonstrated that older patients can successfully be recruited to intervention studies of the treatment of heart failure.[9] [w30]

Inotropes

Data on the use of digoxin in systolic heart failure with normal sinus rhythm are equivocal,[w31] but there is some evidence of benefit for patients with severe heart failure; fewer clinical deteriorations, hospital admissions, and emergency visits have been reported with digoxin.[w32] Digoxin must be used with caution in the elderly because of its narrow therapeutic window,[w33] and it is advisable to monitor blood concentrations especially if circumstances change and the patient develops pre-renal uraemia (influenza, chest infection, dehydration, haematemesis). Other possible inotropes cannot be recommended for routine use in elderly patients at the present time.

Other pharmacological agents

The absence of older patients in the recent studies of β blockers and spironolactone in heart failure make it difficult to assess their benefits in older patients. It is likely, however, that the older heart failure patient will benefit but this requires confirmation. For patients intolerant of ACE inhibitors the usual practice has been to use a combination of hydralazine and isosorbide mononitrate.[w34] [w35] While there are no direct comparisons of hydralazine, isosorbide mononitrate and angiotensin II receptor antagonists, it is likely that the latter will be better tolerated in older patients.

General measures

Bed rest is discouraged in elderly patients because the risk of thromboembolism and physical deconditioning far outweigh any advantages.[10] Compression stockings should be used and anticoagulation should be considered in the immobile patient with severe failure and/or atrial fibrillation to guard against the development of deep venous thrombosis and embolisation.[w36] Hopefully the period of anticoagulation should be limited until mobility is restored. The European Society of Cardiology guidelines stress the importance of general lifestyle measures which are probably of equal benefit in the older patient.[11] Fluid restriction is not usually necessary and may be dangerous, as many elderly patients have poor oral intake when ill. Salt restriction is often difficult as many elderly patients survive on convenience foods in which the salt content is high. The elderly also suffer from "cardiac cachexia"—loss of fat free mass.[w37] The mechanism is unclear, although fat absorption is impaired,[w38] but there is no evidence of gastrointestinal protein loss.[w39] Apoptosis in skeletal muscle is common in patients with heart failure.[w40] It is often not noticed until the oedema has subsided in response to diuretic treatment.

The social burden of heart failure on elderly patients is largely ignored. Many older patients live alone and the onset of heart failure drastically reduces independence. The provision of a home help, a shopper, aids or appliances may substantially improve quality of life and maintain patients in their own homes. These measures are as important as drug treatment of many older patients.

Support clinics

Studies have shown the effectiveness of nurse led, patient focused support clinics for heart failure patients by reducing hospital readmissions, improving compliance with medications, enhancing quality of life, and improving patient education.[w41–43] Our own simple studies of older unselected patients discharged from hospital demonstrate significant improvements in exercise capacity, quality of life, drug adherence, and a 60% reduction in readmissions in the three months after hospital discharge. A more intensive nurse led multidisciplinary intervention in the USA improved quality of life and reduced rehospitalisations of older selected patients with heart failure.[12] Attention to the delivery of support to older heart failure patients may be more beneficial and cost effective than adherence to the latest drug usage guidelines.

"Diastolic" heart failure

The management of heart failure with preserved systolic function is not as clear as that of heart failure in which systolic function is impaired. Treatment objectives should be to improve ventricular relaxation and filling. Attention to aggravating factors (such as hypertension, atrial fibrillation, anaemia, and left ventricular outflow obstruction) is the first step in management. There are no trials of treatment of diastolic heart failure so drug recommendations can only be made on an empirical basis. Certainly patients benefit symptomatically from diuretics. However, hypovolaemia and reduced preload secondary to over vigorous diuresis should be avoided. Thus loop diuretics should be started low and monitored carefully. Digoxin is not indicated and may be harmful.[w33] Agents that may improve ventricular filling in diastole include β blockers, calcium channel blockers, and perhaps ACE inhibitors.[9] Calcium channel blockers have been shown to improve left ventricular diastolic filling, whether impairment is age associated, or caused by ischaemic heart disease or hypertension.[w13 w20 w44] Studies on efficacy in diastolic heart failure of β blockers and ACE inhibitors are awaited.[w45]

Prognosis

Heart failure caused by diastolic dysfunction has a better prognosis in terms of mortality than systolic heart failure.[13] The five year mortality rate with systolic heart failure is about 50%.[w46] In elderly patients and those with severe heart failure the mortality at one year is at least 30%. Older males have higher mortality than females and white men have a 10% greater risk of death than black men.[w47] These figures underscore the importance of secondary prevention strategies and the early detection and treatment of heart failure in older patients. Prognosis also depends on the presence of other cardiovascular comorbidities such as ischaemic heart disease, hypertension, and vascular complications of diabetes.[w48] Additionally older patients suffer multiple pathologies which have to be taken into account when planning management or assessing prognosis.

Congestive heart failure is the most common cause of hospital admission in elderly patients in the USA, with patients subject to frequent readmissions.[w49] Poor compliance with medication, particularly diuretics, is an important factor and has been reported in up to 50% of elderly patients with congestive heart failure.[w50]

Coronary artery disease

Coronary artery disease increases in incidence with aging. Age itself is an independent risk factor for coronary artery disease.[w51 w52] Sixty per cent of all deaths attributed to acute myo-cardial infarction are in patients over 75 years of age.[w53] A necropsy study of patients 90 years of age and over revealed that 70% of subjects had one or more coronary vessels occluded.[w54]

In recent years, coronary artery disease mortality has declined in elderly patients, but to a lesser extent than in younger patients. Risk factors are similar to those in younger patients and equally modifiable.

Myocardial infarction

Older patients may describe the typical central chest pain of myocardial infarction, but are as likely to present with dyspnoea without pain.[w55] As in congestive heart failure, they may also present non-specifically with confusion, syncope, vertigo, or epigastric pains.[w56 w57] In the Framingham study, 42% of myocardial infarctions were noted to be clinically silent (asymptomatic) or unrecognised in men aged 75–84 years compared with only 18% in men aged 45–54 years.[w58] The proportion of unrecognised myocardial infarctions was higher in women. Some studies have reported that up to 60% of myocardial infarctions may be unrecognised in the very old.[w59] Unrecognised myocardial infarction patients are more likely to be hypertensive, have diabetes, and smoke, and have a lower prevalence of preceding angina.[w60 w61]

Risk factors are similar in both sexes, but women have a less favourable psychosocial risk profile, including living alone, which adversely affects prognosis.[w62] Older people and women of all ages present later to hospital.[w63 w64] One study reported that patients over 80 years of age delayed more than 6.5 hours in calling paramedics, compared with a 3.9 hour delay in younger patients.[w65] Older patients are twice as likely as younger patients to have non-Q wave myocardial infarctions.[14] Up to 40% of elderly patients do not have typical ST elevation or Q waves on their ECG at presentation.[w65] Right ventricular infarction is also more frequent in older patients,[15] and mortality rates as high as 75% have been reported in this group.[w66]

Management

Unfortunately, elderly patients have been largely excluded from the randomised controlled trials of treatments for myocardial infarction. Pooled data from several large placebo controlled trials show that the absolute reduction in mortality is at least as great in older as in younger patients.[w67] It is no surprise that elderly patients are less likely to receive thrombolysis than younger patients given the differences in presentation. Contraindications are similar to those for younger patients, but elderly patients are more likely to experience adverse effects from treatment. There is an excess of eight haemorrhagic strokes per thousand in patients over 75 years given thrombolytics, and it may occur more frequently with recombinant tissue plasminogen activator (rt-PA) than streptokinase.[w68] The decision to administer thrombolysis and the choice of agent used must therefore depend on the overall assessment of risk versus the potential benefit.

Aspirin should be administered to older patients as for younger patients. In ISIS-2, the absolute benefit from aspirin was greatest in patients over 70 years of age.[w69] In the absence of contraindications, early use of β blockers reduces mortality post-myocardial infarction at all ages.[w70 w71] ACE inhibitors should be given to haemodynamically stable patients, particularly older patients, within 24 hours if there are any signs of heart failure, and possibly routinely in the presence of a large anterior myocardial infarction.[w72 w73] Other treatments including nitrates and oxygen should be administered as for younger patients. Smaller doses of morphine are recommended for elderly patients.

Evidence to support routine use of unfractionated heparin in acute myocardial infarction is lacking, but its benefit is clear in unstable angina. The low molecular weight heparin, enoxaparin, was superior to unfractionated heparin in reducing recurrent angina, myocardial infarction, and death in patients with unstable angina or non-Q wave infarction.[w70 w74]

In acute infarction the role of primary percutaneous transluminal coronary angioplasty (PTCA) in this age group has not been evaluated, apart from one small study in which mortality compared favourably between PTCA and streptokinase.[16] There are very little data available on the use of intracoronary stents in older people.

Prognosis
Hospital mortality for myocardial infarction patients over 70 years of age is at least three times that of younger patients.[w75 w76] Older patients are at high risk for major cardiovascular complications. Women have a higher crude mortality associated with myocardial infarction.[w77] Poor prognosis in this age group is multifactorial. Numerous studies have shown that the therapeutic approach in older patients is unjustifiably less aggressive than in younger patients and potentially beneficial drugs are underused.[w78 w79]

Secondary prevention
Risk factors should be identified in older patients, and modified if possible. Lifestyle measures such as diet, smoking, and exercise should be addressed whatever the age of the patient. It is surprisingly easy to persuade older patients who have smoked cigarettes for half a century to give up if they are given all the information. Hypertension, especially isolated systolic hypertension, should be treated rigorously while monitoring for adverse drug effects, which are more common in the older patient. Patients should be screened for impaired glucose tolerance or non-insulin dependent diabetes mellitus, and both treated to maintain normal glycaemia. Patients with a raised low density lipoprotein (LDL) cholesterol should receive dietary advice and a statin as for younger patients. Pravastatin reduced coronary events and mortality in patients up to 75 years of age with average cholesterol over a five year follow up period.[17] Cholesterol may be a poorer predictor of coronary events in older people as plasma concentrations are influenced by comorbidity. Patients over 75 years have not been recruited to the major lipid lowering trials. However, because of the accumulation of other perhaps non-modifiable risk factors, intervention is probably still warranted.[w80]

Rehabilitation
All older patients who are not seriously cognitively impaired should have access to cardiac rehabilitation, with the aim of maintaining peak physical functioning and personal independence. Staff in cardiac rehabilitation programmes have to be aware of the patients' comorbidities and modify programmes and support as appropriate. Exercise training programmes have been found to improve endurance and functional capacity in older people after myocardial infarction.[18] In spite of advanced age older patients, rather than healthy subjects, can and will change well-entrenched lifestyles. Even after 20 years relative inactivity, patients can and will increase exercise if given good reasons and "permission" to do so and can be made aware of personal benefits.

Angina
Lifestyle limiting angina has a prevalence of around 16% in people over the age of 65 years.[w81] The diagnosis in older patients can be difficult. It is overdiagnosed because too little attention is paid to obtaining a precise history or the diagnosis is a legacy from many years ago. Many "old old" patients had angina in their 60s which they seem to have outgrown in their 80s. This may be due to almost subconscious avoidance of precipitating factors. It is more acceptable for older subjects to adopt a sedentary lifestyle and thus avoid provoking symptoms on exercise. This may also lead to underdiagnosis of angina. Standard treatment should be followed in this age group as for younger patients but adverse drug effects (postural hypotension, negative inotropism, and oedema) may limit drug options. In this situation, or where patients are resistant to maximal medical treatment, referral for PTCA or surgery is indicated.[w82] While PTCA or surgery confirm no survival benefit, recent evidence suggests that elderly patients benefit from symptom relief more than younger patients with aggressive surgical intervention.[w83] They should therefore, at the very least, be referred for assessment and not denied the potential benefits because of age alone.

Arrhythmias

Atrial fibrillation
Five per cent of people over the age of 65 years have chronic atrial fibrillation (AF)[w84] approximately half of whom do not have associated myocardial disease—so called lone AF. Loss of diastolic filling caused by AF may compromise left ventricular filling to such an extent that it precipitates heart failure. Except in recent onset AF chemical or electrical cardioversion to sinus rhythm is not usually an option because of high relapse rates, though careful

232

selection may improve maintenance of sinus rhythm.[w85] Failing this rate control with digoxin is a less effective alternative,[w86] although the addition of a calcium channel antagonist or β blocker may improve rate control during exercise.[w87]

AF is associated with cerebral embolisation and stroke.[w88] The risk of embolisation increases with the addition of other factors such that cardioversion or anticoagulation becomes warranted. These risk factors include previous transient ischaemic attack/stroke, heart failure, hypertension, diabetes,[w89] and most importantly age over 75 years.[w90] AF associated with any one of these risk factors requires anticoagulation.[w91] The latter risk factor alone causes logistic problems for primary care in the management of long term warfarin treatment in the community.[w92]

Several placebo controlled trials have shown the efficacy of anticoagulation in non-rheumatic AF. More than 1000 patients (mean age 67 years) were entered into a placebo comparison with aspirin or warfarin. The trial had to be stopped prematurely at 29 months because of significant benefits of anticoagulation.[w93] A comparison of warfarin and aspirin by the same group showed similar thromboembolic benefits in patients older than 75 years compared with younger patients.[w94] However, bleeding complications with warfarin were higher in the older patients. Novel ways of delivering anticoagulation treatment need to be explored. While adverse effects and risks from anticoagulation do increase with increasing age, benefits still invariably outweigh adverse effects for carefully selected patients.[w95 w96] It should be appreciated that the majority of old people with AF are not so frail and decrepit that they should be denied the undoubted benefits of anticoagulation. To fail to anticoagulate on the basis of age alone is "ageism" and poor medicine.[w22] Anticoagulation with warfarin is probably not indicated in patients with cognitive impairment sufficient to compromise compliance, in patients subject to recurrent falling, and in patients with a history of recent gastrointestinal bleeding (within three months) or potentially serious drug interactions. In patients where full anticoagulation with warfarin is likely to cause potentially severe adverse effects aspirin will deliver less benefit at less risk.

Bradyarrhythmias

Older patients benefit from appropriate physiological pacing which can be provided at a relatively modest cost.[w97] Unfortunately older people in the UK receive pacemakers at approximately half the rate of similar aged patients in the rest of Europe,[w98] and when they do receive a pacemaker it tends to be a bottom of the range model.[w99] Quality of life benefits, especially improvement in cognitive function of older paced patients,[w100] require primary care physicians and generalists to be alert to possible bradyarrhythmias and refer early for appropriate assessment and treatment.

Table 34.2 *Prevalence of different forms of hypertension in a community sample of people aged more than 65 years*[w102]

Type of hypertension	Screening	
	Visit 1	Visit 2
Isolated systolic	19.1	4.2
Isolated diastolic	5.7	1.0
Combined	9.8	3.9
Total	52.2	10.3

Hypertension

Epidemiology

Blood pressure rises with increasing age. The NHANES III survey showed almost linear increases in systolic and diastolic blood pressures from early adult life through to about 65 years of age.[w101] Thereafter systolic levels continue to rise but less so, especially in women, while diastolic levels tends to fall progressively. Thus isolated systolic hypertension becomes the predominant type of hypertension in the "old old"[w102] (table 34.2). As the latter workers showed, the very high prevalences of raised blood pressure in older people decrease with repeated measurements, presumably because of the "white coat" phenomenon. This confirms that the diagnosis of hypertension in older people should not be based upon a single measurement. More than half the population over 85 years of age will be "hypertensive".[w101]

Raised blood pressure in old people is not a benign condition. Hypertension is the major risk factor for strokes, heart failure, coronary heart disease, and peripheral vascular disease.[w103] Isolated systolic hypertension is particularly related to strokes and less so to coronary events. Diastolic pressures may be inversely related to subsequent mortality, implying that pulse pressure may be the best predictor of the adverse effects of raised blood pressure in old people.[w104] Paradoxically low blood pressure is also associated with high mortality in older people but the relation is only short term—that is, within three years of diagnosis. Thereafter, low blood pressure is a predictor of survival.[w105] Presumably the short term observation is a reflection of comorbidity and increased frailty near death.

Treatment

Meta-analyses have quite clearly demonstrated the benefits of treating old people with any type of hypertension, but especially those with isolated systolic hypertension.[w104 w106] Indeed the number needed to treat to prevent one major cardiovascular event decreases significantly with decreasing age, at least under the age of 80 years. Treatment prevents stroke much more than coronary events.[w104 w107] The target blood pressure should be the same as in younger patients—that is, 140/90 mm Hg—and probably lower in that significant proportion of older patients (25%+) with non-insulin dependent diabetes mellitus.[w108]

There remains the problem of the "old old". No adequately controlled treatment study of hypertensive patients aged more than 80 years has been reported.[w22] Very few "old old" patients have been included in wider age range studies, and where they have the numbers are so small that treatment recommendations cannot be made. There is no reason to believe that "old old" hypertensive patients would not benefit from blood pressure lowering, but it is likely that the increased incidence of adverse drug effects may act as a counterbalance. The results of the HYVET study of hypertensive patients over 80 years of age are eagerly awaited.[w109]

1. **Wei JY, Gersh BJ.** Heart disease in the elderly. *Curr Probl Cardiol* 1987;**12**:1–65.
• *This article is a good introduction to the background of cardiovascular disease in the older patient. Management strategies, not surprisingly, are now dated.*

2. **Olivetti G, Melissari M, Capasso JM,** *et al.* Cardiomyopathy of the aging human heart: myocyte loss and reactive hypertrophy. *Circ Res* 1991;**68**:1560–8.
• *This article differentiates aging changes in the heart from age related ischaemic pathology.*

3. **Fairweather DS.** Aging of the heart and the cardiovascular system. *Rev Clin Gerontol* 1992;**2**:83–103.

4. **Arrighi JA, Dilsizian V, Perronefilardi P,** *et al.* Improvement of the age-related impairment in left-ventricular diastolic filling with verapamil in the normal human heart. *Circulation* 1994;**90**:213–9.

5. **Mair FS, Crowley TS, Bundred PE.** Prevalence, aetiology and management of heart failure in general practice. *Br J Gen Pract* 1996;**46**:77–9.
• *A good description is provided of the epidemiology of heart failure based on a community study in an inner city.*

6. **Wong WF, Gold S, Fukuyama O,** *et al.* Diastolic dysfunction in elderly patients with congestive heart failure. *Am J Cardiol* 1989;**63**:1526–8.

7. **Luchi RJ, Taffet GE, Teasdale TA.** Congestive heart failure in the elderly. *J Am Geriatr Soc* 1991;**39**:810–25.

• *This article gives a very detailed overview of heart failure in the elderly, although the diagnostic criteria are now out of date.*

8. **European Study Group on Diastolic Heart Failure.** How to diagnose diastolic heart failure. *Eur Heart J* 1998;**19**:990–1003.
• *A clear description is provided of criteria to positively diagnose diastolic dysfunction in heart failure.*

9. **Pitt B, Segal R, Martinez FA,** *et al.* Randomised trial of losartan versus captopril in patients over 65 with heart failure (evaluation of losartan in the elderly study, ELITE). *Lancet* 1997;**349**:747–52.
• *This double blind study of a comparison between an ACE inhibitor and an angiotensin II receptor blocking agent surprisingly showed better survival with the latter. The study was not powered for mortality results, however. The importance of this study lies not so much in the results but that it shows the feasibility of carrying out controlled trials in elderly heart failure patients.*

10. **Wei JY.** Mechanisms of disease: age and the cardiovascular system. *N Engl J Med* 1992;**327**:1735–9.
• *This article provides a clear description of normal cardiovascular aging with emphasis on autonomic and neurohormonal changes.*

11. **The Task Force of the Working Group on Heart Failure of the European Society of Cardiology.** The treatment of heart failure. *Eur Heart J* 1997;**18**:736–53.

12. **Rich MW, Beckham V, Wittenberg C,** *et al.* A multidisciplinary intervention to prevent the readmission of elderly patients with congestive heart failure. *N Engl J Med* 1995;**333**:1190–5.
• *This was the first convincing study to show the benefits of better delivery of therapeutic advances in heart failure.*

13. **Vasan RS, Benjamin EJ, Levy D.** Prevalence, clinical features and prognosis of diastolic heart failure—an epidemiologic perspective. *J Am Coll Cardiol* 1995;**26**:1565–74.

14. **Goldberg RJ, Gore JM, Gurwitz JH,** *et al.* The impact of age on the incidence and prognosis of initial acute myocardial-infarction—the Worcester heart attack study. *Am Heart J* 1989;**117**:543–9.

15. **Tresch DD.** Management of the older patient with acute myocardial infarction: difference in clinical presentations between older and younger patients. *J Am Geriatr Soc* 1998;**46**:1157–62.
• *This is a detailed account of the significant differences in presentation of myocardial infarction between younger and older patients.*

16. **Laster SB, Rutherford BD, Giorgi LV,** *et al.* Results of direct percutaneous transluminal coronary angioplasty in octogenarians. *Am J Cardiol* 1996;**77**:10–13.

17. **The Cholesterol and Recurrent Events (CARE) Trial.** Effect of pravastatin on cardiovascular events in older patients with myocardial infarction and cholesterol levels in the average range: results of the cholesterol and recurrent events (CARE) trial. *Ann Intern Med* 1998;**129**:681–9.

18. **Williams MA, Maresh CM, Aronow WS,** *et al.* The value of early outpatient cardiac exercise programs for the elderly in comparison with other selected age-groups. *Eur Heart J* 1984;**5**:113–5.

website extra

Additional references appear on the Heart website

www.heartjnl.com

35 Thyroid disease and the heart

A D Toft, N A Boon

Cardiologists encounter thyroid disorders frequently. Hyperthyroidism causes and may present with atrial fibrillation, while hypothyroidism is a risk factor for coronary artery disease. Moreover, the use of amiodarone may precipitate a variety of thyroid disorders, and severe heart disease, such as left ventricular failure or acute myocardial infarction, can cause confusing disturbances in thyroid function tests.

Hyperthyroidism

Hyperthyroidism is a common condition with a prevalence of approximately 1%; it affects predominantly women aged 30–50 years and is usually (70%) caused by Graves' disease which is characterised by diffuse goitre, orbitopathy, pretibial myxoedema, and the presence of stimulating thyrotrophin (TSH) receptor antibody in the serum. Most of the remaining cases (20%) are caused by autonomous production of thyroid hormones by a nodular goitre.

Effects of thyroid hormones on the cardiovascular system

The thyroid secretes two active hormones: thyroxine (T4) which is a prohormone and tri-iodothyronine (T3) which acts as the final mediator. In hyperthyroidism there is excessive production of T3, owing to hypersecretion by the thyroid gland, and an increase in the peripheral monodeiodination of T4, which leads to profound changes in the cardiovascular system through both nuclear and non-nuclear actions at the cellular level.[1]

The interrelation between the direct and indirect actions of T3 on the peripheral circulation and the heart is shown in fig 35.1.[2] Myocardial contractility is increased as a result of a change in the synthesis of myosin heavy chain protein from the β to the α form, increased transcription of the calcium ATPase gene, and enhanced calcium and glucose uptake. These changes make contraction less efficient and increase heat production. Afterload is reduced, with a reduction of as much as 50–70% in systemic vascular resistance, caused by the direct effects of T3 and the indirect effects of excess lactate production (increased tissue thermogenesis) on vascular smooth muscle. Blood flow, particularly to skin, muscle, and heart, is therefore greatly increased. The preload of the heart rises because blood volume is expanded owing to increases in the serum concentrations of angiotensin converting enzyme and erythropoietin, with resultant increases in renal sodium absorption and red cell mass.

Hyperthyroidism is characterised by a high left ventricular ejection fraction (LVEF) at rest but, paradoxically, by a significant fall during exercise. Restoration of euthyroidism is accompanied by the anticipated rise in LVEF on exercise at the same workload and heart rate.[3] This reversible "cardiomyopathy" could explain the reduced exercise tolerance of patients with hyperthyroidism. Rather than being an intermediate state between normal left ventricular function and left ventricular dysfunction at rest, the failure of LVEF to increase on exercise is perhaps better viewed as a consequence of the additional burden of exercise induced increase in afterload on a heart performing near its maximum capacity.

The characteristic tachycardia is caused by a combination of more rapid diastolic depolarisation and shortening of the action potential of the sinoatrial cells. The refractory period of the atrial cells is also shortened which may explain the well known propensity to atrial fibrillation.

There is a complex interaction between thyroid hormones and the adrenergic system, and many of the clinical features of hyperthyroidism such as tachycardia, increased pulse pressure, and tremor resemble the heightened β adrenergic state of phaeochromocytoma. However, serum and urinary catecholamine concentrations are normal or even low in hyperthyroidism, and there is no good evidence of greater sensitivity to catecholamines despite an increased density of β_1 adrenoceptors in cardiac muscle. It may well be that thyroid hormones and catecholamines act independently at the cellular level but share a signalling pathway. This would explain why non-selective β adrenoceptor antagonists, such as propranolol or nadolol, improve but do not abolish many of the symptoms of hyperthyroidism.

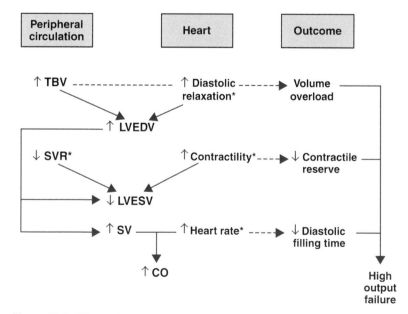

Figure 35.1. Effects of hyperthyroidism on the cardiovascular system and the possible outcomes. TBV, total blood volume; LVEDV, left ventricular end diastolic volume; LVESV, left ventricular end systolic volume; SV stroke volume; SVR systemic vascular resistance; CO, cardiac output; ↑ increased; ↓ decreased. Solid arrows indicate direct effects, and dashed arrows potential outcomes. *Features for which T3 is directly responsible.

A

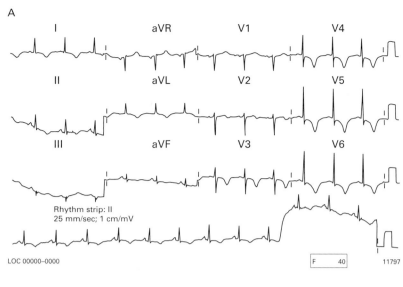

B

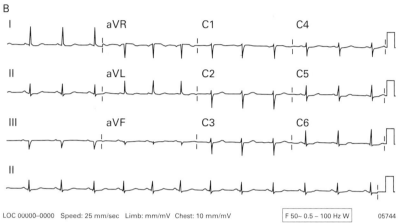

Figure 35.2. (A) ECG in a 48 year old woman in whom there was an exacerbation of hyperthyroidism 72 hours after treatment with iodine[131]. (B) The pronounced ST changes slowly resolved and the tracing was normal three months after the patient became euthyroid.

Clinical features

Most patients with hyperthyroidism complain of palpitations and breathlessness on exertion, although symptoms such as weight loss in the presence of a normal or increased appetite, heat intolerance, and irritability tend to predominate. Established angina may become worse and may, exceptionally, be a new development. Myocardial ischaemia is presumably caused by the increased demands of the thyrotoxic myocardium. However, coronary spasm may be an additional factor and myocardial infarction can occur in the absence of significant atheroma.[4] The ECG is usually normal but in severe hyperthyroidism there may be impressive ST-T wave changes in the absence of ischaemic chest pain (fig 35.2).

Characteristically there is a sinus tachycardia of approximately 100 per minute with a good volume, often collapsing pulse, and a wide pulse pressure. The apex beat is forceful, flow murmurs are common, and there may be a bruit over the enlarged thyroid gland. Mild ankle oedema is common but is rarely caused by cardiac failure and is, in part, a manifestation of the reduced day:night ratio of urinary sodium excretion by the kidneys.

Overt cardiac failure is uncommon in hyperthyroidism and usually occurs in the context of rapid atrial fibrillation in an elderly patient with pre-existing ischaemic or valvar heart disease. Nevertheless, high output failure is a rare but recognised complication of severe thyrotoxicosis.

Atrial fibrillation

A variety of atrial and ventricular tachycardias have been described in hyperthyroidism, but the most common arrhythmia is atrial fibrillation. In unselected series 10–15% of patients with thyrotoxicosis were in atrial fibrillation at presentation; however, the prevalence is probably falling because the widespread availability of accurate tests of thyroid function means that hyperthyroidism is now diagnosed at an earlier stage in its natural history. Atrial fibrillation is rare in patients under 40 years of age unless there is longstanding severe thyrotoxicosis or coexistent structural heart disease. The prevalence increases with age and is higher in men such that in the authors' experience 50% of hyperthyroid males over the age of 60 are in atrial fibrillation at presentation.

In one series, 13% of patients with "idiopathic" or "lone" atrial fibrillation attending a cardiology clinic were found to have overt or subclinical hyperthyroidism; the discovery of atrial fibrillation, in the absence of an obvious cause, should therefore prompt a request for thyroid function testing.[5]

Atrial fibrillation may be the dominant feature of hyperthyroidism in older patients and is not necessarily accompanied by pronounced elevation of the serum concentrations of T3 and T4. Increases of thyroid hormones within their respective reference ranges associated with a suppressed serum TSH concentration (subclinical hyperthyroidism) may be sufficient to trigger atrial fibrillation in susceptible individuals.[6] In the Framingham study, for example, a low serum TSH was associated with a threefold increase in the incidence of atrial fibrillation among clinically euthyroid elderly subjects, 28% of whom developed atrial fibrillation during 10 years of follow up.[7]

Sixty per cent of patients with hyperthyroid atrial fibrillation will revert spontaneously to sinus rhythm within a few weeks of restoration of normal tests of thyroid function; approximately half of the remainder will respond to DC cardioversion if serum TSH concentrations are normal or raised at the time of the procedure. Failure to achieve stable sinus rhythm is most likely in those in whom the diagnosis of hyperthyroidism has been delayed. These are usually patients with mild hyperthyroidism caused by a small multinodular goitre in whom only serum T3 may be elevated (T3 toxicosis) and in whom other useful diagnostic features, such as ophthalmopathy or major weight loss, are missing.

Hyperthyroid atrial fibrillation is typically resistant to digoxin, caused in part by an increase in the renal clearance and the apparent volume of distribution of the drug. It is often necessary to add a non-selective β adrenoceptor antagonist to achieve adequate rate control.

Anticoagulation
Systemic embolisation is increased in hyperthyroid atrial fibrillation, but the risk is difficult to quantify with estimates in cross sectional studies ranging from 2–20%. Patients over 50 years of age with valvar or hypertensive heart disease would appear to be at greatest risk. Whether younger patients with structurally normal hearts benefit from anticoagulation is not known, but a decision to withhold warfarin would be more secure if there was no evidence of atrial thrombus at transoesophageal echocardiography. As the development of a dense hemiplegia complicating a readily reversible metabolic disorder is a clinical disaster, it is our policy to consider anticoagulation with warfarin (target international normalised ratio (INR) 2–3:1) in all patients with hyperthyroid atrial fibrillation. Anticoagulant control may be difficult because hyperthyroidism is associated with an increased sensitivity to warfarin.[8]

Treatment of hyperthyroidism
Radioiodine (iodine[131]) is the treatment of choice in patients over 40 years of age, but in younger patients most centres adopt the empirical approach of prescribing a 12–18 month course of carbimazole and recommending surgery if relapse occurs. There should be a noticeable clinical improvement within 10–14 days, and most patients will be biochemically euthyroid within 4–6 weeks of starting carbimazole 40 mg daily. Patients with Graves' disease are likely to become hypothyroid within a year of treatment with radioiodine, but this is an unusual occurrence in patients with nodular goitre. There may be an exacerbation of hyperthyroidism a few days after treatment with radioiodine, owing to a transient increase in serum thyroid hormone concentrations; in patients with atrial fibrillation and cardiac failure it is therefore good practice to render the patient euthyroid with an antithyroid drug before giving radioiodine.

Hyperthyroidism is associated with an increase in cardiovascular and cerebrovascular mortality, which is most evident in the first year following treatment with radioiodine. For example, a large series from a single centre, based on more than 100 000 patient years of follow up, showed that the standardised mortality ratio, in the year after ablative radioiodine, was 1.8:1 (95% confidence interval (CI) 1.6 to 2:1).[9] At least some of this excess mortality could probably be avoided by earlier diagnosis and more aggressive treatment of the hyperthyroidism and its cardiovascular complications.

Hypothyroidism

Symptomatic thyroid failure is present in 1–2% of the population and tends to affect women. In the absence of previous radioiodine or surgical treatment of Graves' disease, the condition is usually caused by autoimmune mediated atrophy of the gland, or Hashimoto's thyroiditis which is characterised by diffuse firm thyroid enlargement. In contrast to hyperthyroidism, the low serum concentrations of thyroid hormones are associated with a decrease in cardiac output, heart rate, stroke volume, and myocardial contractility, and an increase in systemic vascular resistance. The clinical features are not as dramatic as those of thyrotoxicosis and are usually only evident in patients with profound longstanding thyroid failure in whom there may be a characteristic facies. The cardiac manifestations of hypothyroidism include sinus bradycardia, pericardial effusion, heart failure (fig 35.3), and coronary atheroma.

Ischaemic heart disease
Overt hypothyroidism is associated with hyperlipidaemia and coronary artery disease. Approximately 3% of patients with longstanding hypothyroidism report angina, and a similar proportion report it during treatment with thyroxine. In most patients the angina does not change, diminishes or disappears when thyroxine is introduced; however, it may worsen and up to 40% of those patients who present with hypothyroidism and angina cannot tolerate full replacement treatment. Moreover, myocardial infarction and sudden death are well recognised complications of starting treatment, even in patients receiving as little as 25 μg of thyroxine daily. For these reasons it is customary to begin treatment with thyroxine in patients with symptomatic ischaemic heart disease in a dose of 25 μg daily, increasing by 25 μg increments every three weeks until a dose of 100 μg daily is reached. After a further six weeks, serum free T4 and TSH should be measured and the dose of thyroxine adjusted to ensure that free T4 and TSH concentrations are in the upper and lower parts respectively of the reference range. It should be exceptional not to achieve full replacement treatment.

Subclinical hypothyroidism
Subclinical hypothyroidism (normal serum T4, raised TSH) is usually caused by autoimmune (lymphocytic) thyroiditis, characterised by the presence of antiperoxidase antibodies in the serum, and may be associated with coronary artery disease. For example, in one postmortem study there was histological evidence of lymphocytic thyroiditis in 20% of men and 50% of women with fatal myocardial infarction and only 10% of men and women who died from other causes.[10] Although hyperlipidaemia is common in overt hypothyroidism this may not explain the putative link between subclinical autoimmune thyroid disease and ischaemic heart disease. A meta-analysis of the many studies published between 1976 and 1996 on the effect of thyroxine replacement on lipids in subclinical hypothyroidism showed that restoration of serum TSH to normal reduced total cholesterol by only 0.4 mmol/l, and had little effect on high density lipoprotein (HDL) cholesterol.[11]

Over replacement with thyroxine?
There is some concern that administering thyroxine in a dose which suppresses serum TSH may provoke significant cardiovascular problems, including abnormal ventricular diastolic relaxation, a reduced exercise capacity, an

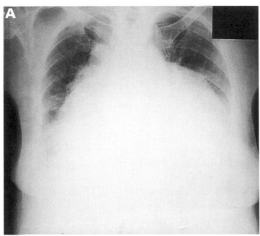

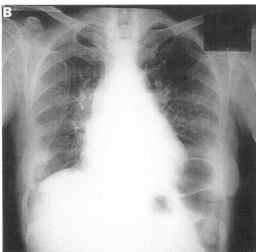

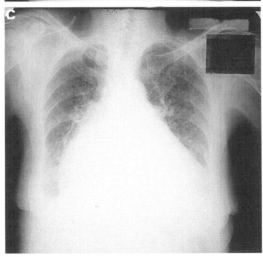

Figure 35.3. Sequential chest x rays from a patient with longstanding hypothyroidism that was complicated by congestive cardiac failure. (A) Before treatment. Cardiomegaly was caused by a combination of dilatation of all the cardiac chambers and pericardial effusion. (B) After treatment with thyroxine for nine months. (C) Seven years later, two years after the patient has stopped taking thyroxine, against medical advice, and had re-presented to the same physician with the symptoms and signs of heart failure. Reproduced from *Davidson's principles and practice of medicine*, 18th ed, p 570, with permission of the publisher Churchill Livingstone.

increase in mean basal heart rate, and atrial premature contractions.[12] Apart from an increase in left ventricular mass index within the normal range, these observations have not been verified.[13] Moreover, there is no evidence, despite the findings of the Framingham study,

that a suppressed serum TSH concentration in a patient taking thyroxine in whom serum T3 is unequivocally normal is a risk factor for atrial fibrillation.

Influence of heart disease on thyroid function tests

The interpretation of thyroid function test results may be difficult in the presence of acute or chronic non-thyroidal illness such as myocardial infarction or congestive cardiac failure for a variety of metabolic and technical reasons. In these situations there is a reduction in the peripheral monodeiodination of T4 to T3, resulting in the so called "low T3 syndrome" and, depending upon the assay employed, a low, normal or raised serum concentration of free T4. Secretion of TSH is inhibited centrally and may also be influenced by drugs such as dopamine, so that concentrations of less than 0.05 mU/l are not uncommon. Conversely, serum TSH may rise into the hypothyroid range during recovery from illness. Moreover, certain inhibitors in the serum, and possibly also the tissues, of some patients with non-thyroidal illness may interfere with binding of thyroid hormones to their carrier proteins, prevent transport of T3 and T4 into cells, and block the attachment of T3 to intracellular nuclear and cytoplasmic receptors. Many of these problems are amplified by the refusal of some commercial kit manufacturers to disclose the exact nature of their products, and by the manipulation of some assay systems in order to provide a result thought to be consistent with thyroid status. As a result low, normal or raised concentrations of free T3 and T4 may be recorded in the same patient using different assays.

The difficulty of relying upon serum TSH measurements to assess thyroid function in ill patients is highlighted by the finding that in a large series of hospitalised patients a low serum TSH concentration was three times as likely to be caused by non-thyroidal illness as hyperthyroidism, and a raised TSH of greater than 20 mU/l was as commonly due to illness as to primary hypothyroidism.[14] The combination of low serum TSH and high free T4 is, therefore, not uncommon in euthyroid patients with significant cardiovascular disease, and some would take the view that thyroid function testing should not be requested unless there is good evidence of thyroid disease, such as goitre, ophthalmopathy or unexplained atrial fibrillation. Even adopting such a counsel of perfection, there will be occasional patients in whom it is not possible to make an unequivocal diagnosis of euthyroidism or hyperthyroidism using the whole panoply of thyroid function testing. In this situation there is little choice but to recommend a trial of antithyroid drugs for three months.

The biochemical changes (that is, low TSH and low T3) associated with illness or starvation are often considered teleologically as an adaptive response to spare calories and protein; however, it is not clear whether chronic disease can, in some circumstances, cause the poten-

Key points

- Serious non-thyroidal illness, such as heart failure, can cause high T4 and low TSH concentrations, suggesting hyperthyroidism.

- Measurements of T3 may help to exclude thyrotoxicosis in this situation but can be inconclusive, and in some situations a trial of antithyroid drugs may be warranted.

- In view of these difficulties thyroid function tests should only be requested in patients with credible evidence of thyroid disease such as goitre or unexplained atrial fibrillation.

tially detrimental entity of "tissue hypothyroidism".[15] Although the present consensus is that thyroid hormone treatment is not indicated in patients with significant non-thyroidal illness, this has become a controversial issue. There are some studies which have shown improvements in cardiac output and systemic vascular resistance in patients with chronic cardiac failure following treatment with intravenous T3 or oral T4.[16]

Amiodarone induced thyroid disease

Amiodarone is a lipid soluble benzofuranic antiarrhythmic drug that has complex effects on the thyroid and may interfere significantly with thyroid hormone metabolism.[17 18] Owing to its high iodine content amiodarone may cause thyroid dysfunction in patients with pre-existing thyroid disease; it can also cause a destructive thyroiditis in patients with an inherently normal thyroid gland. The combined incidence of hyper- and hypothyroidism in patients taking amiodarone is 14–18% and, because of its extraordinarily long half life, either problem may occur several months after stopping the drug.

Effects on thyroid hormone metabolism

Amiodarone administered chronically to euthyroid patients with no evidence of underlying thyroid disease results in raised serum T4 concentrations (free T4 up to 80 pmol/l) with low normal T3. These changes are caused by the potent inhibition of 5'-deiodinase which converts T4 to T3. Serum TSH concentrations may increase initially then return to normal, but in some patients are suppressed at less than 0.05 mU/l. This may make it difficult to decide whether a patient is euthyroid or hyperthyroid, particularly as the antiadrenergic effects of amiodarone can mask the clinical features of hyperthyroidism.

Type I amiodarone induced hyperthyroidism

Each 200 mg tablet of amiodarone contains 25 mg of iodine of which approximately 9 mg is released during metabolism. A patient taking a maintenance dose of 400 mg of amiodarone daily will therefore receive approximately 18 mg of inorganic iodine which is 100 times the recommended daily allowance. Chronic exposure of patients with underlying thyroid autonomy, such as Graves' disease in remission or nodular goitre, to these excessive quantities of iodine may induce hyperthyroidism (type I amiodarone induced hyperthyroidism). This is not necessarily an indication to stop amiodarone because many patients can be managed satisfactorily by introducing concomitant antithyroid medication. However, this form of hyperthyroidism can be difficult to treat, especially in areas with relative iodine deficiency as is the case in much of mainland Europe. Standard doses of carbimazole, methimazole or propylthiouracil are often ineffective and it may be necessary to add potassium perchlorate in an attempt to reduce further the iodine uptake, and therefore hormone synthesis, by the thyroid. Treatment with iodine[131] is not usually advisable because of the relatively poor ability of the already iodine rich gland to concentrate the radioisotope. Total thyroidectomy may be the only method of rapid reversal of the thyrotoxicosis and has been successfully performed in patients with significant heart disease.

Type II amiodarone induced hyperthyroidism

Amiodarone per se may cause a drug induced destructive thyroiditis in patients with no pre-existing thyroid disease (type II amiodarone induced hyperthyroidism). In most cases this will resolve within 3–4 months whether or not amiodarone is discontinued. The disturbance of thyroid function is similar to that found in other forms of destructive thyroiditis, such as de Quervain's (subacute) or postpartum thyroiditis, with a few weeks of hyperthyroidism caused by the release of preformed thyroid hormones, followed by a brief spell of hypothyroidism, and then recovery.

Which type of hyperthyroidism?

Although there are features which help to distinguish between the two types of hyperthyroidism (table 35.1), the differentiation may be difficult and in some patients both mechanisms may be operating. In such circumstances it is sensible to institute a trial of carbimazole and to withdraw the drug after 3–4 months. If the patient remains euthyroid or becomes hypothyroid the diagnosis is likely to be type II hyperthyroidism; evidence of persistent hyperthyroidism suggests a diagnosis of type I hyperthyroidism and the need to maintain carbimazole treatment for as long as the amiodarone is necessary and beyond.

Table 35.1   Features which may help to distinguish between type I and type II amiodarone induced hyperthyroidism

	Type I	Type II
Pre-existing thyroid disease	Yes	No
Goitre	Diffuse or nodular	Uncommon, may be tender
Radioiodine uptake by thyroid	Low normal	Negligible
TSH receptor antibodies in serum	May be present	Absent
Antiperoxidase (microsomal antibodies in serum)	May be present	May be present
Serum IL-6	Normal or slightly elevated	Very elevated
Subsequent hypothyroidism	No	Possible

IL-6, interleukin 6.

Table 35.2 Patterns of thyroid function tests which may occur during treatment with amiodarone

	Euthyroid (effect of amiodarone on thyroid hormone metabolism)	Type I or II hyperthyroidism	Hypothyroid
T3	Normal or low normal	Raised > 3.0 nmol/l	Low or low normal
T4	Raised, may be in excess of 60 pmol/l	Raised	Low, normal
TSH	Raised, normal or low	Low	Raised

Reference ranges: total T3 1.1 to 2.8 nmol/l; free T4 10 to 25 pmol/l; TSH 0.15 to 3.50 mU/l.

Amiodarone induced hypothyroidism

Amiodarone may cause hypothyroidism in patients with pre-existing Hashimoto's thyroiditis. However, the presence of a raised serum TSH concentration before or during treatment is not a contraindication to the use of amiodarone as the thyroid failure is readily treated with thyroxine.

Assessment of thyroid function before and during treatment

In an attempt to minimise the risk of type I hyperthyroidism we recommend that before initiating treatment with amiodarone patients should be examined for the presence of goitre or Graves' ophthalmopathy and measurements made of serum T3, T4, TSH, antiperoxidase (microsomal) and, if possible, TSH receptor antibodies. Clinical evidence of thyroid disease and/or a suppressed serum TSH concentration, particularly if associated with antithyroid antibodies, should prompt a reconsideration of the use of amiodarone, and discussion with an endocrinologist.

Measurement of serum concentrations of T3, T4, and TSH should be made three and six months after starting amiodarone treatment and every six months thereafter, including during the first year after the drug is stopped. Table 35.2 shows the different patterns of abnormal thyroid function test results which may occur. Serum T3 concentration is the best indicator of hyperthyroidism, but in some circumstances a trial of carbimazole for 6–8 weeks may be necessary to establish whether the patient is hyperthyroid or not.

1. **Klein I, Levey GS.** The cardiovascular system in thyrotoxicosis. In: Braverman LE, Utiger RD, eds. *The thyroid*, 8th ed. Philadelphia: Lippincott-Raven, 2000:596–604.

2. **Woeber KA.** Thyrotoxicosis and the heart. *N Engl J Med* 1992;**327**:94–8.

3. **Forfar JC, Muir AL, Sawers SA,** *et al.* Abnormal left ventricular function in hyperthyroidism. Evidence for possible reversible cardiomyopathy. *N Engl J Med* 1982;**307**:1165–70.
   - *Left ventricular ejection fraction measured by radionuclide ventriculography was increased at rest in hyperthyroidism but fell on exercise. This paradoxical response disappeared within a few weeks of the patients becoming euthyroid, raising the possibility of a reversible cardiomyopathy in hyperthyroidism.*

4. **Wei JY, Genecin A, Greene HL,** *et al.* Coronary spasm with ventricular fibrillation during thyrotoxicosis: response to attaining euthyroid state. *Am J Cardiol* 1979;**43**:335–9.

5. **Forfar JC, Miller HC, Toft AD.** Occult thyrotoxicosis: a correctable cause of "idiopathic" atrial fibrillation. *Am J Cardiol* 1979;**44**:9–12.

6. **Forfar JC, Feek CM, Miller HC,** *et al.* Atrial fibrillation and isolated suppression of the pituitary-thyroid axis: response to specific antithyroid therapy. *Int J Cardiol* 1981;**1**:43–8.
   - *The first demonstration that subclinical hyperthyroidism could cause atrial fibrillation.*

7. **Sawin CT, Geller A, Wolf PA.** Low serum thyrotropin levels as a risk factor for atrial fibrillation in older persons. *N Engl J Med* 1994;**331**:1249–52.
   - *Large Framingham community study in which a heterogeneous group of patients with a low serum TSH concentration were shown to be at a sixfold risk of developing atrial fibrillation.*

8. **Kellett HA, Sawers JSA, Boulton FE,** *et al.* Problems of anticoagulation with warfarin in hyperthyroidism. *QJM* 1986;**58**:43–51.

9. **Franklyn JA, Maisonneuve P, Sheppard MC,** *et al.* Mortality after the treatment of hyperthyroidism with radioactive iodine. *N Engl J Med* 1998;**338**:712–8.
   - *Cohort of 7209 patients with hyperthyroidism treated in one centre with iodine[131] between 1950 and 1989, with 105 028 person years of follow up. The risk of death from cardiovascular disease was increased throughout the period of study but most obvious in the first post-treatment year (standardised mortality ratio (SMR) 1.6; 95% CI 1.2 to 2.1).*

10. **Bastenie PA, Vanhaelst L, Neve P.** Coronary artery disease in hypothyroidism. Observations in preclinical myxoedema. *Lancet* 1967;**ii**:1221–2.

11. **Tanis BC, Westendorp RJ, Smelt AM.** Effect of thyroid substitution on hypercholesterolaemia in patients with subclinical hypothyroidism: a re-analysis of intervention studies. *Clin Endocrinol* 1996;**44**:643–9.

12. **Biondi B, Fazio S, Cuocolo A,** *et al.* Impaired cardiac reserve and exercise capacity in patients receiving long-term thyrotropin suppressive therapy with levothyroxine. *J Clin Endocrinol Metab* 1996;**81**:4224–28.

13. **Shapiro LE, Sievert R, Ong L,** *et al.* Minimal cardiac effects in asymptomatic athyreotic patients chronically treated with thyrotropin-suppressive doses of L-thyroxine. *J Clin Endocrinol Metab* 1997;**82**:2592–5.

14. **Spencer C, Eigen A, Shen D,** *et al.* Specificity of sensitive assays of thyrotropin (TSH) used to screen for thyroid disease in hospitalised patients. *Clin Chem* 1987;**33**:1391–6.
   - *Analysis of thyroid function tests measured in a large number of patients with non-thyroidal illness demonstrates the lack of specificity of even the most sensitive assays of TSH in determining thyroid status.*

15. **De Groot LJ.** Dangerous dogmas in medicine: the nonthyroidal illness syndrome. *J Clin Endocrinol Metab* 1999;**84**:151–64.
   - *A comprehensive review of the changes in thyroid hormone metabolism in acute and chronic non-thyroidal illness, the problems of measurement and of deciding thyroid status. The arguments in favour of treating selected patients with thyroid hormone are well developed, although as yet unproven.*

16. **Hamilton MA, Stevenson LW, Fonarow GC,** *et al.* Safety and hemodynamic effects of intravenous triiodothyronine in advanced congestive heart failure. *Am J Cardiol* 1998;**81**:443–7.

17. **Weirsinga WM.** Amiodarone and the thyroid. In: Weetman AP, Grossman A. *Pharmacotherapeutics of the thyroid gland*. Berlin: Springer, 1997: 225–87.

18. **Newman CM, Price A, Davies DW,** *et al.* Amiodarone and the thyroid: a practical guide to the management of the thyroid dysfunction induced by amiodarone therapy. *Heart* 1998;**79**:121–7.

36 Evaluation of large scale clinical trials and their application to usual practice

Andrew M Tonkin

"If it were not for the great variability among individuals, Medicine might be a Science, not an Art"—*Sir William Osler, 1882, The Principles and Practice of Medicine*

It is important to apply current best evidence in making decisions about management of individual patients. While the evidence may be derived from basic and applied research, the findings from large scale clinical trials of interventions are the most relevant. However, in many cases there are uncertainties around the effects of treatments and indeed guidelines can "legitimise" these uncertainties by defining boundaries within which decisions are reasonable. Therefore, the appropriate interpretation of clinical trial results is just as important for those who are charged with the development and implementation of guidelines as they are for the clinician in discussing options with individual patients.

Important aspects relating to trial design and interpretation are discussed, using illustrative examples drawn from various fields of cardiovascular medicine.

The science of clinical trial methodology has been discussed in detail elsewhere,[1] and the application of trial results to individual patients considered by other authors,[2] including overviews of trials of many interventions. However, to date, relatively few relating to cardiovascular medicine have been produced through the Cochrane Collaboration (http://www.epi.bris.ac.uk/cochrane.heart.htm).[3]

Rationale for the trial

The background to the clinical trial should be very clearly stated (and read) in the introduction to the paper which reports a trial result, as it will have a major influence on the trial design and hence its results. The intervention should have a sound biologic and/or pathophysiological rationale. The trial will often test the principal mechanism of action of the intervention. However, drugs often have pleiotropic effects and it needs to be borne in mind that the trial will test the particular drug (often in one dose) and not its mechanism(s); indeed, dose–response relations for different effects may vary.

The hypothesis to be tested will often have been generated from a meta-analysis of previous studies in the area. The recently published HOPE study[4] illustrates the manner in which the hypothesis for the trial can be generated from an overview of studies in more restricted patient populations. While meta-analyses may be very useful in defining likely effects in certain subgroups, by and large such overviews should be regarded as hypothesis generating. However, an example of what may be the unique benefits of meta-analyses is the antiplatelet trialists collaboration,[5] following which the more widespread use of aspirin would likely not have been achieved without an overview of many trials which individually were underpowered to show significant benefit.

The cohort of patients: generalisability of results

The main purpose of large scale trials is to cause widespread appropriate change in clinical practice. Typically, controlled clinical trials examine the effects of an intervention which is administered following tightly specified protocols to patients who are selected and generally compliant. This contrasts to the care of unselected patients by usual practices and practitioners.

It follows that it is important that patients recruited to trials closely resemble those in typical practice. Therefore, evaluation of a trial requires consideration of exclusion as well as inclusion criteria, and, if possible, of baseline characteristics of those patients who were "logged" but not recruited. Typically baseline characteristics are presented in the first table in reports of large scale studies. When the intervention modifies a biomedical risk factor, such as in the case of lipid modifying treatment in patients with known coronary artery disease, the trial has most relevance when the cholesterol concentrations of those studied most represent those of usual patients.

It is also important that trials test the particular treatment on a background of usual accepted practice. Indeed when usual care of study patients does not include general advances in treatment, the trial results must be interpreted with a degree of caution. The management of patients with coronary artery disease is an important example. Many large scale trials of different therapeutic approaches do not embrace the contemporary approach which might include more complete use of arterial conduits during bypass surgery, stent deployment during percutaneous coronary intervention, and an aggressive approach to cholesterol lowering treatment as part of medical management.

In cardiovascular trials the elderly and women are often under represented. The incidence of cardiovascular disease, including coronary heart disease and its manifestations, increases greatly with age. Absolute risk is greater in the elderly and failure to include such patients could lead to underestimation of the benefits of intervention. Alternatively, the true effects of treatment in the elderly may be missed because rates of deleterious outcomes may also be different. Recently published observational data in almost 8000 patients showed that among patients with myocardial infarction receiving thrombolytic treatment, in those over 75 years old who received treatment the mortality rate was 18% in the first month after discharge, compared to 15% in those who did not receive treatment.[6] While some older patients undoubtedly benefit from thrombolytic treatment, others have an increased risk of cerebral haemorrhage and other complications. Comorbidities such as hypertension or previous stroke which may have increased bleeding risk may have been ignored. However, because controlled trials of thrombolysis have been confined to relatively younger patients, a randomised trial of thrombolysis in the "old old" may be appropriate.

The elderly have been notably under represented in trials of treatments for heart failure. Because the average age of patients recruited to heart failure trials is younger than those usually treated, this in turn may also lead to recruitment of fewer females as they develop disease manifestations at an older age.[7] Furthermore, heart failure trials frequently recruit from cardiology departments in the hospital environment, and inclusion criteria may require objective evidence of greater left ventricular dysfunction than is found in usual patients, particularly in the community setting.

Trial design and monitoring

An understanding of the principles and different types of trial design is important. Observational studies are particularly affected by issues of bias and confounding that cast doubts about their validity. Indeed, randomisation is one of the major factors that has increased the relevance of clinical trials. Even then, all attempts must still be made to reduce bias at the time of randomisation. The randomisation process may include stratification for key baseline descriptor(s), but in very large scale studies it is often assumed that baseline risks should be matched between the two groups assigned different therapeutic approaches.

The importance of an adequate (ideally placebo) control group has been demonstrated repeatedly. As one example, without inclusion of a contemporary, placebo group, the important proarrhythmic effect of class 1c antiarrhythmic drugs may not have been recognised in the CAST (cardiac arrhythmia suppression trial) study,[8] as event rates in those randomised to active treatment were similar to those from previous individual patient usage data held by the pharmaceutical company.

A placebo limb may be unethical in certain circumstances—for example, thrombolysis in acute myocardial infarction. In such a context, different "active" treatments should be compared. Because of decreasing mortality rates with general improvements in management, trials which attempt to show superiority of newer agents above standard treatments are increasingly more difficult. The large number of patients needed can be a major problem. As an extension to this, trials designed to demonstrate "equivalence" with narrow confidence intervals actually require more rather than fewer patients compared with "superiority" studies.[9] Because of this, the latest shift has been to "non-inferiority" trials. Then the clinical value of demonstrating that there is no clinically significant difference in outcomes between a new agent and conventional treatment may lie in the lower cost, greater ease of administration, or greater safety of the new agent. These analyses are often undertaken in conjunction with the main trial.

Other design strategies which may be incorporated to increase power in comparative studies are not only to increase the sample size, but to randomise unevenly by including fewer patients in "control" groups, and to deliberately enrol patients at higher risk so as to increase the number of end points.

A further relatively new development has been the possible use of a "cluster" design which allows randomisation of groups of people. This technique is used when the intervention is administered to and can affect entire clusters of people rather than individuals within the cluster, or when the intervention, although given to individuals, may "contaminate" others in the control group so as to weaken any estimate of treatment difference.[10] The methodology can be particularly applied to studies of methods of care. An example could be a telephone based support system for patients when compared to usual outpatient care.

Factorial design (and simplicity) are other methodological approaches that may increase the efficiency of randomised controlled trials. Factorial design not only allows more than one hypothesis to be tested simultaneously, but allows large scale evaluation of some treatments such as dietary supplements that might not otherwise be possible because of difficulty in attracting the necessary funding.

Very large scale clinical trials should have an independent data and safety monitoring board. Their role should be clearly stated. Typically, the board will operate with pre-specified general stopping rules but they should usually be encouraged not to terminate a trial too early. This is because the reliability of data is greater with an increasing number of end points, perhaps euphemistically termed "regression to the truth". Accordingly, the mathematical functions which determine stopping often require more extreme evidence of effect earlier compared with later in the trial. Particularly, trials should rarely be terminated very early on the basis of "futility" because this deduction is unreliable when there are relatively few end points.

Appropriate end points: clinical relevance

One major end point should be clearly specified and used as the basis for power calculations, the estimate of the "reliability" of the result. These power calculations should be presented.

All cause mortality is the hardest end point and allows for inaccuracies in the certification of the cause of death.[11] It usually requires inclusion of a very large number of patients in the study. Increasingly, an expanded end point which is a composite of a number of outcomes is the primary end point. An expanded end point could be a composite of cause specific death, related non-fatal events, and perhaps an index of cost benefit such as a measure of hospitalisation. Each component should be biologically plausible and there should be an attempt to minimise any possibility of "double counting".

Care is prudent before there is wide extrapolation from the results of secondary end point data from smaller trials. As an example, data from the ELITE II study[12] failed to confirm a mortality benefit of an angiotensin receptor antagonist compared to an angiotensin converting enzyme (ACE) inhibitor in heart failure patients, although this had previously been demonstrated in the smaller ELITE I study. The primary end point in ELITE I was renal function rather than mortality, but the somewhat dramatic effect on survival had been sufficient to convince a number of regulatory authorities throughout the world to liberalise indications for angiotensin receptor antagonism.

Trial acronyms
ELITE: Evaluation of Losartan In The Elderly
FRISC: Fragmin during Instability in Coronary artery disease
HOPE: Heart Outcomes Prevention Evaluation
TIMI: Thrombolysis In Myocardial Infarction
VANQWISH: Veterans Affairs Non-Q Wave Infarction Strategies in Hospital

graphy and, possibly, revascularisation with a "conservative" approach based on medical treatment. In the TIMI IIIb, VANQWISH, and FRISC II studies, from 14–57% and 48–73%, respectively, of those patients assigned to a conservative therapeutic approach had cardiac catheterisation while an inpatient or within 12 months.[13] These intervention rates translated to revascularisation approaches by 12 months in 33–49% in those assigned initial conservative treatment compared to 44–78% of those assigned to an initial invasive strategy. This made meaningful conclusions concerning the role of early revascularisation very difficult.

The examples also suggest the potential value of additional presentation of "on-treatment" analyses when this is appropriate.

Methods of analysis

Intention to treat analyses are vital to minimise bias and must always be presented. These analyses present outcomes by treatment assigned at the start of the trial, irrespective of whether there is adherence throughout the period of follow up.

However, it is appropriate to examine the data which are presented for the extent of non-adherence to assigned treatment. The reader should ascertain whether or not there was significant "crossover" to the other treatment limb which was being compared. Crossover between assigned treatments can be a particular problem in trials which compare non-pharmacologic interventions and drug treatment. One example involves the trials in patients with unstable angina which have compared outcomes after early coronary angio-

Net benefit: public health impact

Figure 36.1 shows a schema within which the overall effects of a treatment might be considered.

The distinction between relative and absolute risk (and reduction) is very important. Relative risk is the increase (for a risk factor) or decrease (the typical case for an intervention) in the likelihood of an event compared to a reference group. The odds ratio (OR) is another measure of this, calculated as the ratio of odds (OR = $p \div 1-p$, where p is the probability of the event).

However, it is much more important to examine absolute risks. Absolute risk reduction is the arithmetic difference in rates of outcomes between the experimental and "reference" (control) groups in the trial. The reciprocal of

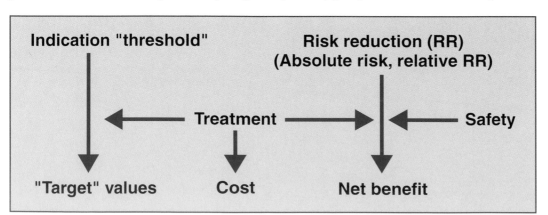

Figure 36.1. A schema within which to consider aspects of a treatment. Information on many of these can be obtained within the context of a large scale trial.

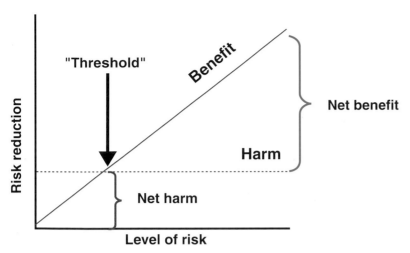

"Threshold" here excludes consideration of costs and inconvenience of therapy

Figure 36.2. Net benefit is a composite of absolute benefit (which will often vary according to baseline level of risk) and harm (which is often independent of the level of risk).

the absolute risk reduction is the number who would need to be treated to prevent one adverse outcome ("number needed to treat"). This takes into account both the relative risk reduction and underlying risk and is often used to gauge the absolute effect of the intervention being tested. To enable comparisons for chronic treatments, the numbers needed to treat are often estimated for five years of intervention.

The thresholds for initiating treatment should reflect the level of absolute risk at which first, the benefits and hazards of treating outweigh those of not treating, and which secondly, justify the associated costs and inconvenience to the patient. As shown in fig 36.2, the risk reduction with an effective treatment should increase, somewhat in proportion to the level of risk of the patient cohort. However, the magnitude of any harmful effects is usually independent of the level of risk for the indication for treatment. A net benefit can then be derived as a composite of these considerations of absolute benefit and harm.

Clinicians need to compare the absolute risk of trial patients with their own patient. If the relative risk reduction is anticipated to be the same, the absolute benefit of an intervention is greatest in the patients at highest risk. Such groups could include the elderly or people with diabetes. These considerations can also be relevant when absolute risk rates are greater in clinical practice than in selected patients recruited to the trial.

An example of the logic outlined above can be found in considering the risk and prevention of stroke in patients with chronic non-rheumatic atrial fibrillation.[14] The overall risk is around 5% per annum but this increases with increasing age, recent congestive heart failure, presence of hypertension or diabetes, a history of previous stroke or transient ischaemic attack, and evidence of left atrial enlargement or left ventricular dysfunction on transthoracic echocardiography. In both primary and sec-

ondary prevention trials, warfarin has been shown to decrease risk by around two thirds, but from a baseline annual risk of 12% in secondary prevention compared to 5% in primary prevention. The same relative risk reduction results in much greater absolute benefit in those who have had previous events, but bleeding risk is no different in the two scenarios. It should be further noted that the rate of bleeding observed in the trials (0.5–0.8% per annum) is much less than that seen in usual clinical practice (around 5% per annum). Therefore, it is important to assess individual patients carefully for comorbidities which could increase risk of bleeding.

Another example concerns primary prevention of coronary heart disease events with lipid modifying treatment. Absolute risk in individuals with similar cholesterol concentrations depends critically on their age, sex, and levels of other established cardiovascular risk factors. On the basis of consideration of multiple risk factors, groups such as the joint European task force have applied multivaried mathematical modelling to enable prediction of an arbitrary risk of events over 10 years and to suggest various "thresholds" at which initiation of treatment may be appropriate.[15]

To establish relative public health benefits, often trials are "lumped" to compare the number needed to be treated in different scenarios. However, because baseline risk often varies widely between trials, care is necessary in pooling of data from multiple trials.[16]

Another note of caution concerns the interpretation of safety data. Few clinical trials extend beyond five years because of factors such as investigator and subject fatigue, and the accumulation of crossovers. This time frame may be inadequate to detect some very important adverse affects such as cancer. As a corollary, the risk:benefit ratio may differ at different time points after the initiation of the treatment.

Cost-benefit analyses

A large part of the direct costs associated with cardiovascular disease relate to hospitalisation, and a disproportionate amount is associated with the care of the elderly. Many regulatory authorities now require formal evaluation of cost–benefit of new treatments and these are often conducted within the clinical trial environment. The findings obviously impact on translation of the outcomes of trials to the clinical context and demonstration of important outcomes can be used to justify the more widespread use, albeit with higher initial costs of some treatments. An example is the value of the implantable cardioverter defibrillator in patients at higher risk of "malignant" ventricular arrhythmias.[17]

Surrogate measures

Because studies which compare two active treatments require much higher numbers to ascertain or exclude differences in treatment effects reliably, "surrogate" measures may be reported. Study of intermediate outcomes for "harder" clinical end points should require appropriate scientific data to suggest the relation is truly a mechanistic one. An association, even a compelling epidemiologic relation, does not necessarily imply a causal relation. Particularly, interventions may have multiple mechanisms of action. Indeed, the relative importance of these different effects may vary according to the criteria which are used to define the patient population under study.

An associated question is whether it is valid to use intermediate outcomes as surrogate measures to deduce a "class" effect among drugs which can differ in their pharmacokinetic and pharmacodynamic properties, and in their spectrum of adverse effects. The argument could apply to ACE inhibitors which, because of differences in tissue binding properties, could have different strengths of action on paracrine ACE systems, or to 3-hydroxy-3-methylglutaryl coenzyme A (HMG CoA) reductase inhibitors which might differ not only in the potency of their lipid modifying effects but also of other potentially relevant mechanisms.

As stated earlier, while the approach is conservative, it is usually sensible to regard large scale trials as testing specific treatments (and in the case of drugs, in particular doses) and not their mechanisms of action. However, guidelines for determining whether or not a drug is exerting (more than) a class effect have been published.[18] One very important example of the potential value of intermediate measures and of substudies was that which established the importance of restoration of TIMI III flow through the infarct related artery for preservation of left ventricular function and long term outcome following myocardial infarction.[19]

Subgroup analyses

Trials are designed to have sufficient power to reliably test the effect of the intervention in the cohort which is defined by the particular inclusion and exclusion criteria. Results in subgroups of the cohort are nearly always less reliable and frequently over interpreted.

The credibility of a subgroup analysis depends on the size of the subgroup, the biologic plausibility of the analysis, and consistency of effects between different trials. Particularly, unless subgroup analyses have been prespecified (both the patient subgroups and the outcomes of interest) and all such prespecified analyses are presented or at least available, bias is frequent if not inevitable, and the selection of subgroup analyses presented might be viewed as "data dredging".

When subgroup analyses are presented, the appropriate statistical test often examines for evidence of heterogeneity between different subgroups—for example, between sex or age groups, or those with or without particular risk factors.

Evaluation of clinical trials: summary

COMPONENT	ASPECTS
The hypothesis	Biologic rationale, meta-analysis
The cohort	Demographics, background treatments
Trial design and monitoring	Appropriate design, independence
Primary and subsidiary end points	Relevance, plausibility
Analysis	Intention to treat, on treatment
Net benefit	Absolute benefit, safety
Affordability	Cost–benefit considerations
Intermediate outcomes	Validity as "surrogate" measures
Subgroup analyses	Whether prespecified

Final comments: patient preferences

Trials of cardiovascular treatments have conclusively shown the efficacy of a wide variety of treatments. Patient outcomes can be improved by appropriate translation of the results of these trials to usual practice.

However, it is appropriate that patients are being further empowered concerning decisions relating to their health. It is worth noting the opinions of different groups in a recent survey to establish a threshold above which it was judged to be appropriate to use antihypertensive drugs. The number of patients with hypertension regarded as appropriate to be treated over five years to save one life was lower for consultants than general practitioners, but particularly much higher among nurses and, notably, the public.[20] In the current environment with increasing application of information management, perhaps in the future the community and patients may also be seeking details relating to trial management and interpretation, rather than taking what to this time has been the relatively passive role of subjects in such trials.

1. **Friedman LM, Furberg C, DeMets DL.** *Fundamentals of clinical trials*, 3rd ed. St Louis: Mosby, 1996.
• *A comprehensive edition devoted to fundamentals of the design, conduct and analysis of clinical trials.*

2. **Dans AL, Dans LF, Guyatt GH,** *et al* for the Evidence-Based Medicine Working Group. User's guides to the medical literature. XIV. How to decide on the applicability of clinical trial results to your patient. *JAMA* 1998;**279**:545–9.
• *Another discussion of the issues—biologic, social and economic, and epidemiologic—that might influence applicability of clinical trial results to an individual patient.*

3. **Cochrane AL.** *Effectiveness and efficiency. Random reflections on health services.* London: Nuffield Provincial Hospitals, Trust, 1972.
• *The Cochrane Collaboration is an international venture which provides overviews of controlled trials for a variety of treatments. It is named after Archie Cochrane, a British epidemiologist who wished people to make more informed decisions about health care, by providing better access to reliable reviews of the relevant evidence.*

4. **The Heart Outcomes Prevention Evaluation Study Investigators.** Effects of an angiotensin-converting-enzyme inhibitor, ramipril, on cardiovascular events in high-risk patients. *N Engl J Med* 2000;**342**:145–53.
• *HOPE is a landmark study which was based on subsidiary analyses of older trials of ACE inhibitors in patients with heart failure or asymptomatic left ventricular dysfunction. It confirmed a reduction in cardiovascular events as the primary end point, but extended this to a wide range of vascular patients, irrespective of their left ventricular function.*

5. **Antiplatelet Trialists' Collaboration.** Collaborative overview of randomised trials of antiplatelet therapy. 1: prevention of death, myocardial infarction, and stroke by

prolonged antiplatelet therapy in various categories of patients. *BMJ* 1994;**308**:81–106.
- *This meta-analysis of antiplatelet treatments enabled conclusions for practice to be drawn which were not otherwise available from individual trials which had been underpowered.*

6. **Thiemann DR, Coresh J, Schulman SP,** *et al.* Lack of benefit for intravenous thrombolysis in patients with myocardial infarction who are older than 75 years. *Circulation* 2000;**101**:2239–46.

7. **Cohen-Solal A, Desnos M, Delahaye F,** *et al* for the Myocardial and Heart Failure Working Group of the French Society of Cardiology, the National College of General Hospital Cardiologists and the French Geriatrics Society. A national survey of heart failure in French hospitals. *Eur Heart J* 2000;**21**:763–9.
- *This observational study characterised heart failure patients in medical and geriatric as well as cardiology departments in 120 French hospitals. Patient characteristics such as age and sex distribution differed significantly from those in patients recruited to recent heart failure trials.*

8. **The Cardiac Arrhythmia Suppression Trial Investigators.** Preliminary report: effects of encainide and flecainide on mortality in a randomised trial of arrhythmia suppression after myocardial infarction. *N Engl J Med* 1989;**321**:406–12.
- *The placebo controlled design of this study allowed recognition of the potential for proarrhythmic effects and worsened outcome with antiarrhythmic drugs. The trial was based on the hypothesis that suppression of ventricular ectopic beats would prevent sudden death, an assumption which has since been shown to be fallacious.*

9. **White HD.** Thrombolytic therapy and equivalence trials. *J Am Coll Cardiol* 1998;**31**:494–6.

10. **Donner A.** Some aspects of the design and analysis of cluster randomised trials. *Appl Stat* 1998;**47**:95–113.

11. **Lauer MS, Blackstone EH, Young JB,** *et al.* Cause of death in clinical research: time for a reassessment? *J Am Coll Cardiol.* 1999;**34**:618–20.

12. **Pitt B, Poole-Wilson PA, Segal R,** *et al.* Effect of losartan compared with captopril on mortality in patients with symptomatic heart failure: randomised trial. The losartan heart failure survival study ELITE II. *Lancet* 2000;**355**:1582–7.

13. **Mehta SR, Eikelboom JW, Yusuf S.** Long-term management of unstable angina and non-Q-wave myocardial infarction. *Eur Heart J* 2000;**2**(suppl E):E6–12.

14. **Atrial Fibrillation Investigators.** Risk factors for stroke and efficacy of antithrombotic therapy in atrial fibrillation. Analysis of pooled data from five randomised controlled trials. *Arch Intern Med* 1994;**154**:1449–57.

15. **Wood DA, DeBacker G, Faergeman O,** *et al* on behalf of the Task Force, Prevention of Coronary Heart Disease in Clinical Practice. Recommendations of the second joint task force of the European Society of Cardiology, European Atherosclerosis Society and European Society of Hypertension. *Eur Heart J* 1998;**19**:1434–503. *Atherosclerosis* 1998;**140**:199–270. *J Hypertens* 1998;**16**:1407–14.

16. **Smeeth L, Haines A, Ebrahim S.** Numbers needed to treat derived from meta-analyses—sometimes informative, usually misleading. *BMJ* 1999;**318**:1548–51.
- *A critical commentary on the caution needed in interpreting pooled data from trials, in this case specifically, numbers needed to treat. Contains examples from various therapies in cardiovascular disease.*

17. **Roberts PR, Betts TR, Morgan JM.** Cost effectiveness of the implantable cardioverter defibrillator. *Eur Heart J* 2000;**21**:712–19.

18. **McAlister FA, Laupacis A, Wells GA,** *et al* for the Evidence-Based Medicine Working Group. Users' guides to the medical literature: XIX. Applying clinical trial results. B. Guidelines for determining whether a drug is exerting more than a class effect. *JAMA* 1999;**282**:1371–7.
- *This interesting article gives examples and discusses level of evidence for determining whether or not drugs are exhibiting a class effect.*

19. **The GUSTO Angiographic Investigators.** The effects of tissue-plasminogen activator, streptokinase, or both on coronary-artery patency, ventricular function, and survival after acute myocardial infarction. *N Engl J Med* 1993;**329**:1615–22.
- *This substudy of the first GUSTO trial compared patency rates and left ventricular function for different thrombolytic regimens. It illustrates how careful substudies may yield very important data on mechanisms of therapeutic effect.*

20. **Steel N.** Thresholds for taking antihypertensive drugs in different professional and lay groups: questionnaire survey. *BMJ* 2000;**320**:1446–7.

Index

Page numbers in **bold** type refer to figures, and those in *italic* refer to tables or boxed material

Index

Index

Index

Citation Index

SECTION I: CORONARY DISEASE

1. Davies MJ. The pathophysiology of acute coronary syndromes. *Heart* 2000; **83**: 361–6.

2. Weissberg PL. Atherogenesis: current understanding of the causes of atheroma. *Heart* 2000; **83**: 247–52

3. Fox KAA. Acute coronary syndromes: presentation – clinical spectrum and management. *Heart* 2000; **84**: 93–100.

4. Timmis A. Acute coronary syndromes: risk stratification. *Heart* 2000; **83**: 241–6.

5. Topol EJ. Acute myocardial infarction: thrombolysis. *Heart* 2000; **83**: 122–6

6. Norris RM. The natural history of acute myocardial infarction. *Heart* 2000; **83**: 726–30

7. Thompson DR, Lewin RJP. Management of the post-myocardial infarction patient: rehabilitation and cardiac neurosis. *Heart* 2000; **84**: 101–5.

8. Windecker S, Meier B. Intervention in coronary artery disease. *Heart* 2000; **83**: 481–90

SECTION II: HEART FAILURE

9. McMurray J J, Stewart S. Epidemiology, aetiology, and prognosis of heart failure. *Heart* 2000; **83**: 596–602

10. Struthers AD. The diagnosis of heart failure. *Heart* 2000; **84**: 334–8

11. Westaby S. Non-transplant surgery for heart failure. *Heart* 2000; **83**: 603–10

SECTION III: CARDIOMYOPATHY

12. Davies MJ. The cardiomyopathies: an overview. *Heart* 2000; **83**: 469–74

13. Elliott P. Diagnosis and management of dilated cardiomyopathy. *Heart* 2000; **84**: 106–12

14. Corrado D, Basso C, Thiene G. Arrhythmogenic right ventricular cardiomyopathy: diagnosis, prognosis, and treatment. *Heart* 2000; **83**: 588–95

SECTION IV: VALVE DISEASE

15. Soler-Soler J, Galve E. Worldwide perspective on valve disease. *Heart* 2000; **83**: 721–5

16. Otto CM. Timing of aortic valve surgery. *Heart* 2000; **84**: 211–18

17. Prêtre R, Turina MI. Cardiac valve surgery in the octogenarian. *Heart* 2000; **83**: 116–21

18. Gohlke-Bärwolf C. Anticoagulation in valvar heart disease: new aspects and management during non-cardiac surgery. *Heart* 2000; **84**: 567–72

19. Iung B. Interface between valve disease and ischaemic heart disease. *Heart* 2000; **84**: 347–52

20. Anderson RH. Clinical anatomy of the aortic root. *Heart* 2000; **84**: 670–3

21. Treasure T. Cardiovascular surgery for Marfan syndrome. *Heart* 2000; **84**: 674–8

SECTION V: ELECTROPHYSIOLOGY

22. Gammage MD. Temporary cardiac pacing. *Heart* 2000; **83**: 715–20

23. Roden DM. Antiarrhythmic drugs: from mechanisms to clinical practice. *Heart* 2000; **84**: 339–46

24. Waldo AL. Treatment of atrial flutter. *Heart* 2000; **84**: 227–32

25. Stevenson WG, Delacretaz E. Radiofrequency catheter ablation of ventricular tachycardia. *Heart* 2000; **84**: 553–9

SECTION VI: CONGENITAL HEART DISEASE

26. Allan L. Antenatal diagnosis of heart disease. *Heart* 2000; **83**: 367–70

27. Järvelin M-R. Fetal and infant markers of adult heart diseases. *Heart* 2000; **84**: 219–26

28. Gibbs JL. Interventional catheterisation. Opening up I: the ventricular outflow tracts and great arteries. *Heart* 2000; **83**: 111–15

29. Gibbs JL. Interventional catheterisation. Opening up II: venous return, the atrial septum, the arterial duct, aortopulmonary shunts, and aortopulmonary collaterals. *Heart* 2000; **83**: 237–40

SECTION VII: IMAGING TECHNIQUES

30. Gibbons RJ. Myocardial perfusion imaging. *Heart* 2000; **83**: 355–60

31. Camici PG. Positron emission tomography and myocardial imaging. *Heart* 2000; **83**: 475–80

32. Feyter PJ de, Nieman K, van Ooijen P, Ouderk M. Non-invasive coronary artery imaging with electron beam computed tomography and magnetic resonance imaging. *Heart* 2000; **84**: 442–8

SECTION VIII: GENERAL CARDIOLOGY

33. Oakley CM. Myocarditis, pericarditis and other pericardial diseases. *Heart* 2000; **84**: 449–54

34. Lye M, Donnellan C. Heart disease in the elderly. *Heart* 2000; **84**: 560–6

35. Toft AD, Boon NA. Thyroid disease and the heart. *Heart* 2000; **84**: 455–60

36. Tonkin AM. Evaluation of large scale clinical trials and their application to usual practice. *Heart* 2000; **84**: 679–84